SURGICAL
Laparoscopy

SURGICAL
Laparoscopy

EDITED BY

Karl A. Zucker, M.D., F.A.C.S.

Associate Professor of Surgery and Director of Surgical Endoscopy,
University of Maryland School of Medicine; Assistant Chief of Surgery,
Baltimore VA Medical Center, Baltimore, Maryland

ASSOCIATE EDITORS

Robert W. Bailey, M.D.

Assistant Professor of Surgery, Department of Surgery, University of
Maryland School of Medicine, Baltimore, Maryland

Eddie Joe Reddick, M.D., F.A.C.S.

General Surgeon, West Side Hospital, Nashville, Tennessee

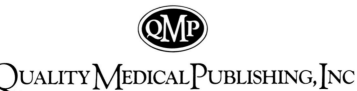

QUALITY MEDICAL PUBLISHING, INC

ST. LOUIS, MISSOURI
1991

Printed in the United States of America.

PUBLISHER   Karen Berger

ASSOCIATE EDITOR   Beth Campbell-Blethroad

PROJECT MANAGER   Carolita Deter

PRODUCTION   Susan Trail

BOOK DESIGN   Susan Trail

COVER DESIGN   Diane M. Beasley

Quality Medical Publishing, Inc.
2086 Craigshire Drive
St. Louis, Missouri 63146

LIBRARY OF CONGRESS CATALOGING IN PUBLICATION DATA

Surgical laparoscopy / editor, Karl A. Zucker ; associate editors,
   Robert W. Bailey, Eddie Joe Reddick.
        p.   cm.
     Includes bibliographical references and index.
     ISBN 0-942219-21-X — ISBN 0-683-14510-X (intnt)
     1. Abdomen—Endoscopic surgery. 2. Biliary tract—Endoscopic
surgery. I. Zucker, Karl A., 1953-   . II. Bailey, Robert W.,
1956-   . III. Reddick, Eddie Joe, 1949-
     [DNLM: 1. Biliary Tract Surgery—methods. 2. Gastrointestinal
System—surgery. 3. Peritoneoscopy—instrumentation.
4. Peritoneoscopy—methods.   WI 575 S961]
RD540.S927   1991
617.5'5059—dc20
DNLM/DLC
for Library of Congress   91-51
                                                                  CIP

ISBN 0-942219-21-X

VT/WW/WW
5   4   3

Contributors

Robert W. Bailey, M.D.
Assistant Professor of Surgery, Department of Surgery, University of Maryland School of Medicine, Baltimore, Maryland

Avram M. Cooperman, M.D., F.A.C.S.
Professor of Surgery, Department of Surgery, New York Medical College, New York, New York

Carlos Fernández-del Castillo, M.D.
Research Fellow in Surgery, Department of Surgery, Massachusetts General Hospital and Harvard University, Boston, Massachusetts

Charles J. Filipi, M.D., F.A.C.S.
Assistant Clinical Professor, Department of General Surgery, Creighton University School of Medicine, Omaha, Nebraska

Robert J. Fitzgibbons, Jr., M.D., F.A.C.S.
Associate Professor of Surgery, Department of Surgery, Creighton University School of Medicine, Omaha, Nebraska

Thomas R. Gadacz, M.D., F.A.C.S.
Professor, Department of Surgery, The Johns Hopkins University School of Medicine; Chief, Surgical Service, Baltimore VA Medical Center, Baltimore, Maryland

Jawad U. Hasnain, M.D., F.A.C.A.
Assistant Professor, Department of Anesthesiology, University of Maryland School of Medicine, Baltimore, Maryland

Peter Hertzmann
Medical Marketing and Management Consultant, Palo Alto, California

Anthony L. Imbembo, M.D.
Professor and Chairman, Department of Surgery, University of Maryland School of Medicine, Baltimore, Maryland

Namir Katkhouda, M.D.
Chargé d'Enseignement, University of Nice School of Medicine; Assistant Chief of Surgery, Hôpital St. Roch, Nice, France

Keith D. Lillemoe, M.D.
Assistant Professor, Department of Surgery, The Johns Hopkins University School of Medicine, Baltimore, Maryland

M. Jane Matjasko, M.D., F.A.C.A.
Martin Helrich Professor and Chairman, Department of Anesthesiology, University of Maryland School of Medicine, Baltimore, Maryland

Jean Mouiel, M.D., F.A.C.S.
Professor of Surgery, University of Nice School of Medicine; Chief of Surgery, Hôpital St. Roch, Nice, France

Henry A. Pitt, M.D.
Professor of Surgery, Department of Surgery, The Johns Hopkins University School of Medicine, Baltimore, Maryland

Eddie Joe Reddick, M.D., F.A.C.S.
General Surgeon, West Side Hospital, Nashville, Tennessee

Giovanni M. Salerno, M.D.
Research Fellow, Department of Surgery, Creighton University School of Medicine, Omaha, Nebraska

William B. Saye, M.D., F.A.C.O.G., F.A.C.S.
Private practice, Marietta, Georgia

William W. Schuessler, M.D., P.A.
Texas Endosurgery Institute, San Antonio, Texas

Mark A. Talamini, M.D.
Assistant Professor, Department of Surgery,
The Johns Hopkins University School of
Medicine, Baltimore, Maryland

Thierry G. Vancaillie, M.D.
Assistant Professor, Department of Obstetrics
and Gynecology, The University of Texas
Health Science Center at San Antonio, San
Antonio, Texas

Andrew L. Warshaw, M.D.
Professor of Surgery, Department of Surgery,
Harvard Medical School/Massachusetts
General Hospital, Boston, Massachusetts

Karl A. Zucker, M.D., F.A.C.S.
Associate Professor of Surgery and Director of
Surgical Endoscopy, University of Maryland
School of Medicine; Assistant Chief of
Surgery, Baltimore VA Medical Center,
Baltimore, Maryland

Foreword

The discipline of surgery is changing. Traditional concepts and approaches to the treatment of surgical illnesses are giving way to a new type of operative intervention variously referred to as minimally invasive surgery, limited exposure surgery, or endoscopic surgery. Several factors have driven this change. The most important impetus has been the heightened awareness of more sophisticated health care consumers. Advanced imaging techniques, improved optics, and new classes of instruments have paved the way for these innovative procedures; this is just the beginning of the technology transfer we are witnessing. Learning new techniques to gain access to a body cavity without the need for external exposure presents an exciting challenge for this and the next generation of surgeons.

This textbook is an important landmark in the evolution of the young and burgeoning field of surgical laparoscopy. The application of minimally invasive surgery is not new, but surgical laparoscopy is just now gaining wide acceptability by general surgeons. Our colleagues in gynecology have had a longstanding interest in laparoscopy, and numerous publications are available to them. Endourologists, peripheral endovascular surgeons, and gastrointestinal endoscopists likewise have at their disposal resources detailing diagnostic and therapeutic approaches. *Surgical Laparoscopy* helps to bridge the gap for the general surgeon.

Clearly, it is the patient who will benefit from these new procedures. As techniques improve, as instruments are refined, and as new technologies are developed, increasingly complex operations can be performed with less debilitating effects on the patient. Successful treatment of complicated illnesses and the expeditious return of the patient to society as a functioning member should be our goal.

Dr. Zucker and his contributors have put together a thoughtful and practical state-of-the-art description of the application of surgical laparoscopy to general surgery. They cover important new advances in both diagnostic and therapeutic intervention using laparoscopic techniques. Comparisons are made to standard open techniques, and appropriate indications and potential risks and complications are fairly presented.

Surgical Laparoscopy clearly shows that we are only limited by our imagination.

Michael J. Zinner
Professor and Chairman
Department of Surgery, UCLA Medical Center
Los Angeles, California

Preface

Although not widely recognized for almost two years, an event occurred in the summer of 1987 that would dramatically change the practice of general surgery. In that year, P. Mouret and his colleagues performed the first laparoscopic cholecystectomy in Lyon, France. What has happened since is without precedent in modern surgery. Despite the scarcity of data in the literature, surgeons throughout Europe, North America, and other areas of the world have eagerly embraced this procedure because of the significant benefits in overall patient care. Already we are seeing innovative clinical investigators adapting laparoscopic technology to other commonly performed abdominal operations such as appendectomy, inguinal hernia repair, and vagotomy.

Surgical Laparoscopy is intended to introduce surgeons to the principles of laparoscopic surgery and to familiarize those already performing laparoscopic cholecystectomy with the newer procedures and instruments that have been developed. Although laparoscopy has proved to be an effective diagnostic as well as therapeutic modality, this book concentrates on actual operative procedures. A number of atlases and textbooks cover diagnostic laparoscopy in depth, but they have not proved useful to surgeons attempting to learn therapeutic procedures. *Surgical Laparoscopy* was intended to serve as a comprehensive and practical reference for surgeons learning these techniques.

Although the focus is laparoscopic biliary tract surgery, we have also included sections on a number of other laparoscopic procedures. We were fortunate that many of those surgeons who have pioneered these operations were willing to contribute to this effort. In sharing their experiences, they emphasize ways to avoid complications that can occur with any new procedures. To avoid interfering with the individual style of each author, we have permitted some repetition in the description of procedures. However, the reader has the advantage of being exposed to a number of different methods of insufflation, trocar insertion, tissue dissection, avoidance of complications, etc.

In a few years medical historians will begin describing the most important achievements affecting surgery during the twentieth century. It is our belief that laparoscopic surgery will be considered a milestone as significant as the discovery of antibiotics, the introduction of blood transfusion therapy, and advances in anesthesia. We hope *Surgical Laparoscopy* will make the transition to this new era of surgical laparoscopy easier and safer.

Karl A. Zucker

Contents

SURGICAL
Laparoscopy

PART ONE

Fundamentals

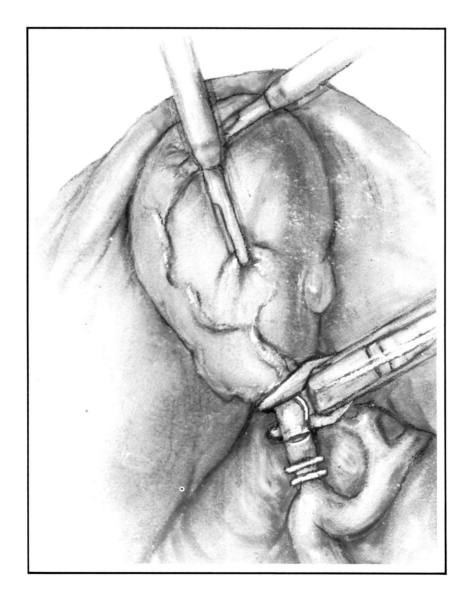

Historical Review: Diagnostic Laparoscopy to Laparoscopic Cholecystectomy and Beyond

Charles J. Filipi, M.D.
Robert J. Fitzgibbons, Jr., M.D.
Giovanni M. Salerno, M.D.

Endoscopic surgery is rapidly becoming a popular alternative to traditional operative procedures for a variety of diseases. Laparoscopic biliary tract surgery, laparoscopic appendectomy, laparoscopic gynecologic procedures, thoracoscopic treatment of pneumothorax and persistent pleural effusions, as well as arthroscopic examination and treatment of joint spaces have all become accepted endoscopic procedures. If conducted safely, endoscopic surgery offers savings in total health care dollars as a result of shorter hospital stays and a more rapid return to work, factors that are appealing to both commercial and governmental health care providers. Public awareness that endoscopic surgery is associated with diminished pain and cosmetic disfigurement as well as quicker resumption of normal activities has accelerated its acceptance by surgeons. This is exemplified by the recent introduction of laparoscopic cholecystectomy, which attracted only minor curiosity when first performed in 1987. Interest in this procedure has grown almost exponentially, largely fueled by patient demands. This chapter provides an historical perspective of the development of laparoscopic surgery and describes the technologic advances that have resulted in the current state of the art.

HISTORICAL MILESTONES

The importance of performing an internal examination of the many compartments of the human body has been recognized for several centuries. The Arabian physician Abulkasim (936-1013) is often credited with being the first to use reflected light to inspect an internal organ, the cervix. Other investigators subsequently developed instruments to examine the nasal recesses and the urinary bladder with the aid of artificial light and mirrors. Endoscopy, as we know it today, was not developed until the problem of thermal tissue injury caused by the illuminating source was solved. The first endoscopes that incorporated an optical viewing component used a glowing platinum wire at one end as the light source. Later, clinical investigators used endoscopes with incandescent light bulbs at the tip of the instrument. It is not surprising, therefore, that cystoscopy, which was developed in the nineteenth century, preceded other forms of endoscopy because of the coolant effect of water on the distal light source. The usefulness of photography to record the endoscopic findings was recognized early, and by 1874 Stein[1] had modified existing cameras to record images of bladder pathology.

In 1901 Kelling[2] reported using a cystoscope to inspect the peritoneal cavity of a dog after insufflation with air. He then coined the term "celioscopy" to describe this technique. The first report of using this procedure in man was by the Swedish physician Jacobaeus[3] in 1910. These early procedures, however, were entirely diagnostic in nature; the exposure obtained and the instruments available did not allow operative intervention. The early pioneers introduced their trocars and cystoscopes directly into the peritoneal cavity; it was another 30 years before pneumoperitoneum was used prior to insertion of the first cannula. Goetz and later Veress developed an insufflation needle for the safe introduction of gas into the abdomen. A spring-loaded obturator was incorporated within the barrel of the needle, which retracted during fascial penetration and then covered the sharp point as it entered the peritoneal cavity.

The introduction of an endoscope through the abdominal wall was initially associated with a number of major and minor complications. The risk of injury to underlying bowel and vascular structures has always been a major concern of clinicians performing this procedure. In 1946 Decker[4] introduced an alternative method of placing the laparoscope into the abdominal cavity in an attempt to minimize this complication. He inserted the scope into the pelvis through the cul-de-sac and named the procedure culdoscopy. For this procedure, the patient was placed in a knee-chest position and given local anesthetics only. Raoul Palmer in Paris advocated placing patients in the Trendelenburg position to bring the air into the pelvic cavity and in 1944 stressed the importance of monitoring intra-abdominal pressure. It was another 20 years, however, before Kurt Semm in Kiel, Germany, developed an automatic insufflation device that monitored abdominal pressure and gas flow. Prior to this time air was introduced into the peritoneal cavity by means of a syringe.

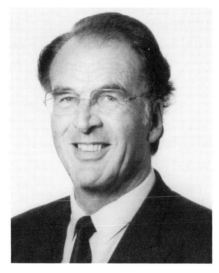

Kurt Semm

With the development of safer insufflation needles as well as instruments for controlling gas flow during pneumoperitoneum, complications such as bowel perforations and injuries to retroperitoneal vessels were significantly reduced.[5] Nevertheless, because laparoscopy was considered a "blind" procedure with an inherent risk of injury to intraperitoneal structures, acceptance was slow throughout Europe and North America.

Perhaps one of the most significant advances in rigid endoscopy was the development of the rod-lens system in 1966 by the British optical physicist Hopkins. His design resulted in vastly improved image brightness and clarity. These same principles are still utilized in laparoscopes today. The introduction of fiberoptic (cold) light sources in the early 1960s eliminated the risk of bowel burns caused by incandescent lighting. Bowel injuries related to unipolar coagulation, however, remained a problem (see Chapters 2 and 16). Such concerns stimulated the development of fallop rings for tubal sterilization, the Hulka clip, and finally a bipolar grasping forceps (Kleppinger forceps). Because of these and other technologic advances, laparoscopy for diagnostic purposes, elective sterilization, and in vitro fertilization procedures was soon popularized. Professor Kurt Semm played a vital role in the development of surgical laparoscopy. To disassociate his procedures from earlier attempts at laparoscopy, which had been fraught with complications, he coined the term "operative pelviscopy" [pelvioscopy]. His pioneering work resulted in a series of technologic advances that led to more complicated therapeutic laparoscopic procedures.[6] To avoid injuries caused by unipolar cautery, he created an innovative heat transfer system, thermocoagulation, for sterilization procedures. Semm found that he could better visualize the pelvic structures using a laparoscope with an angled lens. To provide accurate and easy transection of tissues, he invented the hook scissors, which minimized the problems of using these scissors without the advantages of depth perception. In 1969 he designed a "uterus vacuum mobilizer" for improved manipulation and laparoscopic visualization of reproductive organs. The morcellator shown below was created to safely remove large pieces of benign and even neoplastic tissue.

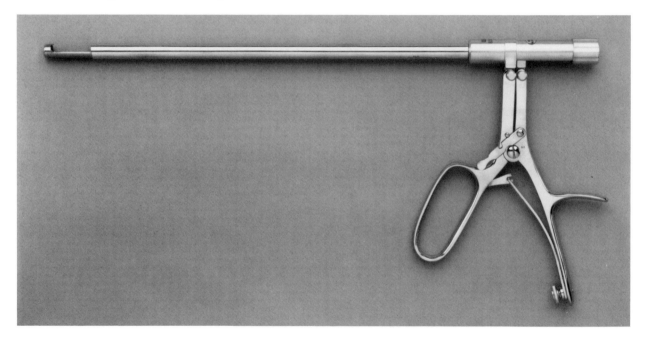

His surgical department was also responsible for perfecting the EndoLoop applicator, a device designed to prevent loss of intraperitoneal insufflated CO_2 when inserting sutures into the peritoneal cavity.

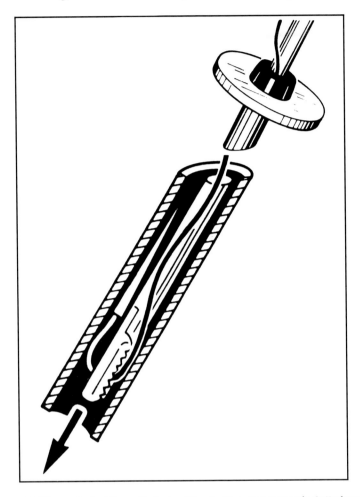

From Semm K. History. In Sanfilippo JS, Levine RL, eds. Operative Gynecologic Endoscopy. New York: Springer-Verlag, 1989.

In the early years of operative pelvioscopy, inadequate hemostasis often necessitated conversion to laparotomy. The pretied suture loop (Roeder loop) alleviated some of these problems. Semm also perfected intra- and extracorporeal knot-tying techniques and the instruments required to perform these maneuvers.[7,8] As more difficult operative procedures were undertaken, it became evident that a high-volume irrigation system to evacuate clots and obtain a clear operative field was desirable. As a result, he developed an irrigation/aspiration apparatus with design modifications to prevent tube clogging.

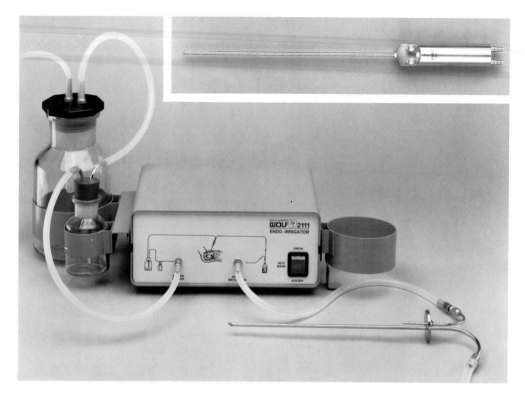

Many other instruments such as needle holders, cone-shaped trocars, microscissors, clip appliers, and atraumatic forceps were conceptualized, created, and first utilized at the University of Kiel. In conjunction with these technical advances, Semm devised a number of laparoscopic surgical procedures to replace conventional open operations, such as direct micro-surgical suturing that allowed laparoscopic management of ectopic pregnancies, often with preservation of the affected tube, tubal sterilization by endocoagulation, salpingostomy, oophorectomy, salpingolysis, tumor reduction therapy, and frimbiolysis. Other laparoscopic procedures he popularized included lysis of omental adhesions, bowel suturing,[9] endometrial implant coagulation, tumor biopsy and staging, repair of uterine perforations, and incidental appendectomy. Semm also facilitated laparoscopic training by creating the Pelvitrainer designed to teach surgeons the hand-eye coordination and suture-tying techniques required for operative laparoscopy.[10]

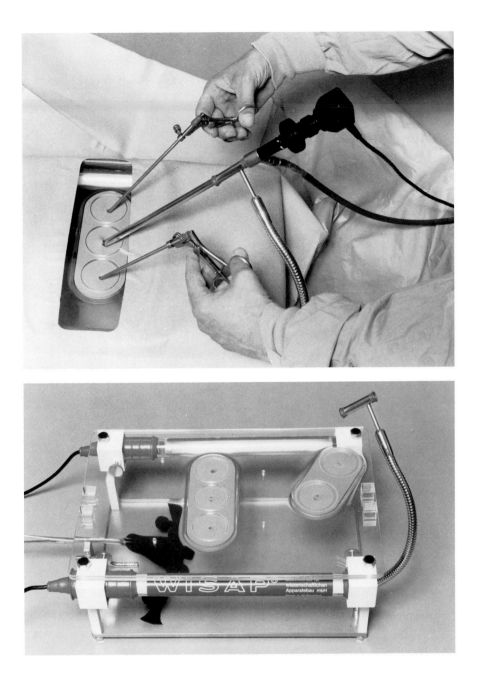

Currently, 75% of all gynecologic procedures are performed under laparoscopic guidance at Semm's clinic. Many of these operations were previously performed via open laparotomy. Over 14,000 total laparoscopic procedures have been performed in Kiel during the past two decades with an overall complication rate of 0.28%.[11] Semm has, therefore, clearly demonstrated that laparoscopic surgery is safe, cost effective, and less traumatic than traditional open surgery.

Because of the 1% complication rate associated with percutaneous or blind trocar entry into the peritoneal cavity, Hasson[12] proposed an alternative method called open laparoscopy, also referred to as the Hasson technique. This method provides direct visualization of the peritoneal cavity prior to trocar insertion. The Hasson technique and the cannula used for this procedure have proved popular with many general surgeons now learning laparoscopic surgery because of their concern about bowel or vascular injuries associated with the percutaneous approach.

Laparoscopic visualization of the abdominal cavity was once restricted to the individual directing the operative procedure, and participation by other members of the surgical team was thus limited. Therefore complicated operative procedures proved to be tedious because of the inability of the assistant(s) to effectively interact with the surgeon. Although articulated attachments containing a series of mirrors could split the laparoscopic image, these proved to be cumbersome and ineffective.

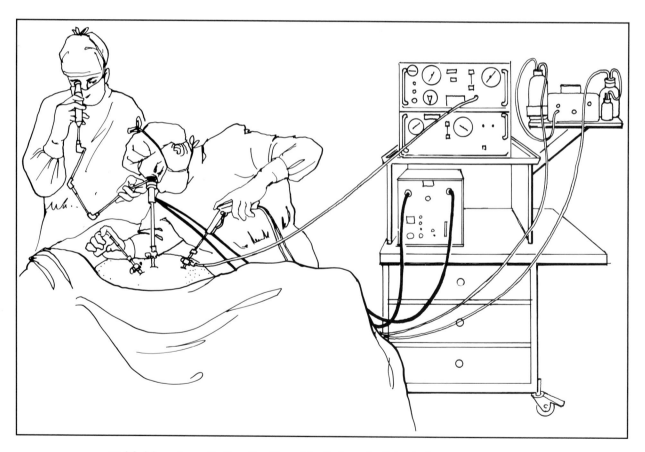

Modified from Semm K. Operative Manual for Endoscopic Abdominal Surgery (Friedrick ER, translator and editor). Chicago: Year Book, 1986.

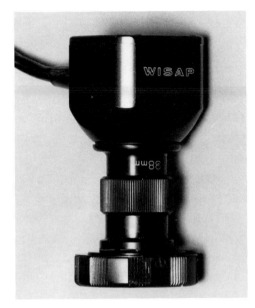

In 1986, however, this problem was solved with the development of a computer chip TV camera attached to the laparoscope.

This began the era of video-guided surgery in which laparoscopic surgical techniques could be used for more complicated gastrointestinal procedures. Video imaging has also facilitated the education of other surgeons and house staff. In addition, videotapes can now be used to document the diagnostic or operative procedure. Rapid developments in the area of video imaging have resulted in higher resolution video monitors affording greater clarity and definition as well as improved magnification of the operative field, making fine dissection of tissue planes easier.

The first surgical lasers were introduced in the mid-1960s. Laser light differs from ordinary light in that it travels in a single direction and consists of only one wavelength (see Chapters 2 and 3). It converts light energy to heat, resulting in a tissue reaction based on wavelength and distance to tissue. Early uses of this energy source by ophthalmologists for retinal detachment and by otolaryngologists for vocal cord surgery suggested its applicability to laparoscopic surgeons. The fear of uncontrolled bowel injuries from monopolar coagulation also prompted many gynecologists to adopt the laser as a dissecting and coagulation device. The first clinical report describing laser energy for operative pelvioscopy was by Bruhat, Mage, and Manhes[13] in 1979. Subsequently, laser light has been used for coagulation and enucleation of endometrial implants,[14] treatment of ectopic pregnancy with preservation of the affected adnexa,[15] adhesiolysis,[16] incision of hydrosalpinx, incision and aspiration of multiple cysts of the ovary (Stein-Leventhal syndrome), and vaporization of uterosacral ligaments for dysmenorrhea.[17] The theoretical benefits of laser treatment are improved hemostasis, greater precision during tissue dissection, and decreased complications from inadvertent burns distant from the operative field. Data to support the superiority of this modality over that of laparoscopic electrocoagulation, however, has not been forthcoming. The issue continues to be debated (see Chapter 16).

With modern technology available, oophorectomy and hysterectomy for benign disease[18,19] have also been performed laparoscopically. Resection of full-thickness bowel wall endometrial implants and conservative endoscopic management of pelvic inflammatory disease have been reported as well.[20] Laparoscopic treatment of tubo-ovarian abscesses vs. antibiotic therapy alone may be superior, but more extensive trials are required.

The introduction of laparoscopy in general surgery was made in an attempt to improve on the diagnosis of acute appendicitis.[21-28] Many general surgeons were first exposed to laparoscopy while assisting gynecologists in the evaluation of young women with atypical right lower quadrant pain. It was soon demonstrated that the appendix could be directly visualized in as many as 90% of patients. Laparoscopic diagnosis of acute appendicitis was based on direct visualization, turbid peritoneal fluid, cecal inflammation, or omental inflammation and adherence in the right iliac fossa. Its diagnostic use was most applicable to young females with equivocal signs of appendicitis, and many centers reported a 50% to 70% reduction in the removal of normal appendices. However, its broader application to all patients has remained debatable.[21,22]

The first laparoscopic procedure performed by general surgeons appears to have been liver biopsies guided under direct vision.[29] Clinical investigators rapidly recognized the versatility of this procedure in obtaining tissue from other areas of the abdominal cavity. Warshaw, Tepper, and Shipley[30] utilized laparoscopy in 1986 for staging of pancreatic carcinoma and demonstrated an overall accuracy rate of 93%. Follow-up studies have continued to document the benefit of this approach for patients with pancreatic cancer and gastric malignancies.[31]

Video imaging, improved instrumentation, and the growing recognition of the potential of laparoscopy for diagnostic and staging procedures made therapeutic laparoscopy for gastrointestinal disease a reality by the end of the 1980s.

LAPAROSCOPIC CHOLECYSTECTOMY

The prevalence of gallbladder disease as well as the prolonged hospitalization, extended recovery time, and pain associated with a major abdominal operation has prompted many investigators to explore alternative methods of treatment. Within the past two decades nonoperative approaches to eliminate gallstones, such as dissolution therapy and lithotripsy, have been introduced. Although these procedures appeared to have a lower morbidity because the need for cholecystectomy was eliminated, the recurrence of symptomatic gallstones was in excess of 50%. Consequently, the expense associated with repetitive procedures and the need for prolonged administration of agents to prevent recurrent stone formation made this approach less attractive. In this setting laparoscopic cholecystectomy was introduced as an endoscopic procedure for removal of the gallbladder without the postoperative pain sequelae of open cholecystectomy.

Laparoscopic cholecystotomy for the purpose of removing gallstones in pigs was performed by Frimdberg in 1978 (personal communication, 1990). Abd El Ghany, Holley, and Cuschieri[32] reported a modification of this approach in experimental animals using laparoscopic guided percutaneous cholecystotomy to introduce human gallstones and a lithotripsy probe into the gallbladder. Electrohydraulic lithotripsy was then used to disintegrate the stones.

Laparoscopic cholecystectomy was first performed in an animal model by Filipi, Mall, and Roosma in 1985.[33] A collapsible retractor attached to the laparoscope provided visibility.

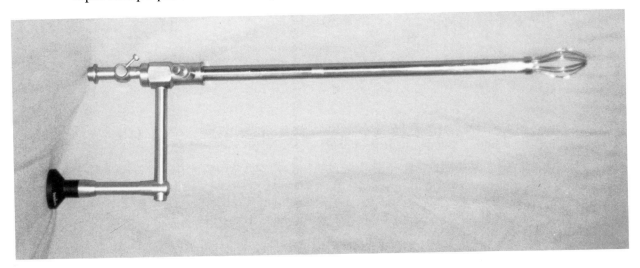

The cystic artery was electrocoagulated, the cystic duct ligated with a tiny rubber band, and the gallbladder removed through one of the puncture sites. Lateral displacement of tissues using this instrument did not provide adequate exposure. Since video systems adaptable to the laparoscope were not available until later, the operative team was unable to assist in a meaningful way. Therefore the technique was considered unsafe and the investigation suspended.

In 1987 the complete removal of a diseased gallbladder in a patient was performed by Mouret in Lyon, France (personal communication, 1990). He exposed the porta hepatis by forceful cephalad retraction of the gallbladder fundus. Dubois, in communication with Mouret, immediately initiated animal laboratory testing and in May of 1988 performed his first clinical laparoscopic cholecystectomy.

Working independently, McKernan and Saye performed the first laparoscopic cholecystectomy in the United States in 1988. Collaborating with McKernan and Saye, Drs. Reddick and Olsen in Nashville, Tennessee, soon began performing this procedure routinely at their institution and developed the technique of laparoscopic cholangiography. Their publication in *Laser Medicine and Surgery News and Advances* was the first clinical report in the English literature on laparoscopic cholecystectomy.[34]

The patient population consisted of five women and one man. An intraoperative perforation of the gallbladder with a blunt instrument in one patient necessitated converting the procedure to an open cholecystectomy. The patient was hospitalized for 4 days but had no adverse effects. The remaining five patients had uneventful recoveries (average length of hospitalization 1.9 days). A customized surgical clip applier was devised by their associate, Wayne Miller, which provided a secure closure of the cystic duct stump and reduced their operative time.

Initially a laser energy modality was used in this country for coagulation and dissection of the gallbladder. Within a short period of time, however, modifications of the technique and the development of new instrumentation proved that this procedure could be performed equally well using electrocautery.[35]

Dubois, Berthelot, and Levard[36] reported a series of 63 patients shortly thereafter in *La Nouvelle Presse Medicale*. He converted three of his first 39 procedures to a mini-cholecystectomy when unsuspected acute cholecystitis was encountered. A fourth patient underwent an immediate laparotomy for uncontrolled cystic artery bleeding.[37] A subhepatic collection of bile was found on the forty-eighth postoperative day in one patient. Exploration revealed no evidence of common bile duct injury or cystic duct leakage.

Initially only good-risk patients who met the following criteria were selected: (1) symptoms consistent with biliary colic, (2) documented stones on ultrasonography or contrast radiography, (3) no evidence of common bile duct disease, (4) the absence of acute cholecystitis, (5) stones <3.0 cm in diameter, and (6) no previous upper abdominal surgery. Subsequently the indications have been greatly expanded (see Chapters 8 and 9), and as many as 95% of patients may now be candidates for this procedure.

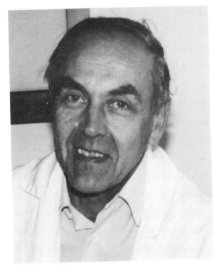

François Dubois

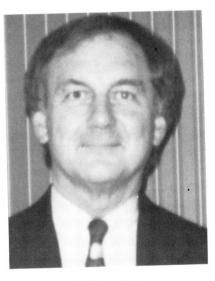

William Saye

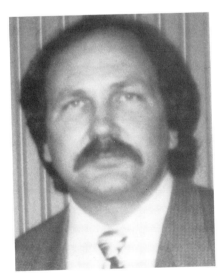

E.J. Reddick

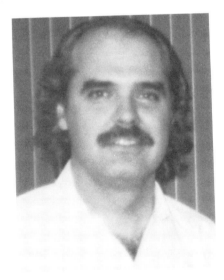

Wayne Miller

Early difficulties deterred many physicians from recommending cholangiography. Schultz in Minneapolis performed laparoscopic cholecystocholangiography by emptying the gallbladder and then slowly injecting contrast material into the gallbladder. Unfortunately this sometimes resulted in the leakage of bile into the peritoneal cavity, and the radiographs obtained were often of poor quality. Fitzgibbons and Petlin both described a technique of direct cholangiography (see Chapter 10). They introduced a cholangiogram catheter through a small opening in the abdominal wall created by a 14-gauge intravenous needle and catheter. The catheter was then guided into the cystic duct and secured in place with a metal clip. Olsen and Reddick developed an innovative instrument that eliminated the need for an additional abdominal puncture. This cholangiogram clamp has a central lumen that allows the surgeon to introduce the catheter into the abdomen. At the end of the instrument are atraumatic grasping forceps that permit the catheter to be guided into an opening made in the cystic duct. The same ring forceps are then used to secure the catheter within the duct and form a watertight seal.

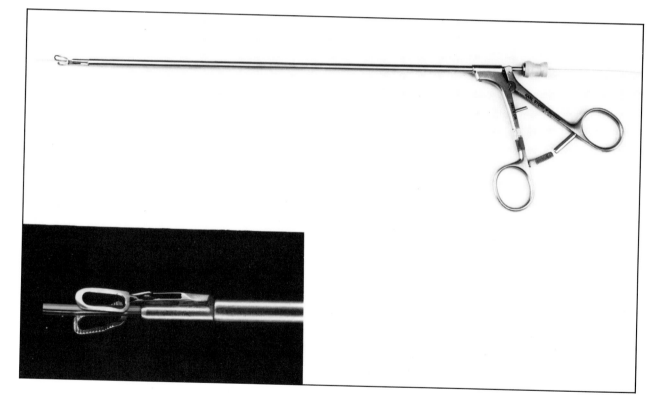

Common duct injuries occurring during laparoscopic guided biliary tract surgery were and remain a major concern of surgeons performing this procedure. Because of the magnification afforded by current high-definition video imaging systems, visualization of the ductal structures may equal or exceed that obtained with traditional open cholecystectomy. The number of reported iatrogenic injuries to the biliary drainage system is quite low at present; however, only a few laparoscopic surgeons have thus far published data detailing their operative complications.[35]

LAPAROSCOPIC APPENDECTOMY

De Kok[38] first performed laparoscopic guided appendectomy in 1977. This procedure, however, required a mini-laparotomy for removing the appendix. In 1983 Semm[39] published the first report on the complete removal of the appendix by laparoscopic means alone. Hemostasis was obtained by passing suture material attached to a small, straight needle through the mesoappendix and tying it extracorporeally. Endoscopic ligation of the appendix was performed using a pretied Roeder loop. Just distal to the proximal point of ligation the appendix was endocoagulated and transected. This operative approach was recommended only for nonacute appendices.

Schreiber[40] performed the first laparoscopic appendectomy for acute appendicitis in 1987. Of the 70 appendectomies he reported, seven were for acute inflammation. In one of these patients a leak from the appendiceal stump was noted postoperatively. This complication was attributed to excessive coagulation of the proximal appendix prior to amputation. At laparotomy a cecal defect was closed, and the patient had an uneventful recovery. Larger series of successful laparoscopic appendectomies for acute inflammation have been reported and will be discussed in Chapter 11.

A larger diameter trocar (20 mm) and sheath have recently been developed to facilitate the laparoscopic removal of very large and inflamed appendices.

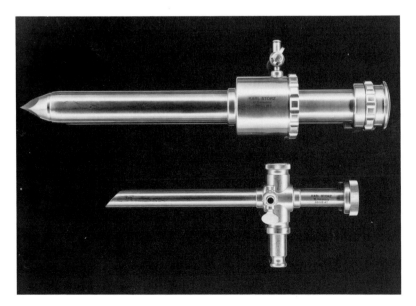

When this device is used, the infected appendix does not come into contact with the abdominal wall, resulting in a lower incidence of wound infections. Additional advantages of laparoscopic appendectomy are diminished pain, less cosmetic disfigurement, and shorter hospitalization. The latter point has been difficult to demonstrate in this country since most patients with appendicitis remain in the hospital for only 2 to 3 days. Most surgeons at present have utilized this procedure only in those patients with atypical symptoms who are undergoing diagnostic laparoscopy. If the patient is found to have acute appendicitis, the laparoscope is used to remove the appendix rather than performing an additional abdominal incision.

LAPAROSCOPIC HERNIORRHAPHY

Isolated reports of laparoscopy for the diagnosis of occult inguinal hernias have been published. Although an accurate diagnostic modality, it remains unclear whether the morbidity may exceed that for simple groin exploration. Ger et al.[41] published an experimental model of laparoscopic inguinal hernia repair in 1990. Twelve experimental animals with congenital indirect inguinal hernias had the internal ring closed with specially designed 15 mm clips. The animals were followed for up to 14 weeks, and no evidence of early recurrence was noted, although one animal developed a contralateral inguinal hernia during this interval. It was mentioned in this report that clinical trials had begun. A video presentation of laparoscopic treatment of inguinal and femoral hernia in patients was shown at the meeting of the American Association of Gynecologic Laparoscopists in 1989. Laparoscopic closure of the internal peritoneal opening in this film was performed by placing interrupted sutures rather than surgical staples. Follow-up results were not made available. Open intraperitoneal hernia repairs by suturing the internal ring alone have been reported previously; however, no meaningful recurrence rates have been determined. Several centers have now initiated investigations into laparoscopic hernia repairs by suturing the peritoneal opening after insertion of a prosthetic mesh plug. This and other forms of laparoscopic hernia research will be reviewed in Chapter 14.

THORACOSCOPIC SURGERY

H.C. Jacobaeus, the first physician to perform clinical laparoscopy, was also the first to introduce diagnostic thoracoscopy. This procedure has since been used as a diagnostic procedure for recurrent pleural effusion, pleural thickening, difficult to localize intrapleural fluid, and lung biopsy. A mortality rate of 0% to 1% has been associated with diagnostic thoracoscopy.

Therapeutic thoracoscopy for division of apical pleural adhesions was also introduced by Jacobaeus in 1921.[42] Thoracoscopic treatment of pneumothoraces was reported in 1974 by Keller, Gutersohn, and Herzog.[43] Talc poudrage, applied through the operative thoracoscope, proved to be effective therapy. Further advances with laser technology have been made in the treatment of this disorder.[44] Low-power laser pulses have been used to coagulate apical blebs and to obliterate the parietal pleura. Thoracoscopic guided drainage of empyema cavities[45] and management of spontaneous esophageal perforation[46] have also been reported. Thoracoscopic lung resections and more intricate diagnostic procedures are soon anticipated with the recently introduced endoscopic stapling instruments. The thoracoscope may prove to be a valuable surgical tool in the near future for a variety of pulmonary disorders.

LAPAROSCOPIC ADHESIOLYSIS

Laparoscopic adhesiolysis has been practiced by Semm and others for many years but was confined to omental and parietal peritoneal adhesions. Subsequently lysis of adhesions involving fimbria was helpful in infertile patients. A few scattered reports of laparoscopic lysis of adhesions for early postoperative bowel obstruction have appeared. With the rapid improvements in laparoscopic technology this approach may become feasible for some patients with early or incomplete small bowel obstruction.

Laparoscopic adhesiolysis for pelvic and abdominal pain has been shown to be beneficial in a recently published series of 261 patients.[47] All patients had well-localized repetitive pain triggered by either position, movement, or food. A 6-month follow-up showed satisfactory results in 215 patients. At present, however, no data are available to show that laparoscopic adhesiolysis is associated with less recurrent adhesion formation than open surgery.

REFERENCES

1. Stein S. Das Photo-Endoskop: Part 3. Berl Klin Wochenschr, 1874.
2. Kelling G. Über Oesophagoskopie, Gastroskopie und Colioskopie. Munch Med Wochenschr 49:21-24, 1901.
3. Jacobaeus HC. Über die Möglichkeit, die Zystoskopie bei Untersuchung seröser Höhlungen anzuwenden. Munch Med Wochenschr 57:2090-2092, 1910.
4. Decker A. Pelvic culdoscopy. In Meigs JV, Sturgis SH, eds. Progress in Gynecology. New York: Grune & Stratton, 1946.
5. Eisenburg J. Über eine Apparatur zur schonenden und kontrollierbaren Gasfüllung der Bauchhöhle für die Laparoskopie. Klin Wochenschr 44:593, 1966.
6. Semm K. History. In Sanfilippo JS, Levine RL, eds. Operative Gynecologic Endoscopy. New York: Springer-Verlag, 1989.

7. Semm K. Tissue-puncher and loop-ligation—New aids for surgical therapeutic pelviscopy (laparoscopy): Endoscopic intra-abdominal surgery. Endoscopy 10:119-127, 1978.

8. Semm K. Advances in pelviscopic surgery (appendectomy). Curr Prob Obstet Gynecol 5(10):entire issue, 1982.

9. Semm K. The endoscopic intra-abdominal suture. Geburtshilfe Frauenheilkd 42:56-57, 1982.

10. Semm K. Operative pelviscopy. Br Med Bull 42:284-295, 1986.

11. Semm K. Endoscopic Intraabdominal Surgery. Kiel, Germany: Christian-Albrects-Universität, 1984.

12. Hasson HM. Open laparoscopy vs. closed laparoscopy: A comparison of complication rates. Adv Planned Parenthood 13:41-50, 1978.

13. Bruhat MA, Mage G, Manhes M. Use of the CO_2 laser by laparoscopy. In Kaplan I, ed. Proceedings of the Third International Congress for Laser Surgery. Tel Aviv: Otpaz, 1979, pp 274-276.

14. Daniell JF, Pittaway DE. Use of the CO_2 laser laparoscope in laparoscopic surgery: Initial experience with the second puncture technique. Infertility 5:15-23, 1982.

15. Daniell JF. Laser laparoscopy. In Baggish MS, ed. Basic and Advanced Laser Laparoscopy in Gynecology. Norwalk, Conn.: Appleton-Century-Crofts, 1985, pp 343-356.

16. Martin DC. Infertility surgery using the carbon dioxide laser. Clin Gynecol Briefs 4(3):1-4, 1983.

17. Feste JR. Laser laparoscopy: A new modality. J Reprod Med 30:413-417, 1985.

18. Reich H. Laparoscopic oophorectomy and salpingo-oophorectomy in the treatment of benign tubo-ovarian disease. Int J Fertil 32:233-236, 1987.

19. Reich H, DeCaprio J, McGlynn F. Laparoscopic hysterectomy. J Gynecol Surg 5:213-215, 1989.

20. Reich H, McGlynn F. Laparoscopic treatment of tuboovarian and pelvic abscess. J Reprod Med 32:747-752, 1987.

21. Whitworth CM, Whitworth PW, Sanfillipo J, Polk HC. Value of diagnostic laparoscopy in young women with possible appendicitis. Surg Gynecol Obstet 167:187-190, 1988.

22. Woodward A, Hemingway D. Which patients should undergo laparoscopy [letter]? Br Med J 296:1740, 1988.

23. Patterson-Brown S, Thompson JN, Eckersley JRT, Ponting GA, Dudley HA. Which patients with suspected appendicitis should undergo laparoscopy? Br Med J 296:1363-1364, 1988.

24. Leape L, Ramenofsky ML. Laparoscopy for questionable appendicitis. Ann Surg 191:410-413, 1980.

25. Anteby SO, Schenker JG, Polishuk, WZ. The value of laparoscopy in acute pelvic pain. Ann Surg 181:484-486, 1975.

26. Spirtos NM, Eisenkop SM, Spirtos TW, Poliakin RI, Hibbard LT. Laparoscopy—A diagnostic aid in cases of suspected appendicitis. Its use in women of reproductive age. Am J Obstet Gynecol 156:90-94, 1987.

27. Clarke PJ, Hands LJ, Gough MH, Kettlewell MC. The use of laparoscopy in the management of right iliac fossa pain. Ann R Coll Surg Engl 68:68-69, 1986.

28. Deutsch A, Zelikovsky A, Reiss R. Laparoscopy in the prevention of unnecessary appendectomies: A prospective study. Br J Surg 69:336-337, 1982.

29. Lightdale CJ. Laparoscopy and biopsy in malignant liver disease. Cancer 50(Suppl 11):2672-2675, 1982.

30. Warshaw AL, Tepper JE, Shipley WU. Laparoscopy in the staging and planning of therapy for pancreatic cancer. Am J Surg 151:76-80, 1986.

31. Possik RA, Franco EL, Pires DR, Wohnrath DR, Ferreira EB. Sensitivity, specificity, and predictive value of laparoscopy for the staging of gastric cancer and for the detection of liver metastases. Cancer 58:1-6, 1986.

32. Abd El Ghany AB, Holley MP, Cuschieri A. Percutaneous stone clearance of the gallbladder through an access cholecystostomy. Surg Endosc 3:126-130, 1989.

33. Fitzgibbons RJ Jr, Schmid S, Santoscoy R, Hinder R, Filipi CJ, Jenkins J, Fitzgibbons RJ Sr. Laparoscopic cholecystectomy: The beginning of a new era in general surgery (submitted for publication).

34. Reddick EJ, Olsen D, Daniell J, Saye W, McKernan B, Miller W, Hoback M. Laparoscopic laser cholecystectomy. Laser Med Surg News Adv Feb. 1989, pp 38-40.

35. Zucker KA, Bailey RW, Gadacz TR, Imbembo AL. Laparoscopic guided cholecystectomy. Am J Surg 161:36-44, 1991.

36. Dubois F, Berthelot G, Levard H. Cholécystectomy par coelioscopy. Nouv Presse Med 18:980-982, 1989.

37. Dubois F, Icard P, Berthelot G, Levard H. Coelioscopic cholecystectomy—Preliminary report of 36 cases. Ann Surg 211:60-62, 1990.
38. De Kok H. A new technique for resecting the non-inflamed not-adhesive appendix through a mini-laparotomy with the aid of the laparoscope. Arch Chir Neerl 29:195-197, 1977.
39. Semm K. Endoscopic appendicectomy. Endoscopy 15:59-64, 1983.
40. Schreiber J. Early experience with laparoscopic appendectomy in women. Surg Endosc 1:211-216, 1987.
41. Ger R, Monroe K, Duvivier R, Mishrick A. Management of indirect inguinal hernias by laparoscopic closure of the neck of the sac. Am J Surg 159:371-373, 1990.
42. Jacobaeus HC. The cauterization of adhesions in pneumothorax treatment of tuberculosis. Surg Gynecol Obstet 32:493-500, 1921.
43. Keller R, Gutersohn J, Herzog H. The management of persistent pneumothorax by thoracoscopic procedures. Thoraxchirurgie 22:457-460, 1974.
44. Torre M, Belloni P. Nd:YAG laser pleurodesis through thoracoscopy: New curative therapy in spontaneous pneumothorax. Ann Thorac Surg 47:887-889, 1989.
45. Hutter J, Harari D, Braimbridge M. The management of empyema thoracis by thoracoscopy and irrigation. Ann Thorac Surg 39:517-520, 1985.
46. Hutter J, Fenn A, Braimbridge M. The management of spontaneous oesophageal perforation by thorascopy and irrigation. Br J Surg 72:208-209, 1985.
47. Mouret P, Marsaud H. Laparoscopic adhesiotomy and preliminary study. Surg Endosc (in press).

CHAPTER 2

Laparoscopic Equipment and Instrumentation

Mark A. Talamini, M.D.
Thomas R. Gadacz, M.D.

Diagnosis and intervention mediated by optical and video technology have been successful in many medical and surgical arenas. As medicine has developed, certain specialties have successfully "adopted" these modalities more quickly and easily than others. General surgery, however, is a conservative discipline, an attribute that once served it well. General surgeons also tend to trust their visual and tactile senses more than "technology." The combination of these factors has caused the treatment of many disease states to slip beyond the province of general surgery (polypectomy via colonoscopy, sphincterotomy via duodenoscopy, etc.).

The growing popularity of a single endoscopic procedure, laparoscopic cholecystectomy, appears destined to usher general surgeons into a new phase of therapeutic technology. For most general surgeons, this will require a significant paradigm shift. We will now be required to trust an image produced on a two-dimensional video screen rather than our three-dimensional vision. We will be required to manipulate and "feel" tissue from a distance of 18 inches. We will need to readjust our senses and develop hand-eye coordination when viewing our movements on a video monitor. All of this will require us to familiarize ourselves with and be dependent on new types of equipment and instruments. With the use of this technology a different and new set of complications will become apparent. Gas embolus and bowel injury due to laparoscopic trocars and lasers (as well as cautery) are just two examples of complications that are unfamiliar to most general surgeons. It is critical that surgeons performing laparoscopic procedures thoroughly understand the purpose, use, and complications associated with the equipment and instruments. It is the goal of this chapter to acquaint the reader with the specialized equipment and instruments necessary to perform surgical laparoscopy, review some of the potential complications of this new technology, and highlight what the future may hold in terms of new equipment and instrumentation.

PLANNING

The sophisticated equipment necessary to perform laparoscopic surgery is expensive (although compared to the cost of a biliary lithotripsy unit it seems quite reasonable). Some key factors other than cost must be considered when planning to purchase equipment and instruments. First, a great many problems can be avoided by ensuring that all equipment is compatible and uniform so that the instruments will fit through the cannulas and the various cables will connect with one another. Unfortunately no industry standards apply to the manufacture of laparoscopic instruments. The diameters of the various dissectors, scissors, clip appliers, etc. vary from one manufacturer to another. This can be frustrating to the novice laparoscopist who will suddenly find that an instrument will not fit through an existing cannula in the abdominal cavity. It is recommended that the surgeon use as many instruments from the same supplier as possible to avoid this problem. Disposable laparoscopic trocars and sheaths are available with converters that can be attached to the cannula, allowing different sized instruments to be used without loss of pneumoperitoneum.

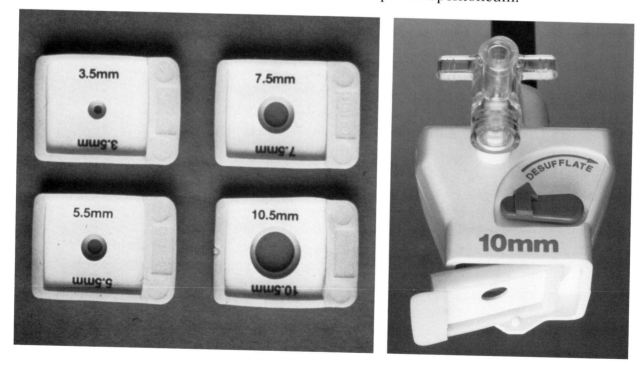

When using these converters it is important to insert a laparoscopic cannula that accommodates the largest instrument to be used since these adapters will permit only the use of smaller devices.

Backup service and technologic support from the manufacturer should also be considered when comparing the price of such systems. Rapid and efficient service from the company's representative and availability of backup equipment are vital to the smooth and uninterrupted performance of laparoscopic surgery.

EQUIPMENT

The technology of endoscopic video equipment is moving forward quickly. In future years we can expect to see new designs with enhanced capacities not yet imagined. Imaging systems incorporating high-definition video cameras and monitors (resolution greater than 1200 lines per inch) are already being field-tested. Most laparoscopic instruments used by general surgeons at present were developed for pelvic surgery. Future developments will undoubtedly include devices designed specifically for cholecystectomy, vagotomy, appendectomy, etc. Equipment falls into two broad categories: those major pieces of equipment that enable the surgeon to perform laparoscopy and those instruments related to the performance of specific tasks or procedures (including electrocautery and laser).

Insufflation Equipment

Visualization within the peritoneal cavity requires "space" in which to shine light and maneuver. In a standard laparotomy this space is created by opening the abdomen and allowing room light and air into the cavity. In laparoscopic procedures this is accomplished by filling the peritoneal cavity with a gas that distends the abdominal wall and provides an area for light and manipulation, a process termed pneumoperitoneum. In the history of laparoscopy many gases have been used for establishing pneumoperitoneum, including room air, nitrous oxide, oxygen, and carbon dioxide. Air and oxygen create a higher risk in terms of air embolism. In addition, they support combustion, which can be an important consideration when using electrocautery or laser energy during therapeutic laparoscopic procedures. Nitrous oxide can be dangerous because of unpredictable and uncontrollable absorption into the bloodstream. CO_2 is the standard gas used for pneumoperitoneum. It can be injected directly into the bloodstream in volumes up to 100 ml/min without serious metabolic effect. It also suppresses combustion and appears to be relatively innocuous to the tissues of the peritoneum. Not only is it the safest gaseous medium currently in use, but it is also readily available, inexpensive, and easy to use.

A means must also be devised for safely initiating and maintaining pneumoperitoneum. It is critical to the safety of the patient that the pressure within the abdomen not rise above 12 to 14 mm Hg to prevent complications such as air embolus, damage to the diaphragms, and hemodynamic instability. In the early days of laparoscopy this was accomplished with a manometer connected to a hand-pumped bulb-valve system with insufflation of room air. Now sophisticated equipment has been developed that automatically delivers CO_2 from a high-pressure tank, through a regulator, and into the patient at predetermined flow rates. These machines constantly monitor the intra-abdominal pressure, stop the flow once a certain intra-abdominal pressure is reached, indicate the rate of flow of CO_2 into the abdomen, and record the total volume of gas delivered from the machine. Rapid CO_2 insufflation into the abdomen is often necessary when a smoke or a laser plume is being evacuated from the abdomen. CO_2 is also lost through leaks around valves and gaskets and during the exchange of instruments. Therefore in laparoscopic general surgery a high-flow insufflator capable of delivering at least 6 L of gas per minute is necessary, but a flow rate of 8 or 10 L/min is preferable. Often this will require the operating room to purchase a new unit. Many of the older insufflators currently used for gynecologic laparoscopy have a maximum flow of 3 L/min. These machines must be frequently inspected to ensure that they are accurately calibrated since there is no backup system for regulating the intra-abdominal pressure.

Insufflators are available in various styles and formats, depending on the manufacturer. Two examples of high-flow insufflators used for laparoscopic cholecystectomy are shown on p. 27.

In addition to the above-mentioned features, the machine should have a clearly readable and understandable set of gauges so that the operating team can observe the intra-abdominal pressure and the gas flow rate continuously. It is also important that the machine have a clearly audible alarm to signal excessive pressures. Some of the causes for high-pressure readings include (1) compression on the abdomen (especially during insertion of the trocar and cannulas), (2) incomplete anesthesia, (3) excessive gas flow from the laser plume (used to cool tip of laser), (4) an empty irrigation reservoir that allows pressured gas to flow through the irrigation channel and directly into the patient, (5) incomplete penetration of the cannula into the abdominal cavity, and (6) kinking of the insufflation tubing.

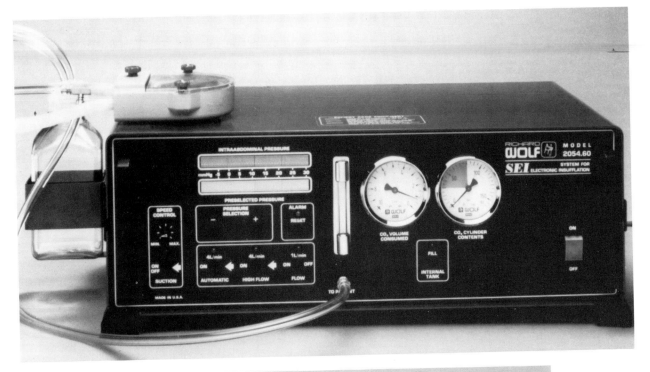

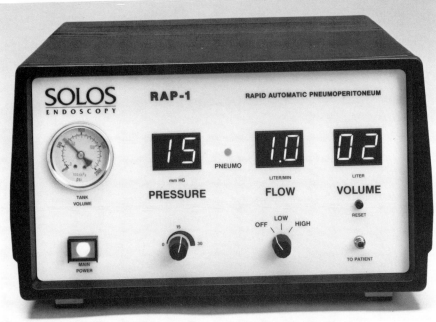

Light Source

The early laparoscopes used an incandescent light source at the tip of the scope with the intensity controlled by a rheostat. As the technology progressed, the light source was moved to the proximal end of the scope. The development of fiberoptics moved both the light source and its controls to a separate and distant unit connected to the laparoscope with a light cord. The physics of light transmission along a quartz rod system, termed total internal reflection, allows the transfer of light through the endoscope with virtually no loss of intensity. The term "cold light" was coined because the actual light source is separated from the fiberoptic cable by a heat shield. Therefore the light maintains its high intensity with a minimum of heat transfer to the tip of the laparoscope.

The quality of the light transmitted into the abdomen is extremely important for the accurate transmission of color and intensity. Variables such as the length, diameter, and quality of the flexible fiberoptic light cable must be exact and meticulously maintained. The quality of the fiberoptic cable can be assessed by holding one end of the cable 1 to 2 inches from any light source. The other end of the cord should light up. Broken fibers within the cable can be seen as black spots on the end of the cord. If more than 20% of the surface is blackened, the cord should be replaced. The sites of cable connections and light interfaces must also be kept clean and free of residue to avoid light loss or color distortion.

Despite the "cold light" source configuration, the intensity of light can produce considerable heat at the end of the fiberoptic light cable or endoscope and must be handled with care. Paper drapes and gowns can be singed or even catch fire. The hot endoscope tip can also burn internal organs if there is prolonged contact within the peritoneal cavity. During any procedure, if the lens becomes cloudy, the laparoscope must be removed and the tip cleaned. If blood and other residue are allowed to accumulate on the end of the laparoscope, the debris will bake onto the surface of the lens and be difficult to remove. Many of the light sources currently available are capable of manual adjustment or the brightness may be controlled automatically by adapting to changes in the video image.

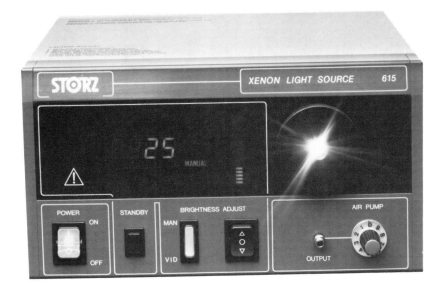

More sophisticated instruments can be equipped with a flash generator for film photography, providing through the lens metering and automatic flash capability. Special mounts that allow a 35 mm camera to be directly joined to the eyepiece of the laparoscope are also available.

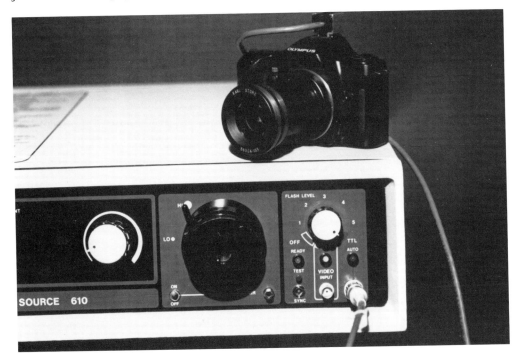

Video Camera

Superb visualization of the operative field is essential to laparoscopic procedures. A one-chip end-viewing camera has 450 horizontal lines per inch of resolution and is, in our opinion, a minimum requirement for adequate imaging.

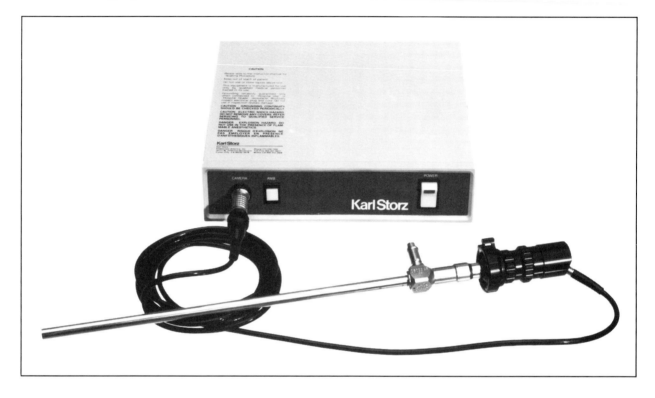

The camera is a small unit representing an optical/electronic interface that is attached to the laparoscope. A cable attaches this unit to a processor that modifies and then transmits the image to a video monitor, recorder, and/or color printer. An end-viewing camera transmits the entire image from the endoscope directly to the camera. This is in contrast to a split-beam camera, which is designed with an eyepiece so that the surgeon can look through the camera as well as have a separate video image. This latter configuration causes part of the image to be transmitted to the camera and part to a lens for direct visualization. This significantly compromises sharpness, detail, and brightness. Since general laparoscopic surgery usually is performed by watching the video monitor, not by direct visualization through the eyepiece of the endoscope, the split-beam camera provides no significant advantage. Prototype three-chip cameras (700 horizontal lines per inch) provide an enhanced video image and will be available in the very near future. This high-tech and high-quality camera maximizes resolution and color accuracy but is expensive (estimated cost approximately $18,000 or more).

The sophisticated video cameras currently available come with various capabilities, some of which are more desirable than others. It is important that they be capable of "color" or "white" balancing. Before use, the camera is aimed at a pure white background, and color balancing is performed to reset the image to absolute white. This allows an accurate spectrum of colors for the procedure and should be done every time the camera is turned on.

Most cameras also have a means for adjusting to variations in light intensity during use. This is usually via an automatic iris that measures the available light and adjusts the iris accordingly. All cameras have a focusing mechanism and some also have a zoom lens. Newer models have buttons mounted on the camera piece itself for adjusting the sensitivity to light or to trigger a video recorder or printer device to save images. Another important feature to be considered is the design of the telescope and the focal length of the lens system. Some laparoscopes require frequent lens adjustments as they are moved in and out of the operative field to keep the operative field in focus. Other laparoscopes can be focused out to infinity and therefore eliminate the need for constant adjustments. A recently introduced feature available from MPVideo (Kirschner Medical Corporation, Hopkinton, Mass.) is a camera and light source system with a high-speed shutter.

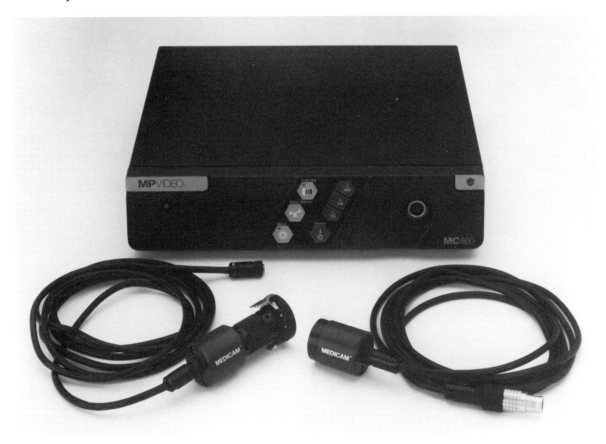

Activation of the shutter mechanism helps reduce glare, which can occur with reflected light off moist surfaces (i.e., visceral peritoneum). Since the camera represents the eye of the procedure and these items are expensive to repair or replace, it is vital that care of this equipment be meticulous and compulsive. Many have seals that allow them to be soaked for sterilization, but doing this will invariably shorten the life of the camera. A sterile plastic bag can also be used to maintain sterility in the operating room. Initially this may be cumbersome to use, but it is less damaging to the camera.

Video Monitors

High-resolution video monitors are essential to take advantage of the current generation of video cameras for laparoscopic general surgery. A standard, medical-grade monitor with a resolution of 400 horizontal lines per inch matches the picture of a one-chip camera, whereas a high-resolution monitor with 700 horizontal lines per inch takes better advantage of the enhanced image of a three-chip camera. The combination of the two elements, camera and monitor, will have the resolution of the least detailed element. For maximal comfort and visibility it is advisable to use two video monitors during a procedure so that the surgeons on each side of the operating table can see the video image along a direct line of sight.

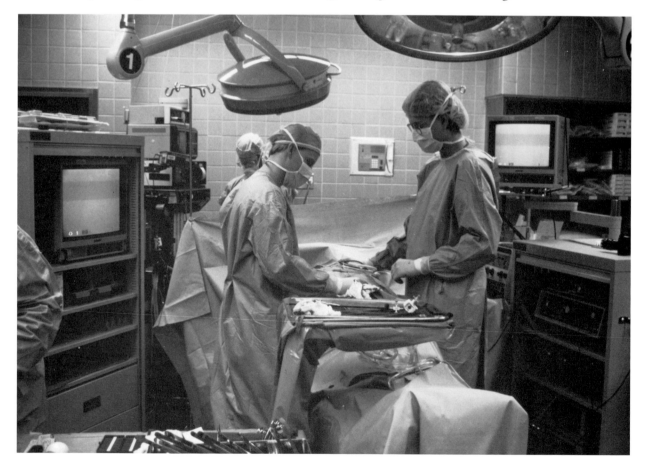

Monitors should be at least 13 inches in size for adequate visibility. Video monitors as well as all the electronic equipment must be grounded and of medical grade for safety in the operating room environment.

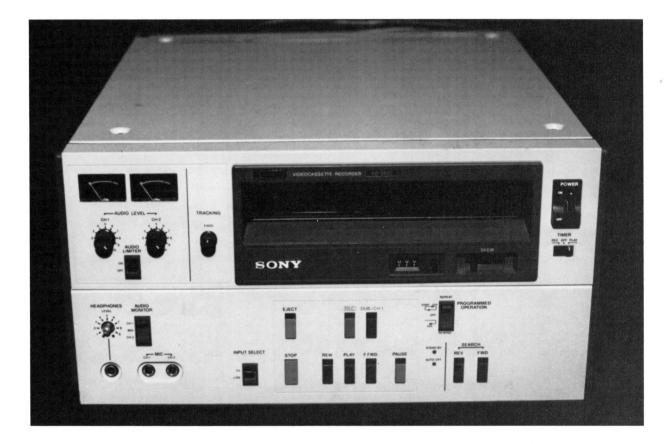

Additional electronic pieces of equipment that may be of benefit are color printers and video recorders to chronicle the images of a procedure. These can be invaluable for teaching purposes or documentation.

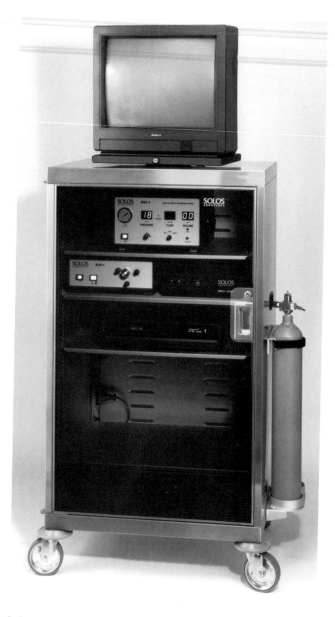

It is also helpful to have a rolling cabinet to contain the electronic components and make them portable as well as secure from inadvertent damage or theft.

Irrigation/Aspiration Devices

There are various types of machines that will instill fluid at a high flow rate. Some of these devices (also called hydrodissectors) have a gauge to regulate the irrigation pressure. The more effective irrigation instruments are powered by pressurized CO_2, which drives fluid from sterile reservoirs of irrigating solution. The device shown below has a switch to allow either reservoir to be used as well as a control knob to adjust the flow of fluid. Two pressure gauges allow for monitoring the status of the pressure in the CO_2 cylinder and the irrigating pressure of the fluid.

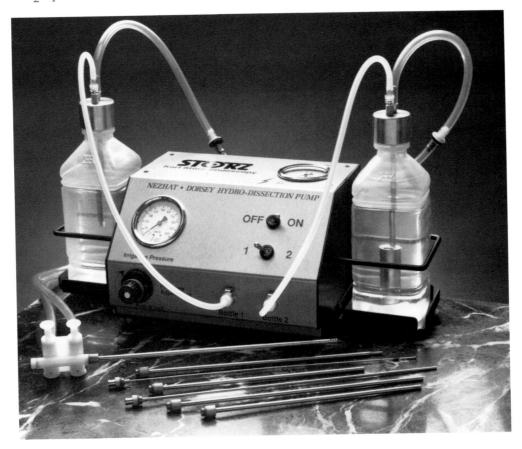

A pressure of 300 mm Hg is usually appropriate for irrigating the abdomen. This allows a relatively rapid flow of fluid that is capable of dislodging loose particulate material (i.e., blood clots) and identifying bleeding points. Irrigation/aspiration probes may have a single channel for both of these functions or separate channels. The latter instruments, therefore, have individual channels approximately 2.0 mm in diameter for either irrigation or suction. This may hinder the ability to remove even small clots from the abdominal cavity. Surgeons using these instruments have often found it necessary to add heparin (5000 units/L) to the irrigation solution to minimize clot formation. Probes with a common 5 mm channel can be connected directly to wall suction and are able to remove even large blood clots. Many of the newer devices are equipped with pool-tipped aspiration probes that also facilitate clot removal. Heparin is usually not necessary with the single-channel irrigation/aspiration probes. Larger irrigation/aspiration devices (10 mm) are currently under development and may prove useful. If the reservoir of irrigation fluid becomes empty, care must be taken not to expose the peritoneal cavity to the full pressure of the CO_2 tank. A high-pressure flow of gas can occur if the reservoir empties and may overflow into the peritoneal cavity. New devices have been designed with a valve to prevent such an occurrence.

Electrocautery/Laser

Electrocautery or laser energy is used to dissect tissue. Either energy modality will also adequately achieve hemostasis of small blood vessels. Electrocautery uses microwave wavelength energy to produce heat that can dissect and coagulate tissue (see Chapter 3). This device is familiar to most general surgeons. The power setting is tested on adjacent tissue (liver, parietal peritoneum) to ensure adequate but not excessive coagulation. A power setting of 20 to 30 watts is usually sufficient. Although a coagulation current is used primarily, a mixed blend of cutting and coagulation may be valuable. A number of different laparoscopic instruments have recently been adapted to incorporate monopolar electrocautery. Electrocautery must be used with caution since a spark-gap effect may cause injury to the bowel. This can be avoided by being sure that the tip of the cautery instrument is in contact with tissue before applying the power. The tip of the electrocautery must also avoid contact with the laparoscopic cannula since injury to other tissues, including the skin, may occur via conduction. This problem is eliminated if disposable cannulas with non-conducting fiberglass sheaths are used instead of the metallic devices.

The laser uses photons to dissect and coagulate tissue. Only the basics of the laser are reviewed here; the use of the laser in laparoscopic surgery is the subject of Chapter 3. A major advantage of the laser is that less lateral tissue damage occurs as compared to electrocautery.

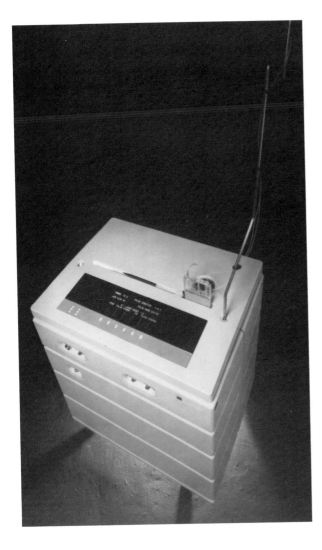

There are two major sources of laser energy used for laparoscopic cholecystectomy: neodymium-doped yttrium-aluminum garnet (Nd:YAG) and potassium-titanyl-phosphate (KTP). The Nd:YAG laser has a wavelength of 1064 nm.

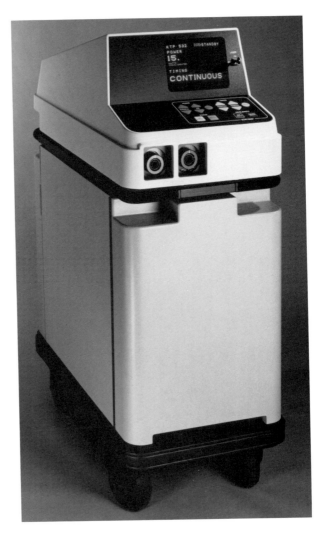

The KTP/532 laser has a wavelength of 532 nm.

Surgical lasers have undergone a dramatic change over the past 5 years. Older instruments were extremely large and required specialized electrical connections as well as direct plumbing attachments to cool the internal components. Newer lasers are much smaller, are easier to transport, utilize standard electrical outlets, and are air cooled.

Laser units currently used in laparoscopic surgery are of two major types—a free-beam and a contact-tip laser. The Nd:YAG can be used either as a free-beam or contact-tip laser. The KTP is a free-beam laser only. The free beam has a maximum power output of 150 watts. It requires careful manipulation of the fiber to control the focal point. The depth of penetration is 3 to 5 mm. Essential structures must not be placed in the path of the beam or major injuries can occur. When dissecting the gallbladder, for instance, the liver must be maintained in the background of the beam to prevent injury to other local organs. It is therefore critical that the surgeon be aware of the path of the beam at all times.

The contact-tip Nd:YAG laser delivers the laser energy to a synthetic sapphire (garnet) tip. The sapphire tip has a penetration depth of 0.2 to 1.0 mm and is not dependent on focal point control. To achieve its effect the sapphire tip must come in contact with the tissue. Various sapphire tips are designed for cutting, coagulation, or a combination of both.

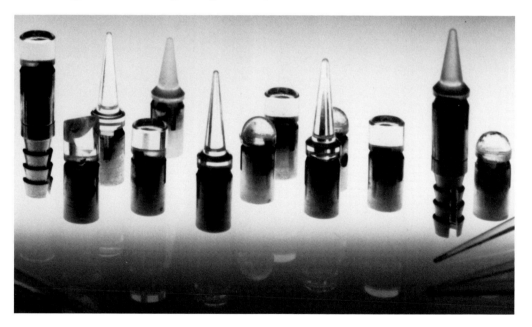

The contact-tip laser is far more effective as a dissecting instrument than as a coagulating device. If bleeding is encountered, it may be necessary to remove the sapphire tip and use the YAG laser free beam to achieve hemostasis. Sapphire tips may be reused; however, they often will only last for two or three surgical procedures. These contact tips cost approximately $400 to replace. In addition, the cost of either laser unit ranges from $70,000 to $150,000, depending on the features desired.

Operating Room Layout

The positioning of the surgeon, assistants, video monitors, anesthesia equipment, and other necessary machines (laser, irrigators, etc.) must all be carefully planned. Placement will vary, depending on the area of focus inside the abdomen. However, some generalizations can be made. Two video monitors are necessary so that the surgeon and his assistant(s) will have an unobstructed view of the operative field. The insufflator and light source should be in direct view of the surgeon or the first assistant so that he may monitor these devices. Specialized laparoscopic carts (see p. 34) allow for compact storage of instruments. Otherwise the numerous electrical cords, gas lines, light cords, etc. obstruct the flow of traffic in the operating room and may even cause an accident involving the patient, operating room personnel, or equipment. Additional instruments such as irrigation/aspiration devices, laser or cautery units, anesthesia carts, and instrument trays must be arranged for surgeon mobility during the operative procedure and to permit the operating room staff to have access to the equipment. A typical laparoscopic operating room layout is shown.

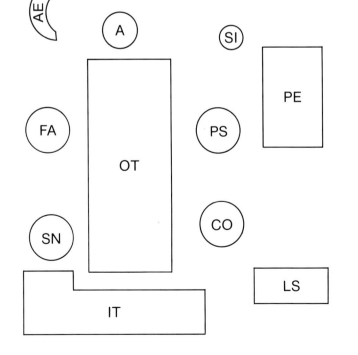

A   – Anesthesiologist
AE – Anesthesia equipment
CO – Camera operator
FA – First assistant
IT   – Instrument tray
LS – Surgical laser and laser safety officer
OT – Operating table
PE – Primary equipment cart
PS – Primary surgeon
SE – Secondary equipment cart
SI   – Suction irrigation device
SN – Scrub nurse

INSTRUMENTS

Most of the instruments currently available for laparoscopy have been designed for use in gynecologic procedures. Although many have been modified for laparoscopic biliary tract surgery, the unique needs of general surgery will undoubtedly result in the development of new and innovative instruments in the near future. Newly developed laparoscopic operations may also require specialized instruments designed for each procedure.

We will review the currently available instruments as well as some of the new devices that have been primarily developed for laparoscopic biliary tract surgery and other gastrointestinal procedures.

Insufflation Needle

Any nonopen technique for establishing pneumoperitoneum involves the percutaneous insertion of a needle into the peritoneal cavity for insufflation of CO_2 prior to the placement of the trocars and cannulas. There are numerous styles of insufflation needles, both disposable (left) and reusable (right), which serve this purpose.

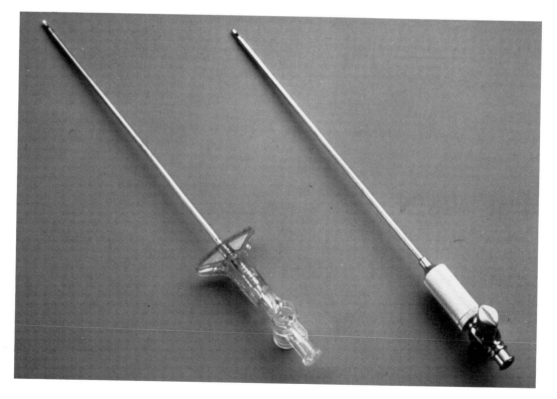

A useful feature of the disposable insufflation needle is that the tip of the needle is always sharp. Reusable instruments often become dull and therefore require a greater force to penetrate the fascia. This may make it difficult for the surgeon to detect exactly when the tip of the needle has entered the peritoneal cavity. Nearly all of these insufflation needles are based on the design of the Veress needle. A common feature is the spring-loaded obturator that advances over the sharp tip as soon as the needle enters the abdominal cavity. This serves to push any loops of bowel out of the path of the sharp tip. The hub of the needle is connected to the insufflating device by means of a sterile length of plastic tubing.

The Hasson trocar system is designed for use with the open technique (see Chapter 5). This approach is particularly useful in patients who have had a previous laparotomy and suspected adhesions near the site of proposed needle insertion. With this instrument a direct cutdown is made into the peritoneal cavity and stay sutures are placed in the fascia. The cannula is placed within the abdominal cavity under direct vision. Two stay sutures are used to secure the cannula in place and maintain pneumoperitoneum. The peritoneal cavity is then insufflated at a high flow rate.

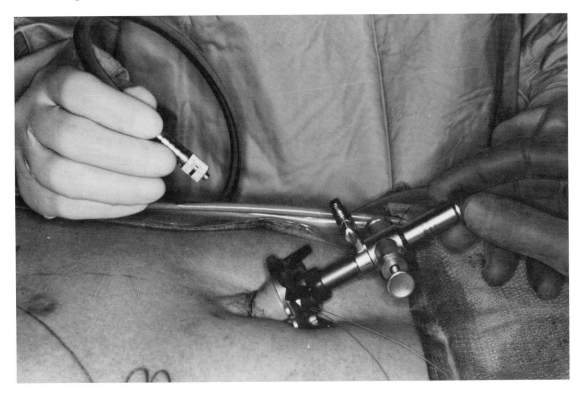

Trocar and Cannula Apparatus

An essential feature of laparoscopic surgery is the establishment of one or more portals of entry into the abdominal cavity. A mechanism for inserting and removing various instruments without loss of pneumoperitoneum is necessary. In general, the size of the cannula sleeve is 1 mm larger in diameter than the corresponding instrument or laparoscope that will traverse it. Laparoscopic cannulas or sheaths are introduced into the abdomen with the aid of a sharp trocar. This device is inserted through the lumen of the cannula as an obturator. Reusable or stainless steel cannulas have a spring-loaded trumpet valve to permit the introduction of instruments into the abdomen and prevent gas from escaping.

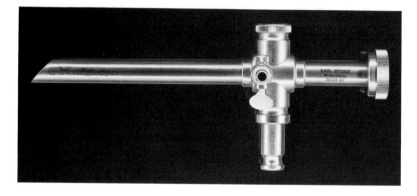

These devices have some disadvantages. The tip of the trocar may become dull after repeated use. This results in the surgeon applying a greater amount of force to penetrate the fascial layers, which may increase the likelihood of an uncontrolled entry into the peritoneal cavity. The trocar tip could then easily lacerate underlying structures. If nondisposable trocars are used, it is important to sharpen the tips on a regular basis so that the amount of force required for entry into the peritoneal cavity remains constant. Reusable trocars and sheaths must be disassembled after each use for sterilization. The reusable devices are radiopaque and may obscure the cholangiogram.

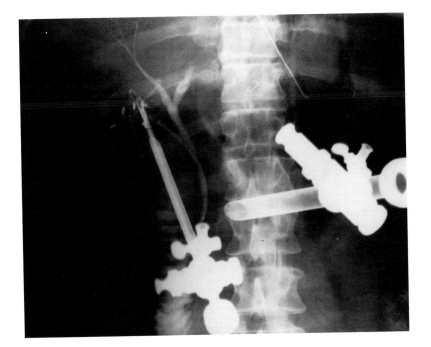

Disposable laparoscopic cannulas and trocars have several unique features: (1) the trocar is always sharp and never dulls from repeated use, (2) the instruments have a protective safety shield that advances over the sharp tip on entry into the peritoneal cavity, and (3) the cannula (fiberglass only) is radiotranslucent and therefore will not obscure the cholangiogram.

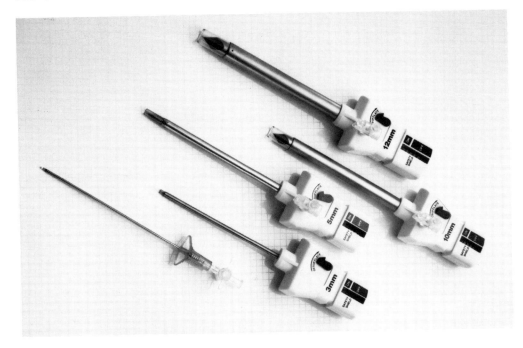

Another useful feature of the disposable sheaths are the gripping devices, which may minimize the risk of inadvertent cannula removal. This may occur as the surgeon or first assistant is repeatedly advancing and withdrawing instruments through the laparoscopic sheath. Sudden removal of the cannula generally results in an immediate loss of pneumoperitoneum and exposure. The SurgiGrip (United States Surgical Corporation, Norwalk, Conn.) attaches over the standard smooth cannula.

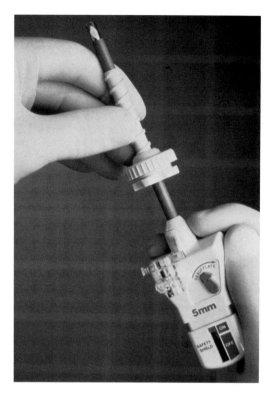

The Endo-Path (Ethicon, Inc., Sommerville, N.J.) incorporates the gripping device in the cannula.

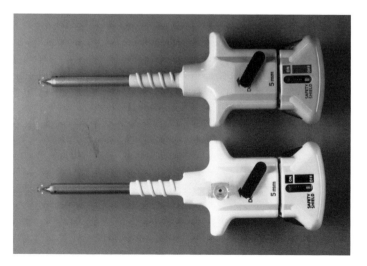

These disposable cannulas have insufflation channels and one-way "flapper" valves to ensure pneumoperitoneum is maintained. The use of disposable trocars and sheaths increases the cost of the surgical procedure; however, factors such as reduced labor for sterilization and maintenance of these devices as well as the diminished risk of bowel and vascular injuries with insertion should be considered.

Laparoscopes

Rigid laparoscopes are unique optical instruments in that they combine certain characteristics of the telescope, the microscope, and the objective lens. The British physicist Hopkins is responsible for the basic optical design used today in nearly all types of laparoscopes. He developed the rod-lens system in which light is transmitted through quartz rods. The system consists of optical fibers for transmitting light down the scope, an objective lens, quartz rod-lens and image reversal system, as well as the eyepiece mechanism. Such a system is able to gather light efficiently (producing brighter images) and provides a large field of vision despite the small diameter of the scope. A variety of designs and types of endoscopes are available for use with laparoscopy. The "operating laparoscope" incorporates both an optical lens system and an adjacent working channel, both through a single 10 mm instrument.

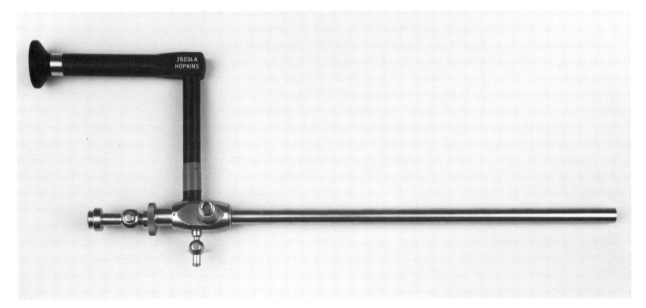

The image is transmitted through a right-angled lens to allow parallel viewing. The disadvantage of this type of instrument is a reduction in aperture size, light intensity, and image quality. It is also difficult to see accurately what is being manipulated when the instrument is in the same line of sight as the telescope. Since most surgical laparoscopic procedures require multiple punctures, the advantages of this type of laparoscope are diminished. Most general surgeons prefer a dedicated viewing laparoscope because of the superior image it produces (see p. 30).

Nonoperating laparoscopes are designed with a variety of angled lenses and diameters. The most commonly used lens for laparoscopic cholecystectomy is a zero-degree laparoscope (also called an end-viewing or forward-viewing laparoscope). An endoscope with a 30- to 45-degree angled lens, however, offers far more versatility in viewing the peritoneal cavity. This laparoscope can be used to see over a distended transverse colon or duodenum as well as around corners to visualize areas of the abdominal cavity not readily accessible from a straight-on approach. This type of laparoscope is more difficult to use initially because the camera operator must orient both the viewing lens and the axis of the video camera. Once mastered, many surgeons prefer the greater versatility afforded by the angled lens.

The diameters of the laparoscopes also vary, but they are usually 10, 7, or 5 mm in size. It is prudent to have several laparoscopes that will fit into any of the cannulas being used (usually 5 and 10 mm for laparoscopic cholecystectomy). This gives the option of viewing the abdomen through a smaller cannula during the operative procedure. This may be necessary if there is a need to reinsert the larger cannula, a different viewpoint is desired, or the larger sheath is needed for the insertion of a special laparoscopic instrument.

A common problem encountered by laparoscopic surgeons is fogging of the distal lens after entering the abdominal cavity. This results from rapid changes in temperature and humidity. Specialized telescope warmers will preheat and humidify the instruments and thus minimize this problem. An alternative is to simply apply a small amount of sterile anti-fogging solution to the end of the laparoscope.

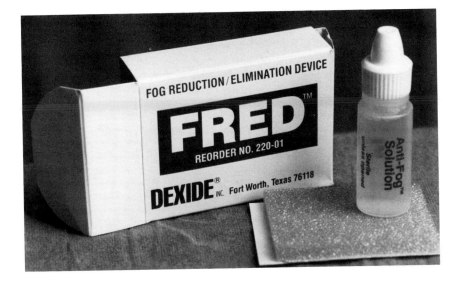

Forceps and Grasping Instruments

Any instrument currently used for grabbing and retracting tissues within the peritoneal cavity, regardless of its original intention, will probably carry the label of a grasping instrument. Different types of these instruments are shown.

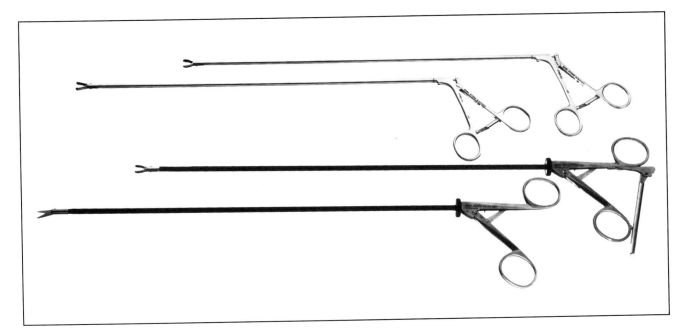

Some type of spring or ratchet mechanism may prove helpful to keep the jaws closed on the tissue. This will prevent fatigue of the assistant, who otherwise will have to manually close the handle of the instrument for the duration of the procedure. The variables in the usefulness of such instruments are the amount of tissue trauma the tool inflicts as well as the potential for perforating the target tissue (bowel graspers are far less traumatic than forceps with teeth). This has to be weighed against the instrument's ability to grab and hold onto tissue. Having available a variety of designs in terms of length and breadth of the jaws as well as sharpness of the teeth is useful since tissues will vary. For example, the gallbladder may be easy or hard to hold and more or less likely to perforate when grasped based on the extent of inflammation, the number of stones, and the amount of distention.

A unique grasping tool is the penetrating or "claw" forceps, which is used for removing tissue from the abdominal cavity (e.g., pulling the gallbladder out through the umbilical fascial opening). This is a 11 mm instrument with large penetrating jaws that firmly hold tissue.

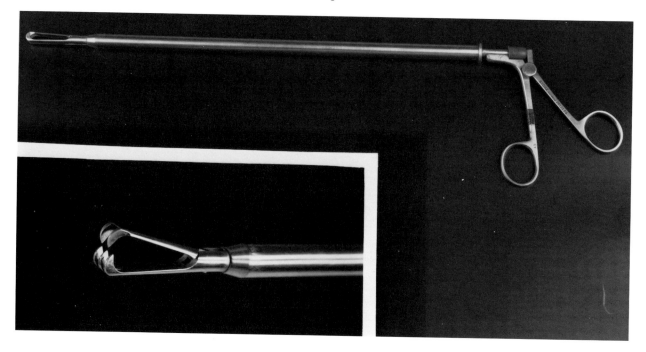

The primary advantage of this instrument is that the surgeon is much less likely to lose control of the gallbladder during extraction. This may occur if less traumatic instruments are used, and it may prove difficult for the surgeon to retrieve the gallbladder if it has dropped into the pelvis or behind loops of bowel.

Dissectors

Perhaps the most important tools in the general surgeon's armamentarium are the blunt and sharp dissectors. Such instruments take on many sizes and shapes for spreading, separating, and dividing tissue. During open procedures, surgeons previously have used such instruments as Metzenbaum scissors, tonsil clamps, Kittner dissectors, or even the sucker tip for these purposes. At present only a few laparoscopic instruments may serve as dissecting tools. These include laparoscopic needle holders and straight grasping forceps. The best instrument is a curved, atraumatic forceps (Maryland dissector; American Surgical Instruments, Pompano, Fla.) that has been specially designed for dissecting the cystic duct and artery.

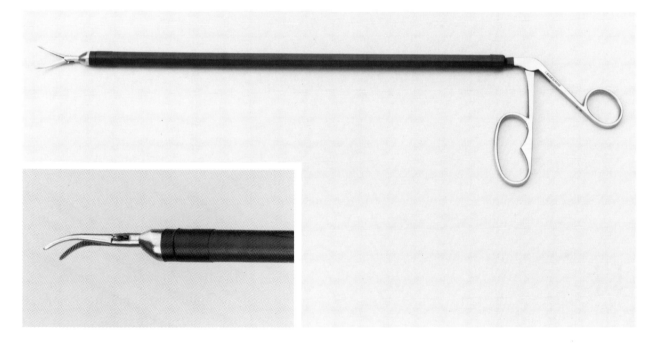

This is a 10 mm instrument that is inserted through the upper midline cannula. It is electrically insulated and may be attached directly to a cautery unit. This allows the surgeon to cauterize small blood vessels or lymphatics encountered during the dissection without the need to exchange instruments. General surgeons adapt easily to its use because it is a familiar and comfortable tool. There are many such instruments under development, and personal preference will play a strong role in an individual's choice for these essential tasks.

Scissors

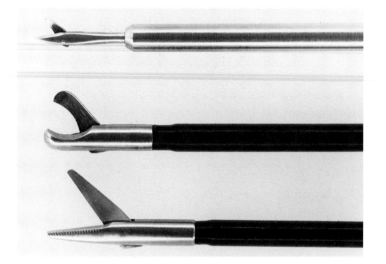

Various instruments are available for intra-abdominal cutting. Hook scissors are designed so that the tips come together first, making tubular structures easy and safe to divide. A structure to be cut can be grasped with the tips of the scissors and then pulled out of the operative field to ensure that adjacent structures are not injured. This is especially important with procedures performed under video imaging because the surgeon lacks the depth perception to ensure that the tips of the scissors are free from the surrounding tissues.

Straight scissors come in either 5 or 10 mm diameters and should only be used for cutting when the tips can be clearly seen and the tissue being cut precisely identified. Microscissors have very small, straight or curved cutting surfaces with sharp tips. These are useful for making controlled, accurate cuts such as in the cystic duct for placement of a cholangiocatheter.

Presently the hook and curved laparoscopic scissors are all 5 mm in diameter and become dull rapidly. Their small size makes them difficult to resharpen. A 10 mm curved and hook scissors that should remain sharp and be easier to maintain will be available soon from American Surgical Instruments. Since they are usually inserted through the 10 mm upper midline cannula during laparoscopic cholecystectomy, adapters or reducing sleeves will not be necessary.

Laparoscopic Clip Appliers and Staplers

The clip applier is a crucial instrument because it provides the simplest, quickest, and most effective means of occluding structures such as small vessels and ducts. Reusable clip appliers dispense individual clips that are approximately 6.0 mm in length. They are durable and economical, but require removal and reloading of the instrument after each clip is applied. This may prolong the operative procedure since the laparoscope and camera must also be pulled back and then reoriented within the operative field each time the instrument is removed. In addition, these clips may become dislodged as the applier is inserted through the cannula and past the trumpet or flapper valve. An automatic clip applier is also available (Endo-Clip applier; United States Surgical Corporation, Norwalk, Conn.).

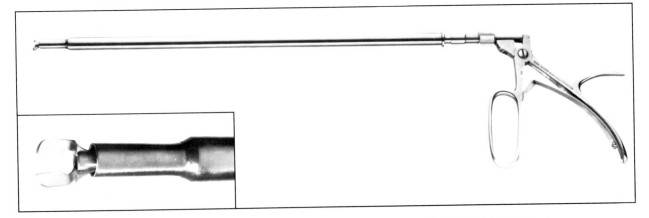

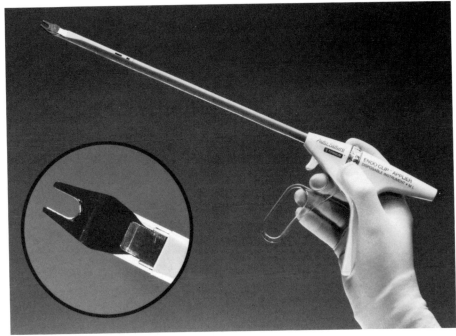

This instrument is disposable and contains 20 titanium clips in 6.0 and 9.0 mm lengths. Each clip can be loaded into the jaws without removing the instrument from the operative field. Surgical clips can be applied to the duct and artery rapidly and sequentially, thus saving valuable time in the operating room.

A disposable GIA stapling device (Endo GIA; United States Surgical Corporation, Norwalk, Conn.) is currently being field-tested and will undoubtedly be available soon.

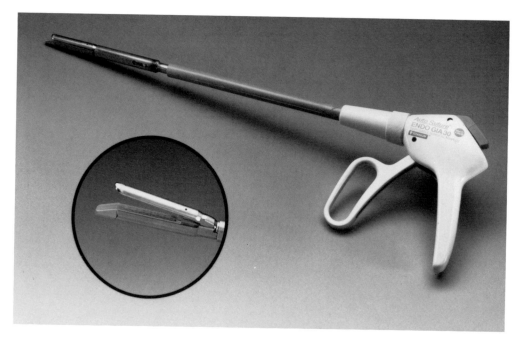

This instrument fires two triple rows of staples and then divides the tissue within its jaws. It performs very much like the stapling instruments currently used in open procedures. It is manufactured in 30 and 60 mm lengths and is inserted through a 12 mm laparoscopic cannula. It is anticipated that this instrument will greatly expand the number of laparoscopic surgical procedures that can be performed, such as intestinal and pulmonary resections.

Electrocautery Instrumentation

Virtually any laparoscopic instrument can be easily modified to incorporate electrocautery. This is usually as simple as applying an insulated coating to the shaft of the instrument and then applying current to the metal handle. Many of the scissors and grasping forceps currently available have a direct attachment allowing them to be used with monopolar cautery. A hook dissector and a blunt-tip spatula have been designed specifically for monopolar cautery dissection. Both instruments have been improved with the addition of smoke-evacuation channels. The hook-type instrument allows the surgeon to loop and hold tissues away from the underlying structures prior to cauterization. The spatula device is used for blunt dissection and electrocauterization of the gallbladder from the liver.

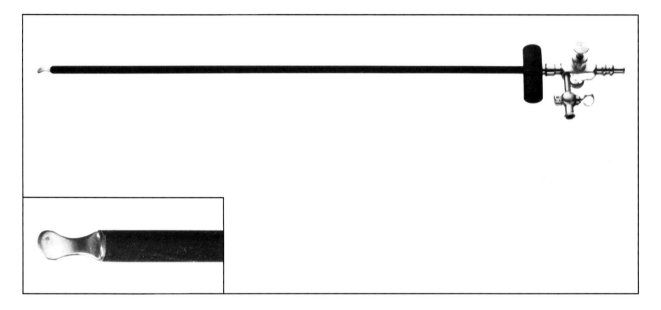

There has been great concern in the past regarding the safety of monopolar cautery in the closed abdominal cavity. Reports of inadvertent bowel burns from arcing of the electrical current in the early 1970s have been carefully reviewed by contemporary clinical investigators. It was determined that many of these injuries were probably mechanical in nature.[1] Fear of uncontrolled electrical discharges apparently has been largely exaggerated. Although there are inherent dangers of bowel, diaphragm, and vascular injuries, these are probably more a reflection of procedural errors made by the surgeon. Indeed, large series of laparoscopic cholecystectomies have been performed without reported electrical injuries.[2]

Specialty Instruments

A multitude of specialty instruments will be developed and marketed as laparoscopic procedures proliferate. A good example of an instrument designed for a single operative procedure is the Olsen cholangiography fixation clamp (Karl Storz Endoscopy, Culver City, Calif.). It has a central lumen for introducing a catheter into the abdominal cavity. In addition, it has two atraumatic ring forceps that extend beyond the lumen to direct the catheter into the duct as well as maintain a watertight seal around the duct and catheter.

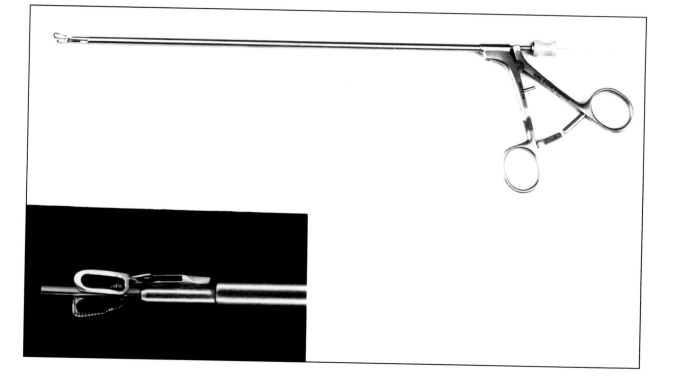

A number of devices are available that aid in the suturing of tissues via the laparoscope. The majority of these techniques have been developed for gynecologic laparoscopic surgery. Pretied laparoscopic sutures (Endo-Loop; Ethicon, Inc., Sommerville, N.J.) are made of plain and chromic catgut and may be used on tissues not suitable for surgical clips (inflamed and edematous ducts, large arteries, etc.).

Most general surgeons, however, have been reluctant to use catgut sutures because of their rapid absorption. Nonabsorbable and more durable absorbable laparoscopic sutures are currently being developed. Sutures and instruments for use through the laparoscope to facilitate the external tying of knots (extracorporeal) as well as the application of suture ligatures are also available. All of these methods require practice before a consistently successful result can be obtained.

•   •   •

We have outlined the equipment and instruments necessary for the successful performance of laparoscopic general surgery. Established companies as well as many new corporations are rapidly developing unique and innovative instrumentation for laparoscopic surgery. General surgeons have had little exposure to the technology that has made procedures such as laparoscopic cholecystectomy possible. Therefore it is imperative that surgeons learning such procedures become familiar with the specialized equipment and instruments they will use.

REFERENCES

1. Soderstrom RM, Levy BS. Bowel injuries during laparoscopy: Causes and medicolegal questions. Contemp Obstet Gynecol 27:41-47.
2. Zucker KA, Bailey RW, Gadacz TR, Imbembo AL. Laparoscopic guided cholecystectomy. Am J Surg 161:36-44, 1991.

Thermal Instrumentation for Laparoscopic General Surgical Procedures

Peter Hertzmann

Within the new field of laparoscopic general surgery, and more specifically the procedure of laparoscopic cholecystectomy, a host of instruments have been developed to accomplish numerous individual specific functions during the surgical procedure. Possibly the most interesting of the instruments are those developed for dissection of tissue. In addition to sharp and blunt dissection performed by means of a laparoscope in a manner similar to standard open procedures, there are special laser and electrosurgical devices specifically designed for laparoscopic application.

Since first being described by Harvey Cushing in 1928, electrosurgery has become a standard operating modality over the years. Lasers were first developed in the late 1950s but only became common in the operating room in the last decade. Both surgical lasers and electrosurgical devices use thermal energy to produce a surgical effect. Thus it is appropriate to discuss them in parallel with respect to their theory and application to laparoscopic general surgery.

Any discussion of lasers and electrosurgical instruments can be broken into four basic topics: how the energy is created, how it is transported from the generator to the tissue site, how the energy interacts with the tissue, and finally, what happens to the environment in which the system is working.

What is a laser? In a surgical sense a laser is not *l*ight *a*mplification by *s*timulated *e*mission of *r*adiation. That is simply the acronym for the device. To surgeons, a laser is an instrument that can *cut, coagulate,* and *vaporize* tissue. The key word is "instrument." The laser is just a tool. And, similarly, the hooks, paddles, and knives used with electric current by means of a laparoscope are also just tools. Electrosurgery uses electrons to cut or coagulate (fulgurate or desiccate, depending on the application) tissue, whereas lasers use photons to cut, coagulate, and vaporize tissue. Lasers and electrosurgical devices both cut by removing tissue rather than by splitting tissue like a scalpel. They actually produce a kerf similar to a saw.

Only thermal lasers will be discussed in this chapter. There are other special lasers used for various medical treatments that do not produce a thermal reaction. These produce either photochemical effects or shock wave effects and tend to have highly specialized applications. Likewise, only high-frequency electrosurgical instruments enter into this discussion. Devices that use electricity to simply heat a probe (e.g., the Semm Endo-coagulator) will not be included.

Although technically lasers produce light that is *coherent* (wavelengths are in phase), *monochromatic* (one wavelength or color), and *collimated* (all photons traveling in one direction), this is really a myth when it comes to surgical lasers. The lasers designed for surgical use produce a thermal effect. They are not coherent, especially after the light has passed through a waveguide or a fiberoptic. They are monochromatic, although some lasers produce more than one color. Tissue sensitivity does not require the extremely narrow color spectrum that a laser produces. Finally, surgical lasers are not designed to be absolutely collimated because this would reduce their efficiency. This aspect of collimation is very important and will be discussed later.

HOW THE THERMAL ENERGY IS CREATED

The basic theoretical laser consists of three elements. The *active medium* is the actual material where the lasing occurs. The *energy source* is the supply of energy to produce the lasing action. The *oscillation cavity* consists of two or more mirrors that bounce the light back and forth so that only rays traveling along one path are reflected.

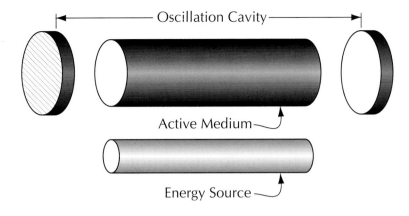

The lasing action is started by activating the energy source. In surgical lasers this means that the system is plugged into the hospital power and the system energized. The electricity either flows directly into the active medium or is used to energize a powerful arc lamp, which in turn produces photons that flow into the active medium. The arc lamp is called the pump source.

In the atomic model of the active medium the electrons orbiting are normally at rest. When a photon from the pump source strikes one of these orbiting electrons, the electron is temporarily raised to a higher energy level. The electron then drops back to its original level, releasing a photon. This process is termed spontaneous emission.

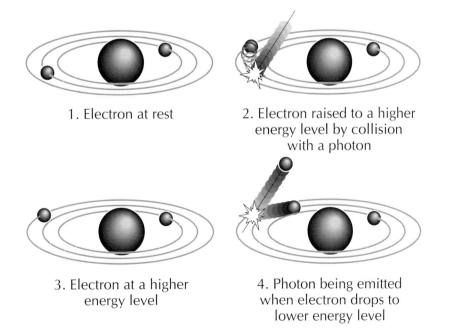

1. Electron at rest

2. Electron raised to a higher energy level by collision with a photon

3. Electron at a higher energy level

4. Photon being emitted when electron drops to lower energy level

If an additional photon strikes an electron when it is at a higher energy level, when the electron drops to its lower energy level, it will release two photons of the exact same color as the photon that struck it. The new photon also will travel in the same direction as the original photon; thus where there was one before the collision, now there are two. This process is termed stimulated emission.

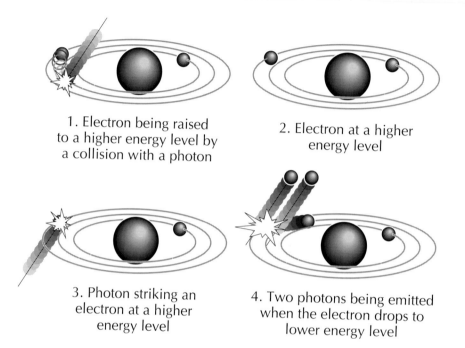

1. Electron being raised to a higher energy level by a collision with a photon

2. Electron at a higher energy level

3. Photon striking an electron at a higher energy level

4. Two photons being emitted when the electron drops to lower energy level

Because there are millions of photons from the pump source raising millions of electrons to higher energy levels, some of the photons emitted by spontaneous emission will strike one of the mirrors of the oscillation cavity in such a way that the photon is reflected back into the active medium causing stimulated emission. Since the photon produced by the collision is traveling in the same direction as the original photon, there are now two photons traveling together. Because of the mirrors, these photons are redirected back into the active medium until they collide with other electrons raised to a higher energy level, and two additional photons are released. Now there are four photons traveling in the same direction. This continues until a large number of photons are produced—the amplification aspect of the laser acronym. One of the mirrors of the oscillation cavity is slightly transmissive, allowing a small portion of the light inside the cavity to leak out. It is this leakage that is used to produce a surgical effect.

The electrons from an electrosurgical generator are produced by means of a solid-state electrical power supply. A radio frequency between 100 kilohertz and 4 megahertz could be used, but most systems commercially available today produce a current in the range of 500 and 750 kilohertz. At frequencies below 100 kilohertz, muscles and nerves are stimulated by the current. At the higher end of the frequency spectrum, capacitance and inductance make it difficult to confine the current strictly to the path defined by the electrical circuitry (wires).

Commercially available electrosurgical generators produce current in three separate waveforms: cut, coag, and blend. The *cut* waveform is a continuous sine wave. The *coag* waveform consists of thousands of short bursts of sine waves. The *blend* waveform consists of bursts of alternating high and low voltage.

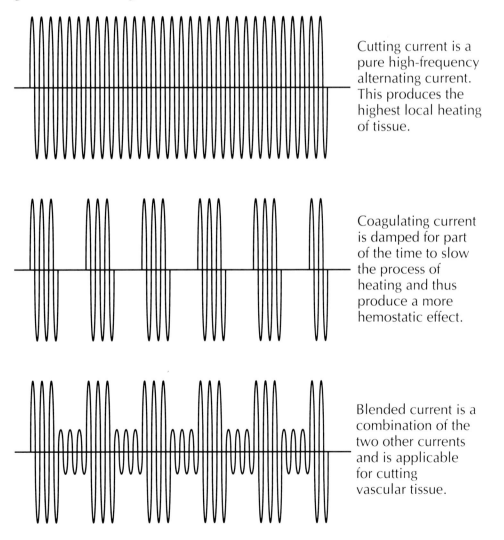

Cutting current is a pure high-frequency alternating current. This produces the highest local heating of tissue.

Coagulating current is damped for part of the time to slow the process of heating and thus produce a more hemostatic effect.

Blended current is a combination of the two other currents and is applicable for cutting vascular tissue.

Electrosurgical generators manufactured in the United States use a fixed ratio of cut and coag to create a blended current and are activated through the cut side of the generator only. Units produced in Europe occasionally allow the surgeon to modify the ratio by adjusting the individual cut and coag dials on the generator.

Just as there are different types of electric current, there are different types of lasers that produce different physical characteristics. One type of laser is a solid-state laser, in which the active medium is a solid material. The neodymium-doped yttrium-aluminum-garnet (Nd:YAG) laser is a typical example of a solid-state laser.

Another type of laser uses gas as an active medium. A typical gas laser would be the carbon dioxide (CO_2) laser or the argon ion (Ar^+) laser. In the case of the Ar^+ laser the gas is held in an old-fashioned vacuum tubelike shell, which is prone to leakage and instability. Older style CO_2 surgical lasers used flowing gas from gas bottles that had to be changed periodically. The newer style CO_2 lasers are sealed.

If a crystal such as potassium-titanyl-phosphate (KTP) is placed in the path of certain laser beams, the color of the beam is changed. This is called frequency doubling. The KTP/532 laser (Laserscope, San Jose, Calif.) is an example of this type of laser. It also is a solid-state laser. In addition, there are lasers that combine the principles of two separate lasers to produce two different sets of laser output. An example of this is the KTP/YAG laser (Laserscope, San Jose, Calif.).

All lasers produce monochromatic light, that is, light of a single color. The Ar^+ laser produces up to 11 single monochromatic colors at the same time. The fact that laser light is monochromatic is relatively unimportant. Coagulation reactions in tissue are somewhat more color dependent than vaporization. Having a very narrow color output is not as important as the actual portion of the electromagnetic spectrum the wavelength is in.

All lasers produce coherent light, that is, all the wavelengths are in phase. The actual mode of this coherent light is very short lived in surgical lasers because no attempt is made to hold the mirrors at an exact distance from each other over small changes in temperature or minor vibrational movement. The coherence is totally unimportant in surgical lasers and has no effect on tissue. In fact, even if a laser produces coherent light, passing it through a fiberoptic or hollow waveguide destroys the coherence.

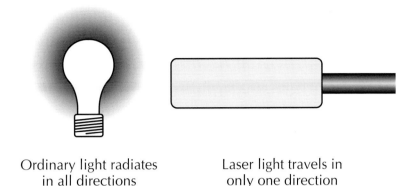

Ordinary light radiates
in all directions

Laser light travels in
only one direction

All lasers produce light that is highly directional. It is not truly collimated, but it is much closer than other artificial light sources. This aspect of lasers allows the light to be focused to a very small spot and to be delivered to the tissue by flexible fiberoptics. This aspect of surgical laser is relatively important.

TRANSPORTING ENERGY FROM GENERATOR TO TISSUE

Since electrical energy must have a complete circuit to function, an electrosurgery generator requires two wires to connect it to the patient's body. For laparoscopic general surgical procedures, a monopolar system (one in which the patient's body is part of the circuit) is common. With monopolar systems, electrical energy is delivered via a single wire attached to the electrosurgical instrument and the return wire is attached via a large surface to the patient, normally at the thigh.

For electrosurgery instrumentation, transporting the electrical energy from the generator to the instrument at the tissue is a matter of using the proper size wires and connectors. Without the proper connection, neuromuscular stimulation will occur. For lasers, in which light energy has to get to the proper surgical site with the maximum amount of safety, the obstacle is a bit more demanding. There are two basic ways to deliver the laser light to tissue: articulated arms and fiberoptic waveguides. Since light travels only in straight lines, it can be transmitted through air and bent by mirrors, the function of the articulated arm. Or light can be delivered in other media such as glass, where it still travels in straight lines. The coating on the fiberoptic redirects the light so that it cannot escape from the sides of the glass.

Articulated arms are rigid and stiff. They require some distal means of concentrating the laser light, such as a lens. Being mechanical devices they are subject to mechanical misalignment, and their weight often restricts free movement. Articulated arms are used in CO_2 lasers, and for this reason this type of laser has not proved popular among many laparoscopic surgeons. Fiberoptics are flexible and cannot be misaligned. They provide the highest accessibility to remote tissue sites because of their small size. They do not require a lens to use them on tissue. Therefore they are easily adaptable for use in laparoscopic surgery or through flexible endoscopes.

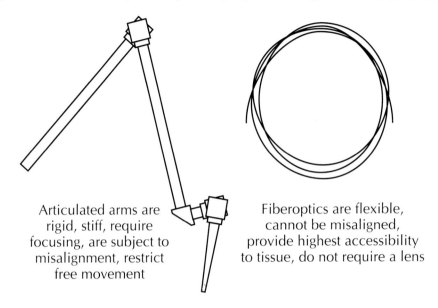

Articulated arms are rigid, stiff, require focusing, are subject to misalignment, restrict free movement

Fiberoptics are flexible, cannot be misaligned, provide highest accessibility to tissue, do not require a lens

Light from a fiberoptic diverges as it moves away from the fiber tip, and the spot size on the target tissue is a function of the fiber-to-tissue distance. Most surgical laser fibers have an angle of divergence of about 15 degrees. This means that the spot size will grow about 1 mm in diameter for each 4 mm of distance the fiber is moved from the tissue.

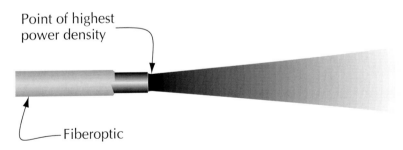

Point of highest power density

Fiberoptic

Some CO_2 lasers use a hollow waveguide connected to the articulated arm instead of a focusing lens. Light from these devices also diverges in a manner similar to the flexible fiberoptic of the other lasers. Although not totally rigid, the waveguides do not provide the same freedom that a true fiberoptic system does. They still require the articulated arm for some of the laser energy transportation, and they cannot be used in contact with tissue like a bare glass fiberoptic. To remain clear of debris and smoke, waveguides require a constant flow of clean gas. When used in the closed abdominal cavity during laparoscopy, this can cause problems with insufflation and abdominal pressure.

When a conical tip is added to the fiber in the form of a separate sapphire tip or by adding a conical or ball tip to the fiber itself, the tip converts the light energy to heat energy. The heat energy then provides the surgical effect, similar to a hot knife. Although these devices cut relatively well, they are poor coagulators. To achieve greater hemostasis the surgeon may remove the sapphire tip and direct the free laser beam to specific bleeding points. As we will discuss later, as more energy is used to produce a cutting effect, less energy is available to transmit slowly through the tissue to provide hemostasis.

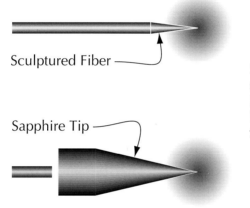

Sculptured Fiber

Sapphire Tip

Sculptured fibers and sapphire tips convert the light energy from a laser into heat energy, and thus become *hot knives*

With electrosurgical instrumentation, tip configuration can also influence the surgical effect. This will be discussed in the next section.

With lasers, means of delivering the energy to the tissue, be it a bare fiber or one with a tip, have been designed by the various manufacturers to be single-use, disposable devices. This has been done because fiber performance will degrade after multiple sterilizations. Additionally, these devices tend to be a bit more fragile than standard surgical instruments and can easily be damaged during cleaning and handling. Many of the electrosurgical instruments currently available for laparoscopic use are reusable. It is wise to have a spare set available in the operating room since these instruments can also be damaged due to handling. The noninsulated tips of some of the electrosurgical instruments can also be damaged during procedures.

ENERGY-TISSUE INTERACTION

In some ways electrosurgical and laser instruments interact with tissue in the same manner. The ultimate effect of cutting vs. coagulation will be a function of the rate that energy is delivered to the tissue and the size of the area it is delivered over.

For laser light, as with any light that hits tissue, a combination of four effects will be produced: reflection, absorption, scatter, and transmission. The combination of these four effects results in the conversion of light energy into heat energy. Of all of these effects, scatter is the most important. The light scatters, or bounces, around the tissue until it is eventually absorbed. The size of the scatter pattern helps determine how each wavelength interacts with tissue and what the extent of the lateral thermal damage will be.

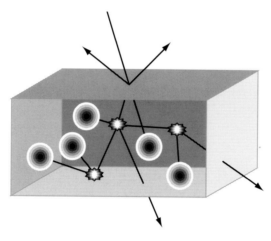

Reflection, absorption, refraction, and transmission combine to form scatter

Light scatters in tissue until the light energy is converted by absorption into heat energy

The lateral thermal damage produced by a particular wavelength is relative to the amount of scatter produced. The CO_2 laser produces the least scatter, the Nd:YAG the most, and KTP and Ar^+ in between. If there is no scatter there is no lateral thermal damage, and hence no hemostasis.

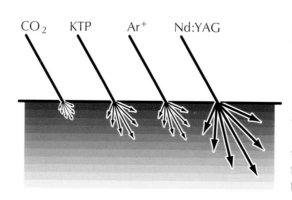

Lateral thermal damage is relative to the amount of scatter produced by a particular wavelength

If there is no scatter there is no hemostasis, if there is too much then the lateral thermal damage is too great

Similarly, with electrosurgical devices, electrical energy is converted to heat energy due to the resistance of the tissue. The greater the local resistance or the more energy applied to the local area, the greater the heat rise.

When tissue is vaporized, some of the heat that produces the vaporization dissipates into the tissue, producing lateral thermal damage in the form of necrosis and coagulation. This is true whether a laser or electrosurgical device is used.

If the interaction of various laser wavelengths with two major tissue components is plotted, the water absorption of the CO_2 laser is high, whereas for the other wavelengths it is low. If the hemoglobin absorption is plotted, the Nd:YAG laser is poorly absorbed and the other wavelengths are highly absorbed. It is interesting to note that the best coagulating wavelength, that of the Nd:YAG laser, is absorbed the least. The worst coagulator is the CO_2 laser, which is absorbed the most. Thus the coagulation ability of a wavelength is relative to how much the wavelength is absorbed by the tissue.

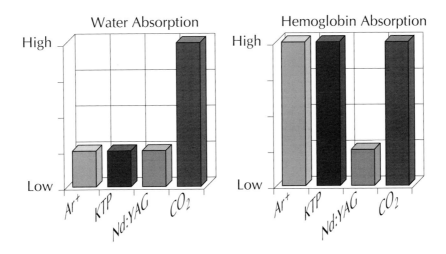

Laser wavelengths that transmit easily through water but not blood can use this effect to their advantage when coagulating bleeding sites. The laser energy can be delivered through a spray of irrigation, keeping the blood off the surface to be coagulated as well as providing additional cooling to ensure that the laser energy simply coagulates the tissue. Because water is an excellent conductor of electrical energy, electrosurgical devices cannot be used effectively through water since the water may act to dissipate the electricity over a broader area of treatment.

Surgical dosage for lasers is described in terms of the amount of power delivered, the length of time it is delivered, and the size of the exposed area on the tissue. Just as a drug dosage is described as so many milligrams per kilogram of body weight so many times per day, the surgical dosage of a laser exposure can be described as so many watts over a particular spot size times the number of seconds the power is on. Mathematically, this would be represented as:

$$\text{Surgical dosage} = \frac{\text{Power} \cdot \text{Time}}{\text{Spot size}}$$

Of the three elements, power is set to a level and then usually left alone for the remainder of a laparoscopic procedure. Spot size is adjusted by changing the fiber-to-tissue distance, and time is adjusted by modulating the rate the fiber is moving with respect to the tissue. By controlling distance and movement speed the surgeon is able to easily alternate between cutting and coagulation with a bare fiber system. If the fiber has been modified with a tip, then the tip will dominate the effect, and it must be changed to modify the surgical effect of the device.

Because electrosurgical devices generally have shapes that produce a contact area relative to the effect desired, cutting or coagulating, the surgical dosage with these devices can be considered similar to the laser dosage. Since the spot size is fixed, the effect is usually modified by changing power at the generator or by changing the time that the energy is applied.

Varying the surgical dosage changes the tissue effects produced by the laser. The greater the surgical dosage, the greater the effect. As the temperature of the tissue increases, the effect changes from no effect to denaturation to coagulation to necrosis to vaporization.

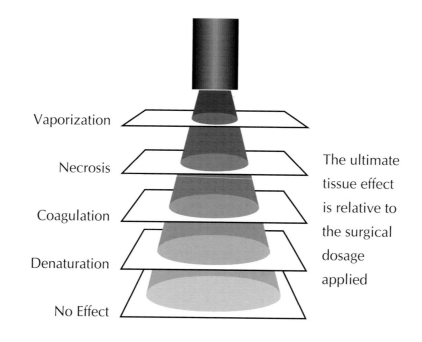

Vaporization

Necrosis

Coagulation

Denaturation

No Effect

The ultimate tissue effect is relative to the surgical dosage applied

With electrosurgical devices, variations in the surgical dosage can also change the ultimate tissue effect. Broad surface area devices with high voltage combined with high wattage will produce mostly coagulation, whereas sharp, fine, small surface devices with low voltage and high wattage will produce cutting effects.

When a bare fiberoptic is used in contact, it will usually produce a cutting effect. When backed away slightly so that it is in near-contact, the effect is mostly vaporization. When moved into a totally noncontact mode, the effect is purely coagulation. With conical-shaped contact tips, whether sapphire tip or sculptured fiber, only a cutting effect is obtainable. The tip must be in contact to work, which can increase the difficulty of using these devices.

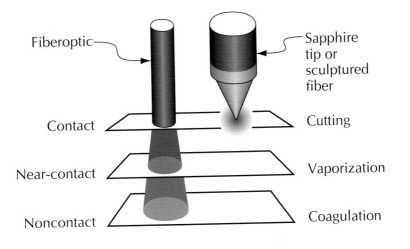

Before attempting to tie all the tissue interactions together, it is necessary to look at the effect in a different way. First of all, there are a couple of effects that occur if the temperature of the tissue is increased even more than required for vaporization. Carbonization occurs when the water is driven from the tissue. Incandescence occurs when the tissue temperature is raised to a point where it actually glows quite brightly. The temperature scale represented by all of the tissue effects is not linear, but the order of the effects is consistent with experience. The horizontal scale represents an increasing surgical dosage (see p. 70). The diagonal line is the rate of work described by a particular wavelength. Three zones are illustrated on the surgical dosage scale. First is a region where the dosage is too low to produce a surgical effect. Second is a region of coagulation. Third is a region of vaporization. The width of the region of coagulation represents the degree of control available with a particular wavelength. A narrow region means that it will be difficult to produce a coagulation effect. A wide region means that the wavelength may not be able to deliver enough dosage to produce vaporization.

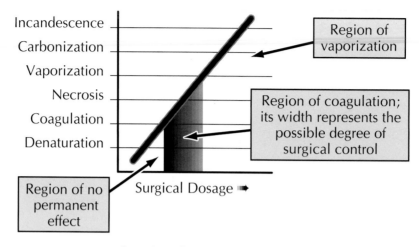

Explanation of rate of work schematic.

When the four lasers are plotted, it can be seen that the CO_2 laser requires less dosage than other lasers to produce an effect. Also, it is difficult to produce coagulation effects with this laser. The Nd:YAG laser requires a very high dosage to produce vaporization, but it has a very wide region over which it can produce coagulation. The KTP laser and the Ar^+ laser can both produce a controllable amount of coagulation, but the KTP laser requires less dosage to produce the desired effects. Since the Ar^+ laser is power limited, its ability to produce effects is often limited.

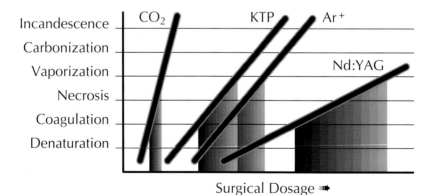

Rate of work for various laser wavelengths.

As stated earlier, variation in surgical effect with electrosurgical devices is partly a function of the physical configuration of the device. Electrosurgical devices for laparoscopic general surgical applications are shaped like hooks, spatulas, or knife blades. These devices are used for dissecting (cutting) tissue. Additionally, blunt grasping instruments are supplied with insulated handles and shafts so that they may be used for coagulation of bleeding sites.

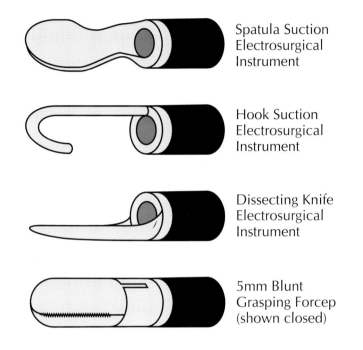

Spatula Suction Electrosurgical Instrument

Hook Suction Electrosurgical Instrument

Dissecting Knife Electrosurgical Instrument

5mm Blunt Grasping Forcep (shown closed)

When tissue is coagulated with the electrosurgical device in direct contact, no spark is created. This is termed desiccation. When tissue is coagulated by near-contact with sparking present, the coagulation is termed fulguration. Desiccated tissue has a relatively soft, light brown eschar, whereas fulgurated tissue is characterized by a hard, black eschar. In both cases the reaction will proceed until either the surgeon releases the foot pedal or the water is driven from the tissue, making it a poor conductor of electrical energy.

The goal of electrosurgical cutting is to raise the temperature of the tissue rapidly, causing the steam created to vacuolate the cell matrix. Because the tissue is heated swiftly, there is insufficient time for the heat to dissipate through the adjacent tissue. Thus, although a cutting effect is achieved, hemostasis may be lacking. Sparking is also present in true electrosurgical cutting. Once the spark is established between the electrosurgical device and the tissue, the tissue is heated by its resistance to the electric current at the point where the spark hits the tissue. The energy dissipated in the spark itself also causes some tissue heating. The two types of heating in tandem and in high concentration cause the cells to explode, producing a cutting effect. Some cutting-like effects of electrosurgical instruments are produced by using the device in direct contact so that no sparking occurs and the tissue is desiccated and softened. The instrument then mechanically breaks apart the tissue.

USING THERMAL ENERGY SAFELY IN THE OPERATING ROOM

The greatest risk associated with either laser or electrosurgical devices is electrical shock. As long as the console's panels are left in place, there is no significant electrical risk for anyone in the operating room. These devices should never be operated unless all panels are properly in place. Only factory-trained personnel should open a laser or electrosurgery system.

Fire is another major concern with either laser or electrosurgical devices. They must never be activated unless directed properly at target tissue. Additionally, lasers should always be placed in the standby mode when not actually in use. Drapes surrounding open surgical sites should be covered with moistened towels. Endoscopic procedures, however, do not require damp towels around the cannulas. When electrosurgical devices are used, care should be taken during procedures to ensure that combustible gases are not allowed to build up under barrier drapes.

Most surgeons who use lasers are generally aware of the risk of eye injury. Appropriate eye protection measures must be used. However, too much eye protection can also prevent safe and proper surgery. At a certain level all laser wavelengths become safe because laser light is not ionizing radiation. Only at high levels of exposure does laser light become unsafe. Eye protection during laparoscopic use consists at the most of adding a filter in the path between the laparoscope and the camera. Care is taken so that the laser is only enabled after the fiber is inserted in the abdomen and placed in the *standby mode* prior to removing it. If a surgeon is planning to directly view a laser exposure through the laparoscope eyepiece, it is necessary to provide protection specific to the wavelength of the laser being used.

Skin injury is the last risk. For a patient, skin burns are usually secondary to fires. For surgeons, skin burns are usually secondary to carelessness. Care must be exercised when using monopolar electrosurgery instruments to ensure that the patient return plate is properly attached to prevent a burn to the patient's thigh.

It is a common misconception that there are specific laws governing the use of laser instruments in the operating room. As a regulator of medical device manufacturers, the Food and Drug Administration mandates various safety features for all surgical lasers, but they do not specify any regulations for the safe use of lasers. The American National Standards Institute (ANSI) has promulgated a standard for the safe use of lasers in hospitals, but this standard is not law.

Good communication is essential to a safe operating environment. Most accidents resulting from electrosurgical or laser devices are attributable to either poor communication or poor training. All communication should be a two-way process. Nothing should ever be assumed.

Proper training is essential. Both users and operators of surgical lasers or electrosurgery devices should have appropriate training for the particular system they are using. Refresher training should be given regularly within the hospital to ensure that everyone is up to date.

TRAINING REQUIREMENTS FOR SAFE LASER USE

Surgeons

Didactic lecture on both laser and clinical applications
Hands-on experience with live laboratory animals
Preceptorship with experienced operators

or

Residency training

Support Staff

Didactic lecture on both operation of the laser and its safe use
Operational training with return demonstration

Safety measures for patients undergoing laser surgery include:

1. Appropriate eye protection must be provided for the type of surgery being performed and the anesthesia used.
2. Open surgical sites should be surrounded by wet towels to protect the drapes and thus the patient.
3. If laser surgery involves the airway, the endotracheal tube must be *laser safe* for the wavelength being used.

Safety measures for patients in whom electrosurgical devices will be used include:

1. Good contact between the return electrode and the patient's skin must be ensured.

2. Insulation on graspers, hooks, spatulas, and other devices to be used in a procedure should be checked to ensure that the spark will only jump from the proper place on the instrument and nowhere else.

3. The surgeon must be careful to ensure that the area of the device being used for cutting or coagulating is in fact the only one in contact with the tissue. If the backside of a electrosurgical instrument is in contact or closer to the tissue than the intended point of contact, burns can occur in surrounding tissue. Worse yet, it can produce a burn unrecognized by the surgeon and result in delayed complications after the procedure (e.g., a bowel burn).

Recommended safety measures for operating room personnel involve clear communication, use of appropriate eye protection (if a laser is being used), use of removable door signs (if a laser is being used), effective smoke evacuation, proper training, and efficient room setup. Door signs should only be in place during the procedures where the laser is actually in use. Signs that are permanently fixed to doors become ignored because they are always there. Effective smoke evacuation is a matter of personal comfort as well as a safety issue. Efficient room setup means that equipment can be operated in a safe manner without hindering movement within the operating room.

For open procedures, appropriate eye protection, designed specifically for the wavelength laser being used, is required for all viewers within the nominal hazard zone. Each laser manufacturer addresses appropriate eye protection in their operating manuals. For closed procedures, eye protection is required for anyone looking directly at the surgical site with an optical system such as an endoscope. Video cameras may need protection from bright laser light as well, but personnel viewing the video monitor do not require eye protection because they are by definition outside of the nominal hazard zone. In a laparoscopic procedure the nominal hazard zone is totally contained within the abdomen.

All laser light is simply a higher brightness, monochromatic version of ordinary light. As such, it is termed electromagnetic radiation. This radiation is not ionizing radiation and poses no health threat to any individual in the operating room. All surgical lasers are required by the Food and

Drug Administration to have a label stating, in part, that the laser produces electromagnetic radiation. This simply means that the laser produces light. It is no more dangerous than any other device that produces light.

The Food and Drug Administration also classifies all lasers that produce more than 500 milliwatts of power as class IV lasers. It does not distinguish between lasers that produce kilowatt levels of power designed to blast tanks on a battlefield from 20-watt lasers designed for surgical applications. Fears about the safety of these devices in the surgical suite are totally unfounded.

CONCLUSION

With many thousands of laparoscopic cholecystectomies having been performed in the United States since the summer of 1988, it has been shown that both laser and electrosurgical instruments can be used safely and effectively in the closed abdomen under laparoscopic control. Lasers have also been safely used in the performance of appendectomy and lysis of bowel adhesions. Additional work is being performed to demonstrate the ability of the laser to be an effective general dissector in the abdomen in procedures such as lymphadenectomy. Electrosurgical instruments have also been used for laparoscopic vagotomy.

An appropriate surgical effect can be achieved with any of these instruments if the surgeon is familiar with the various aspects of each device and has a clear image of his surgical goal.

ADDITIONAL READING

American National Standard for the Safe Use of Laser in Health Care Facilities Z136.3 (1988). New York: American National Standards Institute, 1988.

Borten M. Laparoscopic Complications, Prevention and Management. Toronto: BC Decker, 1986.

Electrosurgical Theory Applied to the Force Generators. Boulder: Valleylab, Inc., 1989.

Hulka JF. Textbook of Laparoscopy. Orlando: Grune & Stratton, 1985.

Reddick EJ, Hertzmann PS. Course Notes in Laparoscopic General Surgery. San Jose: Laserscope, 1990.

Semm K. Operative Manual for Endoscopic Abdominal Surgery. Chicago: Year Book, 1987.

Practical Anesthesia for Laparoscopic Procedures

Jawad U. Hasnain, M.D.
M. Jane Matjasko, M.D.

Operations that once required long hospitalizations and were associated with severe postoperative pain are now in many cases performed on an outpatient or short-stay basis with minimal postoperative discomfort. This has mandated a change in anesthetic technique with emphasis on minimal intraoperative anesthesia and short-acting pharmaceuticals that will allow the patient to awaken quickly and experience few side effects so that he can be discharged from the hospital quickly.

The anesthesiologist's goals are hemodynamic and respiratory stability, appropriate muscle relaxation, and control of diaphragmatic excursion. The latter is especially important, for example, when cannulating the cystic duct for cholangiography as well as for dissection near the cystic and common bile duct junction. Anesthetic and adjuvant drugs are chosen so as not to delay early ambulation or discharge from the hospital. A detailed discussion among team members regarding the perioperative plan and special concerns and considerations is of great benefit if the patient's condition is complex and fragile.

SYSTEMIC CHANGES DURING LAPAROSCOPIC SURGERY
Respiratory System

Conventional gynecologic laparoscopy usually requires much higher insufflation pressures (20 to 40 mm Hg) for pneumoperitoneum than cholecystectomy (10 to 14 mm Hg), vagotomy, appendectomy, etc. The higher pressures used for gynecologic laparoscopy result in a significant decrease in total lung compliance as well as increases in central venous pressure (up to 10 cm H_2O change), arterial CO_2 (Pa_{CO_2}) (up to 10 mm Hg change), and alveolar CO_2 (up to 8 mm Hg change).[1] These changes are much less evident during laparoscopic cholecystectomy, presumably because of the lower insufflation pressures used.

Traditional laparotomy and cholecystectomy, which involve a large upper abdominal incision, are associated with dramatic changes in pulmonary function (vital capacity, FEV_1, functional residual capacity, and PaO_2) that do not return to baseline levels for at least 3 or more days following surgery.[2,3] However, the postoperative effects of laparoscopic cholecystectomy on respiratory function are minimal. Although no data regarding the changes in pulmonary function during or following laparoscopic cholecystectomy have been published to date, clinical observation supports the fact that respiratory dysfunction is minimal. This is probably a reflection of the much smaller abdominal incision and the reduction in postoperative pain.

During laparoscopic procedures performed under general anesthesia, controlled ventilation is often recommended to prevent hypercapnia, which can result from a combination of factors (e.g., narcotic analgesics, mechanical impairment of ventilation from CO_2-induced abdominal distention (pneumoperitoneum), and systemic absorption of CO_2 from the peritoneal cavity).[4,5] During regional anesthesia with heavy sedation, spontaneously ventilating patients may show an increase in $PaCO_2$ levels reaching as high as 75 mm Hg.[6] Controlled ventilation, however, can effectively maintain a normal $PaCO_2$ under such circumstances. During lower abdominal laparoscopy using epidural anesthesia and without heavy systemic narcotic administration, patients maintain adequate alveolar ventilation by increasing their minute ventilation and respiratory rate.[7] If patients have a limited pulmonary reserve, the necessary increase in respiratory work may not be obtainable and respiratory failure may occur. The increase in $PaCO_2$ cannot be prevented if high doses of sedatives are given because of central respiratory depression.

Continuous monitoring of peripheral O_2 saturation is advisable in all patients since hypoxemia can occur from elevation of the diaphragm (loss of functional residual capacity) as a result of pneumoperitoneum. This is more likely to occur during spontaneous ventilation rather than controlled mechanical breathing.

Carbon Dioxide Embolus

CO_2 is commonly used for laparoscopic surgery because it has a relatively innocuous effect on peritoneal surfaces and is highly soluble in the bloodstream. Intravascular entry of small amounts is generally not hazardous because CO_2 is rapidly absorbed via the splanchnic vascular bed. However, excessive intra-abdominal pressures or anesthetic techniques that reduce splanchnic blood flow may reduce its absorption and increase the likelihood of symptomatic gas embolus. If large amounts of CO_2 gain access to the venous circulation, a "gas lock" may form in the right atrium or ventricle. This leads to obstruction of the venous return to the right heart and a profound drop in cardiac output. Gas bubbles may also advance into the pulmonary circulation, resulting in acute pulmonary hypertension and right heart failure. In most circumstances a small CO_2 embolus is rapidly absorbed without evidence of hemodynamic impairment. However, if this event goes unrecognized and there is continued insufflation of CO_2, cardiac arrest and death may ensue. The presenting signs of CO_2 embolus include a sudden, profound fall in blood pressure, dysrhythmia, mill wheel or other heart murmurs, cyanosis, and/or pulmonary edema. End-tidal CO_2 ($etCO_2$) may increase abruptly as CO_2 embolizes. If the gas embolus is large, the $etCO_2$ increase may be followed by an abrupt decrease if right heart dysfunction is severe and blood is no longer delivered to the lungs. An important etiologic factor in the development of CO_2 embolus is high insufflating pressures. Fortunately this pressure is kept low during laparoscopic procedures such as cholecystectomy and vagotomy. Another predisposing factor is the presence of open venous channels, usually resulting from surgical trauma. Excessive bleeding should alert the anesthesiologist to the possibility of a CO_2 embolus. Continuous monitoring of heart sounds, systemic blood pressure, and $etCO_2$ will assist in making an early diagnosis. Precordial Doppler monitoring is another sensitive monitoring modality for the detection of gas embolus. Immediate deflation of the pneumoperitoneum will prevent progression of hemodynamic decompensation. If gas lock does occur within the right heart, cardiac arrest may occur quickly. A steep reverse Trendelenburg position, as used for laparoscopic cholecystectomy, may actually make gas lock more likely. In this case the patient needs immediate cardiopulmonary resuscitation, placement in the Durant position (left lateral decubitus position with head down), and insertion of a central venous catheter for gas aspiration. Other causes of cardiovascular collapse must also be ruled out, such as hemorrhage, pulmonary embolism, myocardial infarction, pneumothorax, pneumomediastinum, excessive intra-abdominal pressure, or a profound vasovagal reflex.

Cardiovascular System

The reverse Trendelenburg position required for laparoscopic cholecystectomy may result in decreased venous return, cardiac output, and blood pressure. In addition, CO_2 insufflation of the abdominal cavity leads to an increase in total peripheral resistance, particularly if intra-abdominal pressures are high and the aorta is compressed. Compared to gynecologic laparoscopy, these hemodynamic changes should be less severe during upper abdominal laparoscopy mainly because of the lower insufflation pressures used. The effect of patient positioning and pneumoperitoneum on venous return and blood pressure is largely dependent on the patient's intravascular volume status prior to insufflation of CO_2. Volume loading with 10 to 20 ml/kg crystalloid solution prior to positioning minimizes these cardiovascular changes. Laparoscopic surgery probably has a minimal effect on cardiac function in healthy patients. However, studies have shown that in healthy young women placed in the Trendelenburg position, stroke work and cardiac indices are reduced, even if intra-abdominal pressures are kept to 14 mm Hg or less.[8] Debilitated patients may respond unpredictably to these effects and will require appropriate invasive monitoring for effective management.

Cardiac dysrhythmia can occur during laparoscopy. Respiratory acidosis and the resultant sympathetic stimulation are thought to be the primary etiologic factors. Hypoxia and vagal stimulation may be other contributing causes.[9] Of the inhalation anesthetics, enflurane and isoflurane have a lower incidence of dysrhythmia than halothane, which increases endogenous catecholamines.[10] During general anesthesia with controlled ventilation, cardiac dysrhythmia can be prevented by carefully regulating the Pa_{CO_2}. If thoracic epidural anesthesia and minimal systemic narcotics are used, the increase in minute ventilation in the awake patient will maintain a normal or slightly decreased Pa_{CO_2}. However, heavy sedation will interfere with the increase in minute ventilation and may increase the risk of dysrhythmia. Patients with chronic obstructive pulmonary disease may not have the respiratory reserve to increase minute ventilation and therefore may not be suitable candidates for regional anesthesia.

Gastric Reflux

Gastric reflux is a significant concern when laparoscopy is performed using regional anesthesia. Predisposing factors include obesity, hiatal hernia, increased intragastric pressure, excessive pneumoperitoneum, and aerophagia. The incidence of reflux and aspiration pneumonitis in high-risk patients can be minimized by careful selection of the anesthetic technique, prophylactic antacids, and H_2 blockers.[11,12] In patients with suspected delayed gastric emptying (obese patients and those with hiatal hernia or diabetes mellitus), preoperative administration of metoclopramide, 10 mg orally or intravenously, increases lower esophageal sphincter tone and gastric emptying and may reduce the likelihood of reflux. Ranitidine, 150 mg orally or 50 mg intravenously, will raise the gastric pH and minimize untoward effects if the patient does aspirate. Pulmonary aspiration of gastric contents can also occur during endotracheal general anesthesia, but the chances are minimal. Several studies have shown that prolonged with-holding of oral fluids does not improve gastric volume or pH and may, in fact, worsen them.[13,14] Within 2 hours of ingestion, 150 ml of water is almost completely emptied from the stomach, even when followed 1 hour later by a narcotic-atropine preanesthetic medication. Healthy patients undergoing elective surgery may be permitted to take small amounts of oral fluids until 2 to 3 hours prior to surgery.

To reduce the risk of injury to the stomach and to facilitate the laparoscopic procedure, a nasogastric or orogastric tube is inserted after the induction of general anesthesia. An orogastric tube may be less traumatic and cause less postoperative discomfort. The gastric tube is removed at the end of the procedure after the stomach is decompressed. Since the patient is awake during epidural anesthesia, an oro- or nasogastric tube adds to the discomfort and may be poorly tolerated. In addition, the gastric tube can induce nausea or vomiting in the awake patient or predispose to passive gastric reflux in the anesthetized patient. Therefore selected patients undergoing laparoscopic cholecystectomy with a regional anesthetic may do better without a gastric catheter provided distention of the stomach does not occur.

SELECTION OF ANESTHETIC TECHNIQUE

The general principles and considerations regarding the choice of anesthesia for traditional open procedures also apply to laparoscopy. It is also important to consider that approximately 5% to 10% of individuals undergoing laparoscopic procedures may require conversion to an open laparotomy. As with any operative procedure, success depends on team cooperation and commitment. No special monitoring is required simply because the procedure is being performed under laparoscopic guidance. More sophisticated monitoring is necessary only if the patient's medical condition warrants it.

Perioperative use of narcotics, including morphine, meperidine, and fentanyl, can cause spasm of the sphincter of Oddi.[15] Although this effect is inconsistent, it may on occasion result in difficulty visualizing the distal common bile duct and demonstrating contrast flow into the duodenum during intraoperative cholangiography. The spasm appears to occur equally often with each drug. Its incidence may be decreased by administering small incremental doses of narcotics to achieve the desired anesthetic effect. The narcotic-induced spasm can be readily reversed by administering intravenous increments of naloxone (minimum 0.04 mg) or glucagon (1.0 mg).[16,17]

The choice of the anesthetic technique should be commensurate with the goal of returning patients to their normal life-style as rapidly as possible. The anesthetic effects should dissipate shortly after the end of the procedure. This can be readily accomplished using the short-acting agents available today.

Postoperative pain control and nausea and vomiting are less significant factors than when performing open procedures. If the patient is prone to postoperative nausea and emesis, a small dose of droperidol, 0.25 mg, may be given at the onset of anesthesia.[18] However, larger doses of droperidol, >0.5 mg, may cause delayed (12 hours) extrapyramidal side effects such as disorientation, dissociative states, movement disorders, anxiety, or restlessness.[19] These can be successfully treated with parenteral diphenhydramine, 50 mg.[20] Transdermal scopolamine has also been used in an attempt to minimize postoperative nausea and vomiting.[21] The 1.5 mg scopolamine patch is applied to the posterior auricular skin prior to surgery and removed 48 hours postoperatively. This method of administration does not appear to induce the undesirable side effects of parenteral scopolamine such as confusion, psychotomimetic reactions, disturbed behavior, and cycloplegia.

General Anesthesia

General anesthesia is advantageous because the cardiorespiratory status can be better controlled. Continuous $etCO_2$ monitoring allows appropriate adjustments of minute ventilation to maintain normal $Paco_2$ levels and facilitates the rapid detection of CO_2 embolus.[22] A transient but rapid increase in $etCO_2$ suggests a CO_2 embolus. Controlled ventilation may reduce the incidence of dysrhythmia in comparison to spontaneous ventilation, particularly in the presence of central nervous system depressants and respiratory acidosis.

Endotracheal intubation offers optimal protection of the airway. Appropriate depth of anesthesia and the use of muscle relaxants minimize motion within the operative field and may shorten the operative time. Cannulation of the cystic duct for laparoscopic cholangiography often requires short periods of apnea, which can be accomplished with either a general or a regional anesthetic. The latter, however, requires considerable patient cooperation, which may prove difficult in the sedated or uncooperative individual.

Evidence points to decreased postoperative morbidity when controlled ventilation and muscle relaxation are used instead of spontaneous ventilation in intubated patients.[23,24] In the studies cited there was an increased incidence of postoperative throat discomfort in the spontaneous ventilation group. Presumably this was due to the fact that these patients manifested more movement of the endotracheal tube against the pharyngeal structures. Overall, there is little difference in morbidity related to the method of ventilation as long as arterial CO_2 remains normal. Spontaneous ventilation during general anesthesia is usually insufficient to deal with the increased $PaCO_2$ load and the respiratory consequences of a pneumoperitoneum, especially in the presence of high concentrations of inhalation or intravenous anesthetic agents.

Regional Anesthesia

Recently the respiratory changes occurring in healthy women undergoing laparoscopic oocyte removal performed under lumbar epidural anesthesia with a T2-5 sensory level have been examined. In these patients there was a significant increase in minute ventilation from 9 to 12 L/min. $PaCO_2$ remained unchanged but $etCO_2$ decreased, suggesting that dead space ventilation had increased. This appears to be an effect of the elevated intra-abdominal pressure reducing the venous return and causing an increase in overall pulmonary ventilation in relation to perfusion. All patients were able to maintain normocarbia because of their ability to increase minute ventilation.[7]

Thoracic epidural anesthesia with the appropriate nerve segments blocked (T2-L1) is an acceptable technique for laparoscopic cholecystectomy and other procedures. However, careful patient selection and the cooperation of the surgical team are needed to ensure appropriate conditions for this type of anesthetic. For a continuous thoracic epidural, bupivacaine, 0.5% (6.0 ml), is used following an appropriate test dose of 1.5% lidocaine with epinephrine (3 ml of a 1:100,000 solution). Appropriate top-up doses are used as needed. The advantages of a regional anesthetic are that the patient is awake and has intact airway protective reflexes. It is essential, however, to use only minimal amounts of intravenous sedation for supplementation; otherwise airway protection cannot be ensured and depressed ventilation will result in an excessively high $PaCO_2$.[11] Heavy sedation may cause severe cardiovascular depression because of the additive effect of the sympathetic blockade from the epidural and baroreceptor depression from the sedative. The cardiovascular depression may be exaggerated even more if general anesthesia is given in addition to the epidural.

The concentration of local anesthetics must be carefully considered. Early ambulation and discharge may be delayed with bupivacaine concentrations >0.5%. If the epidural anesthetic is segmental, the patient may actually be able to sit and ambulate before sensation fully returns. In addition to the usual complications of epidural or spinal anesthesia, patients may complain of significant nausea and/or vomiting during critical portions of the operative procedure. There is no anesthesia for the bladder or gastric catheterization. Many patients experience referred shoulder pain from the diaphragm after insufflation of the peritoneal cavity. This is believed to be the result of excessive stretching or a direct irritation of the diaphragmatic surface from the CO_2 and is difficult to treat. If patient discomfort is excessive, potent narcotics or a general anesthetic may have to be given. Slow insufflation of the abdominal cavity (1.0 to 1.5 L/min) as well as maintaining a lower pressure (<10 mm Hg) will help minimize this referred pain.

Subarachnoid (spinal) block can also be used for this procedure. Concerns and considerations are as described for epidural anesthesia. The use of very small gauge needles (26 gauge) for subarachnoid block will reduce, but not eliminate, the incidence of postdural puncture headache (about 2%). Continuous spinal anesthesia may be required to ensure the appropriate duration of anesthesia. During continuous spinal anesthesia the dural hole is larger than that created by a 26-gauge needle alone, so the incidence of headache may indeed be higher. Although an epidural blood patch has a very high success rate in treating persistent headache, a thoracic epidural is probably preferable because of the lesser chance of cephalgia and a more controllable speed of onset and extent of the block.

Intercostal Nerve Blocks

Bilateral intercostal blocks offer effective relief of pain related to surgery, relaxation of abdominal muscles, a reduced need for systemic narcotics, and the patient remains awake.[25] Patient cooperation is a major issue since this block involves multiple injections in patients who are anxious and have little premedication. Additional concerns are related to the possibility of pneumothorax and a systemic toxic reaction to the anesthetic since there is increased absorption from the vascular intercostal injection sites. A segmental thoracic epidural block is preferable because it produces optimal conditions with less toxicity and less patient discomfort.

Local Anesthesia

Local anesthesia with minimal sedation has been used for gynecologic laparoscopies.[26,27] However, this method is useful only in procedures of very short duration, primarily those of a diagnostic nature. Conditions for more involved surgery would likely be inadequate despite patient motivation and cooperation. We believe that local anesthesia is not an appropriate choice for major laparoscopic procedures because of the high degree of patient discomfort.

CONCLUSION

The minimally invasive nature of most laparoscopic procedures allows the choice of anesthetic techniques that provides maximum patient comfort intraoperatively and postoperatively without compromising the goal of early ambulation and hospital discharge. With careful management and monitoring of physiologic changes in the pulmonary and cardiovascular systems and the management of gastric reflux, laparoscopic procedures can be safely performed on a short-stay basis.

REFERENCES

1. Versichelen L, Serreyn R, Rolly G, Vanderkerckhove D. Physiopathologic changes during anesthesia administration for gynecologic laparoscopy. J Reprod Med 29:697-700, 1984.
2. Hamilton WK, McDonald JS, Fischer HW, Bethards R. Postoperative respiratory complications. Anesthesiology 25:607-612, 1964.
3. Latimer RG, Dickman M, Day WC, Gunn ML, Schmidt CD. Ventilatory patterns and pulmonary complications after upper abdominal surgery determined by preoperative and postoperative computerized spirometry and blood gas analysis. Am J Surg 122:622-631, 1971.
4. Doughty A. Anesthesia for operative obstetrics and gynecology. In Churchill-Davidson HC, ed. A Practice of Anaesthesia. Philadelphia: WB Saunders, 1978, pp 1389-1391.
5. Marshall RL, Jebson PJR, Davie IT, Scott DB. Circulatory effects of carbon dioxide insufflation of the peritoneal cavity for laparoscopy. Br J Anaesth 44:680-684, 1972.
6. Lewis DG, Ryder W, Burn N, Wheldon JT, Tacchi D. Laparoscopy—An investigation during spontaneous ventilation with halothane. Br J Anaesth 44:685-691, 1972.
7. Ciofolo MJ, Clergue F, Seebacher J, Lefebvre G, Viars P. Ventilatory effects of laparoscopy under epidural anesthesia. Anesth Analg 70:357-361, 1990.
8. Johannsen G, Andersen M, Juhl B. The effect of general anaesthesia on the haemodynamic events during laparoscopy with CO_2 insufflation. Acta Anaesthesiol Scand 33:132-136, 1989.
9. Harris MNE, Plantevin OM, Crowther A. Cardiac arrhythmias during anaesthesia for laparoscopy. Br J Anaesth 56:1213-1216, 1984.
10. Hodgson C, McClelland RMA, Newton JR. Some effects of the peritoneal insufflation of carbon dioxide at laparoscopy. Anaesthesia 25:382-389, 1970.
11. Arandia HY, Grogono AW. Comparison of the incidence of combined risk factors for gastric acid aspiration. Anesth Analg 59:862-864, 1980.
12. Coombs DW, Hooper D, Colton T. Preanesthetic cimetidine alteration of gastric fluid volume and pH. Anesth Analg 58:183-188, 1979.
13. Maltby JR, Sutherland AD, Sale JP, Shaffer EA. Postoperative oral fluids: Is a five-hour fast justified prior to elective surgery. Anesth Analg 65:1112-1116, 1986.
14. Maltby JR, Koehli N, Ewen A, Shaffer EA. Gastric fluid volume, pH, and emptying in elective inpatients. Influence of narcotic-atropine premedication, oral fluid, and ranitidine. Can J Anaesth 35:562-566, 1988.
15. Radnay PA, Brodman E, Mankikar D. The effect of equianalgesic doses of fentanyl, morphine, meperidine and pentazocine on common bile duct pressure. Anaesthetist 29:26-29, 1980.
16. McCammon RL, Viegas OJ, Stoelting RK. Naloxone reversal of choledochoduodenal sphincter spasm associated with narcotic administration. Anesthesiology 48:437, 1978.

17. Jones RM, Fiddian-Green R, Knight P. Narcotic-induced choledochoduodenal sphincter spasm reversed by glucagon. Anesth Analg 59:946-947, 1980.
18. Millar JM, Hall PJ. Nausea and vomiting after prostaglandins in day case termination of pregnancy. The efficacy of low dose droperidol. Anaesthesia 42:613-618, 1987.
19. Melnick B, Sawyer R, Karambelkar D, Phitayakorn P, Lim NT, Patel R. Delayed side effects of droperidol after ambulatory general anesthesia. Anesth Analg 69:748-751, 1989.
20. Schreibman DL. Treatment of a delayed reaction to droperidol with diphenhydramine. Anesth Analg 71:105, 1990.
21. Jackson SH, Schmidt MN, McGuire J. Transdermal scopolamine as a preanesthetic drug and postoperative antinauseant and antiemetic. Anesthesiology 57:A330, 1982.
22. Shulman D, Aronson HB. Capnography in the early diagnosis of carbon dioxide embolism during laparoscopy. Can Anaesth Soc J 31:455-459, 1984.
23. Skacel M, Sengupta P, Plantevin OM. Morbidity after day case laparoscopy. A comparison of two techniques of tracheal anaesthesia. Anaesthesia 41:537-541, 1986.
24. Collins KM, Docherty PW, Plantevin OM. Postoperative morbidity following gynaecological outpatient laparoscopy. A reappraisal of the service. Anaesthesia 39:819-822, 1984.
25. Nunn JF, Slavin G. Posterior intercostal nerve block for pain relief after cholecystectomy. Br J Anaesth 52:253-260, 1980.
26. Shane SM. Conscious Sedation for Ambulatory Surgery. Baltimore: University Park Press, 1983, pp 35-42.
27. Beilin B, Vatashsky E, Aronson HB. "Conscious sedation" for laparoscopy. Isr J Med Sci 22:346-349, 1986.

CHAPTER 5

Open Laparoscopy

Robert J. Fitzgibbons, Jr., M.D.
Giovanni M. Salerno, M.D.
Charles J. Filipi, M.D.

Establishment of pneumoperitoneum with gas is required for all laparo-scopic procedures to provide a working space in the normally collapsed abdomen. Pneumoperitoneum is accomplished using one of two tech-niques. In the open technique a mini-laparotomy is performed at the umbilicus, and access to the free peritoneal cavity is confirmed by visual and/or digital exploration. A cannula is then passed, through which gas is insufflated and the laparoscope introduced. In the closed technique an insufflation needle is passed transabdominally or transuterinely for pre-liminary gas instillation; then a large-bore trocar is introduced over which a laparoscopic cannula has been threaded (see Chapter 8).[1] An increas-ingly popular modification of the closed technique eliminates the prelimi-nary insufflation; the intra-abdominal trocar and laparoscopic cannula are inserted directly without first establishing pneumoperitoneum.[2-7] This modification is gaining acceptance because many of the complications of laparoscopy such as omental and abdominal emphysema or gas embolism are related to gas instillation with an insufflation needle. Direct trocar insertion permits visualization of the abdominal contents by passing the laparoscope through the trocar sleeve before beginning gas insufflation. Finally, the development of disposable trocar/cannula systems with built-in spring-loaded safety shields, which immediately cover the sharp point of the trocar as soon as peritoneal penetration has been accomplished, has made the direct trocar method safer.

CLOSED VS. OPEN LAPAROSCOPY

The advantage of the closed technique is that less soft tissue damage occurs because minimal dissection is needed. It is widely believed that it is a faster procedure, although this is questionable once the surgeon has become accustomed to the open technique. The major disadvantage is that it is a blind technique, which increases the possibility of vessel or organ injury.

The exact incidence of complications of closed laparoscopy is difficult to determine because most injuries are rare, isolated events and thus go unreported. Based on large surveys from France and the United Kingdom, it has been estimated that between 3 and 10 major vessel lacerations per 10,000 procedures are caused by the insufflation needle or the trocar.[8,9] The incidence of organ penetration during closed laparoscopy is difficult to quantitate because most series include sterilization procedures and do not specify whether the complication was related to the peritoneal access procedure or to the sterilization procedure. However, Loffer and Pent[10] in 1975 reviewed 56,106 closed laparoscopies and noted 87 cases of organ penetration, which occurred during peritoneal access. Sixty-two of the cases involved the uterus and the remainder the stomach, the small intestine, or the urinary bladder. Riedel et al.[11] have reported the complications of laparoscopy from 1983 through 1985 in nearly 250,000 procedures in the Federal Republic of Germany. The authors note 427 complications serious enough to require laparotomy or repeat laparoscopy. Injuries to the intestine as a result of trocar or Veress needle accidents accounted for 38%. Major blood vessel injury by the same mechanism occurred in 23.3%. Other complications of closed laparoscopy include abdominal wall insufflation, inability to establish pneumoperitoneum (failed pneumoperitoneum), omental or mesenteric emphysema, and gas embolus.[2,3]

The advantage of the open technique is that access to the free peritoneal cavity can be unequivocally established before insufflation is begun or laparoscopic instruments are introduced into the abdomen. The technique virtually eliminates the most feared complication of laparoscopy, that is, major vessel injury with its potentially fatal consequences.[8] The risk of bowel or other solid organ injury is minimal, but should it occur, it does so under direct vision; such injuries are readily recognizable and repaired, making significant sequelae unlikely. Finally, the possibility of abdominal wall or omental emphysema, gas embolism, or failed pneumoperitoneum is diminished because access to the peritoneal cavity is confirmed before beginning insufflation. A disadvantage of the open technique is that more dissection at the umbilicus is necessary, theoretically resulting in an increased rate of local complications. To date, data are not available to support such a contention. Maintenance of adequate intraperitoneal pressure because of gas leak at the cannula insertion point has been stated to be a potential problem with the open technique. However, in over 150 open laparoscopies we have never encountered this problem. It would appear that modern high-flow insufflators eliminate this difficulty.

THE CANNULA

Open laparoscopy can be performed using a standard laparoscopic cannula if a purse-string suture is placed circumferentially around the fascial opening.

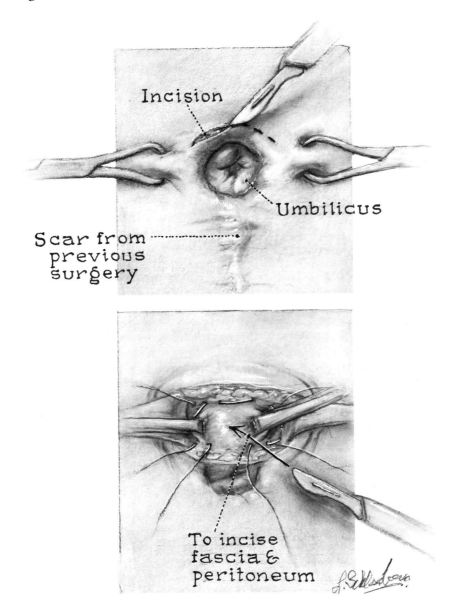

The purse-string suture secures the cannula and prevents gas escape. The technique is effective but requires a relatively large skin incision and a considerable amount of dissection to gain adequate exposure of the fascia to place the purse-string suture. Massive obesity significantly compounds the difficulty encountered in placing the suture.

In the early 1970s Hasson[12] developed a modified laparoscopic cannula that has greatly simplified open laparoscopy. There were three components to this modification. First, an olive-shaped sleeve was placed over the shaft of the cannula, which was designed to be firmly approximated to the skin and fascial opening of the abdomen to prevent gas escape. The olive sleeve could be adjusted up and down the shaft of the cannula so that the length of cannula in the abdominal cavity could be varied. Second, suture wings were added to allow fascial sutures to be attached tautly to the cannula. This was crucial in achieving a tight seal between the skin, fascia, and olive sleeve to prevent gas escape. Third, the sharp trocar was replaced with a blunt obturator to facilitate passage of the device through the mini-laparotomy incision.

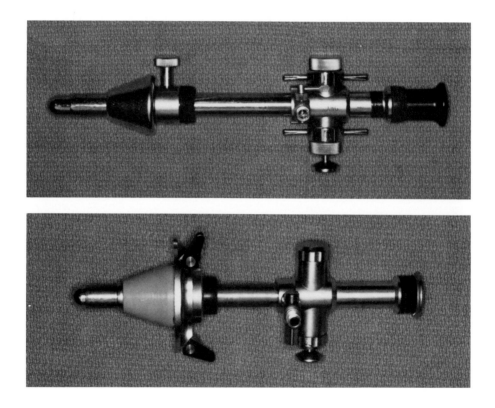

The Hasson cannula (top) is compared to a modified cannula (bottom). The suture wings of the Hasson cannula can be seen attached at the level of the trumpet valve. The olive sleeve can be moved up and down and then fixed to the shaft of the cannula with the metal screw. The location of the olive sleeve is determined by the thickness of the abdominal wall. Although the modified cannula is similar to the original Hasson cannula, it has the advantage of having the suture wings attached to the olive sleeve instead of the shaft of the instrument. This modification allows the length of cannula to be adjusted in the abdomen after initial placement without having to resecure the sutures holding it in place.

TECHNIQUE

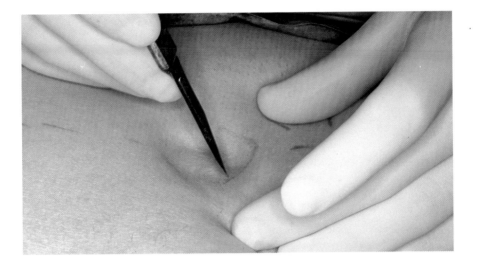

No special preoperative preparation is required. The umbilical skin incision is the same as would be used for closed laparoscopy. A vertical incision is preferred if there is an appropriate skin fold to conceal the scar. A transverse incision is used in this patient because no skin fold exists. The incision is made in the lower border of the umbilicus using a No. 11 scalpel blade.

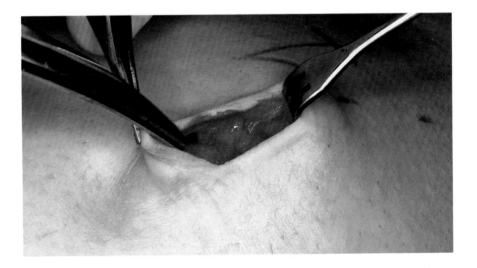

Dissection down to the fascia should proceed very close to the skin of the umbilicus. A curved Mayo scissors facilitates this dissection. Traction on the superior umbilical skin flap anteriorly and cranially will result in a palpable, vertically oriented raphe of tissue between the undersurface of the umbilicus and the deeper abdominal wall. This represents fascial tissue as it fuses at the umbilicus. Even in morbidly obese individuals this raphe of tissue will be palpable just below the skin of the umbilicus.

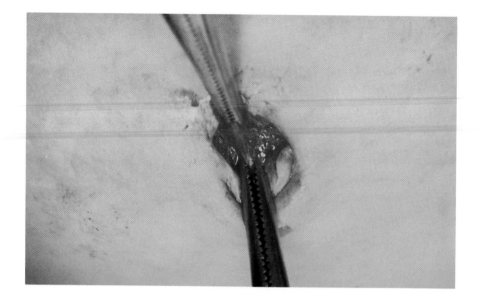

The palpable raphe of fascial tissue should be grasped with two Kocker clamps placed in tandem vertically. The most superior Kocker clamp should be placed as close as possible to the skin of the umbilicus without compromising it.

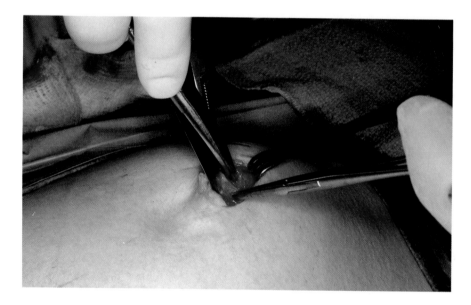

The fascia is incised with curved Mayo scissors. Commonly, access is gained to the preperitoneal cavity as soon as the fascia is opened. However, if a layer of preperitoneal fat and peritoneum remains, it can be grasped with hemostats and opened.

This is the most difficult step in open laparoscopy. Excessive dissection in preperitoneal space will result in separation of the peritoneum from the overlying fascia, making the peritoneum difficult to incise.

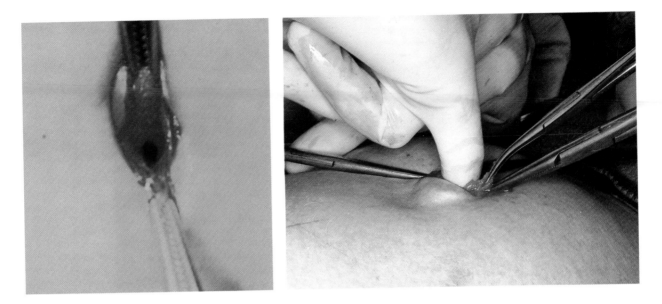

Access to the abdominal cavity is confirmed by visual inspection and digital palpation.

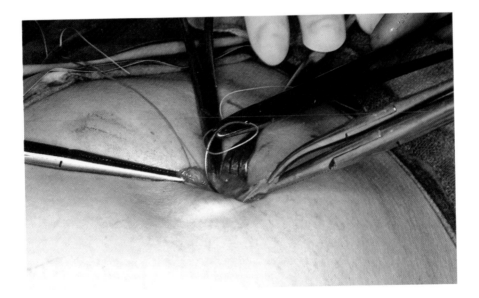

A single 0 or 00 suture is placed on both sides of the fascial defect. The peritoneum can be included in this stitch, but this is not necessary. The choice of suture material depends on the surgeon's preference for fascial closure since these two sutures will ultimately be tied together to close the fascial defect.

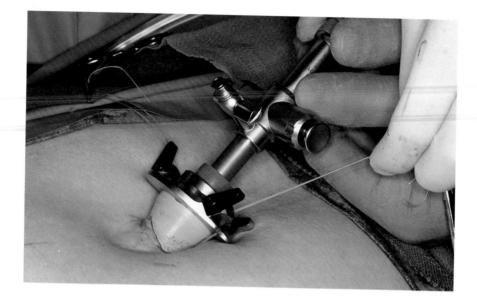

The modified laparoscopic cannula with a blunt obturator is introduced into the abdominal cavity. The previously placed sutures are attached under tension to the suture wings, firmly securing the olive sleeve at the skin and fascial defect.

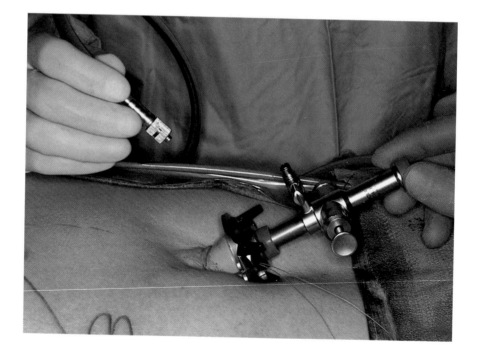

A CO_2 gas conduit is attached to the cannula. There is no need to use preliminary low-flow CO_2 gas insufflation because access to the abdominal cavity has been confirmed. Thus pneumoperitoneum can be established rapidly.

Some surgeons believe that initial rapid insufflation may result in undue stretching of the abdominal wall, resulting in increased abdominal pain postoperatively, but we have not observed this to be the case.

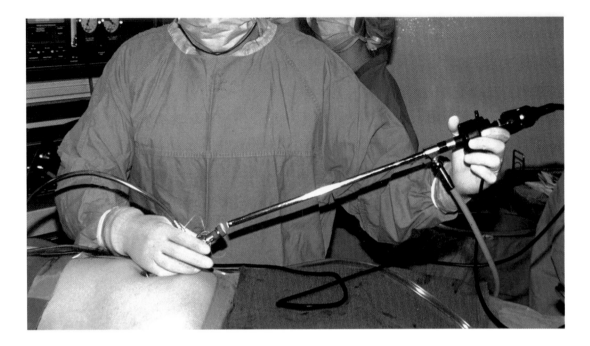

The laparoscope is introduced into the abdomen.

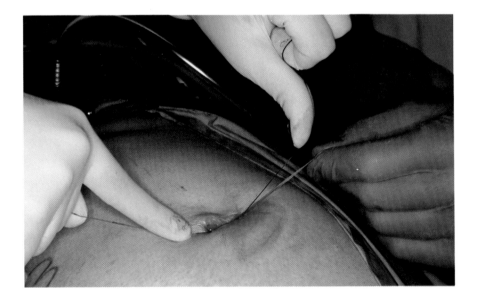

At the conclusion of the procedure the sutures are detached from the modified cannula wings and the cannula withdrawn. These same sutures are used to close the fascial defect.

CONCLUSION

Despite the safety afforded by open laparoscopy, a survey by the American Association of Gynecological Laparoscopists regarding laparoscopic procedures performed in 1982 disclosed that 96% were performed using the closed technique and only 4% using the open technique.[13] Because most gynecologists have been trained in the closed technique and since individual surgeons have rarely experienced a significant number of complications, it has been postulated that they believe there is little reason to alter their routine.[9] In addition, the perception is that the closed technique is faster. Finally, the bulk of laparoscopic procedures reported has been performed by gynecologists, who are less familiar with operations about the umbilicus. Therefore it is not surprising that the closed technique has remained popular.

At the present many laparoscopists reserve the open technique for patients whom they consider likely to have dangerous periumbilical adhesions. This represents a relatively small number of patients since most gynecologists do not believe that a prior laparoscopy, cesarean section, or other abdominal procedure in which the incision is not in close proximity to the umbilicus places the patient at excessive risk. They are, therefore, content to use the closed technique in these situations.[4] This leads to a situation where many laparoscopists fail to gain significant experience with the open technique, and thus they are uncomfortable when this approach is indicated. This problem could be corrected if laparoscopists would use the open technique more often and thus develop familiarity with it.

We have performed over 150 open laparoscopies at the Creighton University School of Medicine affiliated hospitals. There have been no complications related to trocar entry. Approximately 50% of these procedures were performed in patients with prior abdominal incisions near the umbilicus. In this group of patients the percutaneous approach is clearly associated with a greater risk of complications. Since the open technique is routinely performed at our institution, insertion of the Hasson cannula now takes approximately 5 minutes or less. If open laparoscopy is indicated because of underlying adhesions, this procedure can be completed rapidly and safely. Hence, in experienced centers, open laparoscopy should not result in an undue prolongation of the operative procedure. It is our belief that because of the safety and ease of this technique, general surgeons beginning laparoscopic surgery should become adept at open laparoscopy.

REFERENCES

1. Wolf WM, Pasic R. Transuterine insertion of Veress needle in laparoscopy. Obstet Gynecol 75:456-457, 1990.
2. Jarrett JC. Laparoscopy: Direct trocar insertion without pneumoperitoneum. Obstet Gynecol 75:725-727, 1990.
3. Byron JW, Fujiyoshi CA, Miyazawa K. Evaluation of the direct trocar insertion technique at laparoscopy. Obstet Gynecol 74:423-425, 1989.
4. Kaali SG, Vartfai G. Direct insertion of the laparoscopic trocar after an earlier laparotomy. J Reprod Med 33:739-740, 1988.
5. Saidi MH. Direct laparoscopy with prior pneumoperitoneum. J Reprod Med 31:684-686, 1986.
6. Pine S, Barke JI, Barna P. Insertion of the laparoscopic trocar without the use of carbon dioxide gas. Contraception 28:233-239, 1983.
7. Copeland C, Wing R, Hulka JF. Direct trocar insertion at laparoscopy: An evaluation. Obstet Gynecol 62:655-659, 1983.
8. Baadsgaard SE, Bille S, Egeblad K. Major vascular injury during gynecologic laparoscopy. Acta Obstet Gynecol Scand 68:283-285, 1989.
9. Penfield AJ. How to prevent complication of open laparoscopy. J Reprod Med 30:660-663, 1985.
10. Loffer FD, Pent D. Indications, contraindications and complications of laparoscopy. Obstet Gynecol Surv 30:407-427, 1975.
11. Riedel HH, Willenbrock-Lehmann E, Mecke H, Semm K. The frequency of distribution of various pelviscopic (laparoscopic) operations, including complication rates—Statistics of the Federal Republic of Germany in the years 1983-1985. Zentralbl Gynäkol 111:78-91, 1989.
12. Hasson HM. Modified instrument and method for laparoscopy. Am J Obstet Gynecol 110:886-887, 1971.
13. Phillips JM, Hulka JF, Peterson HB. American Association of Gynecologic Laparoscopists' 1982 membership survey. J Reprod Med 29:592-594, 1984.

PART TWO

Clinical Applications

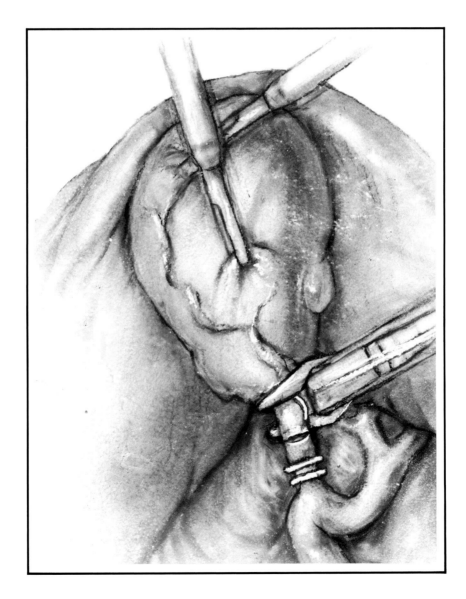

Laparoscopy in Preoperative Diagnosis and Staging for Gastrointestinal Cancers

Andrew L. Warshaw, M.D.
Carlos Fernández-del Castillo, M.D.

Diagnostic laparoscopy in gastroenterology and general surgery has been used primarily for the assessment of chronic liver disease and for the differential diagnosis of ascites.[1] Other indications have included evaluation of patients with abdominal trauma and acute abdomen,[2] staging for lymphoma,[3] and detection of suspected intra-abdominal malignancies.[4] In the past few years we have been interested in the application of laparoscopy in the study of pancreatic cancer[5,6] and have found it to be a useful tool in the diagnosis and staging of this neoplasm. This chapter will review the rationale, technique, and results of laparoscopic examination of patients with this disease and describe its application in the study of other gastrointestinal tumors.

PANCREATIC CANCER
Rationale

The incidence of pancreatic cancer in the United States in 1987 was 9.0 per 100,000.[7] This makes it the second most common gastrointestinal malignancy following colorectal cancer, which affects five times as many individuals. Although the 5-year survival rate for colorectal cancer is over 50%, the rate for pancreatic cancer is only 3.1%; over 85% of patients die within 1 year of diagnosis. Notwithstanding this dismal outlook, it is interesting to note that survival of patients with this malignancy has increased over the past 15 years.[7] Selected series have described survival rates as high as 18% in patients undergoing resection for cure[8] and even 30%[9] when only tumors <2 cm are considered. This means that some patients *can be cured,* and this, at least in part, relates to earlier diagnosis and better preoperative staging.

Traditionally, most patients with pancreatic cancer have undergone surgical exploration, even though only about 5% were treated via pancreatoduodenectomy. This approach was justified because surgery provided the opportunity to confirm the diagnosis histologically and to palliate the biliary and/or gastric obstructions present in many patients. These premises are no longer valid because it is possible to diagnose a malignancy percutaneously and because excellent results are achieved with a biliary endoprosthesis placed endoscopically or by the transhepatic route.[6] There also has been a dramatic reduction in the mortality and morbidity rates associated with pancreatoduodenectomy when performed in specialized centers. Although postoperative mortality rates of over 25% were not uncommon 15 years ago,[10] several major institutions in the United States and Europe now have rates well under 5%.[11] An emerging concept in the treatment of patients with pancreatic cancer is that only individuals with a resectable tumor or those requiring gastrojejunostomy because of duodenal obstruction should be operated on. Patients with a resectable tumor are probably best served if treated in specialized centers. The remainder are best spared an operation that will not affect their short survival or their already jeopardized quality of life.

To achieve this goal, accurate preoperative staging is mandatory. Ultrasonography, CT, and angiography have been primarily used for this purpose in the past. We believe that laparoscopy significantly contributes to the staging process and that it should be considered in all patients with pancreatic cancer who are potential candidates for resection. In addition, cytologic examination of peritoneal tissue, which is generally obtained by peritoneal washings during laparoscopy, appears to provide additional prognostic information and, in the future, may prove to be another unique element for preoperative staging evaluation.

Technique

Laparoscopy can be performed in either an inpatient or an outpatient setting as long as provisions are made for postlaparoscopy admission in the event a complication occurs. Absolute contraindications to laparoscopy include uncorrectable coagulation defects, peritonitis, substantial intestinal distention, and large ventral hernias. Marked obesity increases the risks associated with the procedure but is not a contraindication in itself. Previous intra-abdominal surgery, particularly cholecystectomy, may preclude adequate exploration of the liver surfaces and thus be a limiting factor.

A thorough exploration of the entire abdominal cavity is required to search for metastases, which dictates that 4 to 5 L of CO_2 must be used to achieve adequate insufflation. Many patients cannot tolerate this amount of insufflation under local anesthesia because of pain and respiratory impairment. For this reason we prefer to use general anesthesia with endotracheal intubation and assisted ventilation.

The patient fasts overnight, receives a cleansing enema, and empties the bladder just before the procedure. The abdomen is prepared and draped as for laparotomy, and the site for insertion of the instrument is selected, usually in the midline just below the umbilicus or just above it and slightly to the left to avoid the round ligament and the epigastric vessels. The right lateral border of the rectus sheath is an alternative insertion site when there are previous periumbilical incisions.

A 1.0 cm incision is made through the skin, and the Veress needle is inserted into the peritoneal cavity in a plane directed toward the pelvic hollow to avoid the major vessels of the retroperitoneum. Two characteristic "pops" can be felt as the needle punctures the fascia and then the peritoneum. An attempt is made to verify that the needle tip is truly in the peritoneal cavity by assessing its lateral rotatory movement and by confirming a negative intra-abdominal pressure (a drop of saline solution is placed in the open end of the needle, the abdomen is lifted, and the drop is sucked down). Insufflation with CO_2 is then begun. Flow should be unrestricted and allowed to continue until the abdominal wall is relatively tense and the intra-abdominal pressure reaches 15 mm Hg (generally 4 to 5 L). At this point the anesthesiologist may note decreasing compliance and increased difficulty in ventilating the patient. The needle is then removed, and a trocar and subsequently the laparoscope are inserted along the same plane.

Visual examination of the lower abdomen and pelvis is completed first. The laparoscope is then rotated to inspect the upper abdomen. Examination of the liver surfaces is particularly relevant. It is necessary to insert a rod through a second, smaller trocar (5 mm) in the right upper quadrant of the abdomen. The rod is used to lift areas of the liver so that the undersurface can be inspected or to push other viscera away from the area that the surgeon wishes to see.

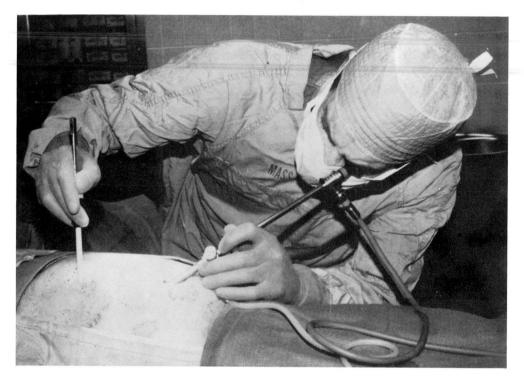

The optimal location for the second trocar is chosen by pressing a finger down on the proposed location and assessing its suitability by noting the point of depression through the laparoscope.

Specimens of peritoneal or omental nodules can be taken for biopsy with forceps inserted through the second trocar. Nodules in the liver are most easily sampled with a cutting needle (such as Tru-Cut) inserted directly through the abdominal wall. Nodules <1 mm in diameter can be accurately sampled under direct vision. Samples of nodules on the pelvic peritoneum also can be taken with a cutting needle; however, because of the location of the nodules, it is sometimes necessary to insert another trocar in the lower midline for the biopsy forceps. Enlarged lymph nodes can be successfully sampled with the cutting needle or by fine-needle aspiration.

If ascitic fluid is present, it should be collected by direct abdominal wall puncture or via a tube inserted through the second trocar. If there is no ascitic fluid, we routinely instill 100 ml of normal saline solution into the subhepatic space. Dispersion of the solution throughout the peritoneal cavity is facilitated by tilting the operating table and agitating the abdominal wall. The fluid is then aspirated under direct vision. The aspirates are examined by making direct smears of the fluid as well as concentrated cell blocks after centrifugation.

In patients with suspected pancreatic cancer, laparoscopy permits visualization of the pancreas by using either a supragastric approach (through the lesser omentum) or entering below the stomach (through the gastro-colic omentum or the mesocolon). This procedure, which has also been called pancreatoscopy, was first proposed by Meyer-Burg[12] and was further developed by Ishida[13] and Cuschieri, Hall, and Clark.[14] For the supra-gastric approach,[13] the operating table is raised to about 30 degrees, and the lesser omentum under the left lobe of the liver is exposed by elevating the latter with the tip of the scope. Next a forceps is inserted into the peritoneal cavity from the right upper part of the abdomen, and a lesser omentotomy is performed. The laparoscope is then inserted through this opening, the pancreatic body is visualized, and a sample is taken for biopsy.

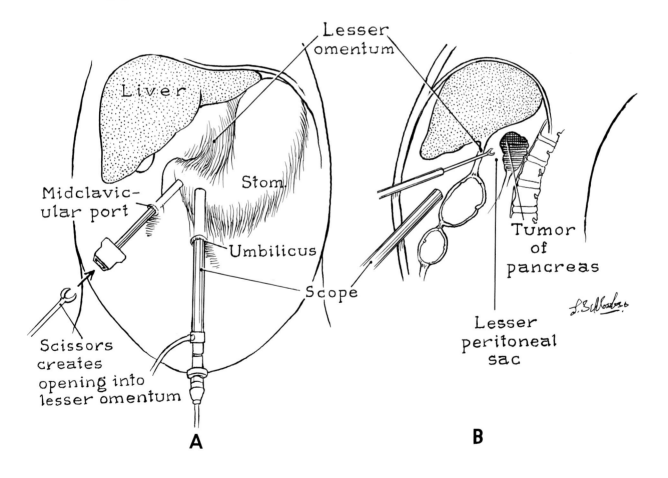

Lesser omentum

Liver

Stom.

Midclavic-ular port

Umbilicus

Scope

Scissors creates opening into lesser omentum

Tumor of pancreas

Lesser peritoneal sac

A　　　　　　　　　　　**B**

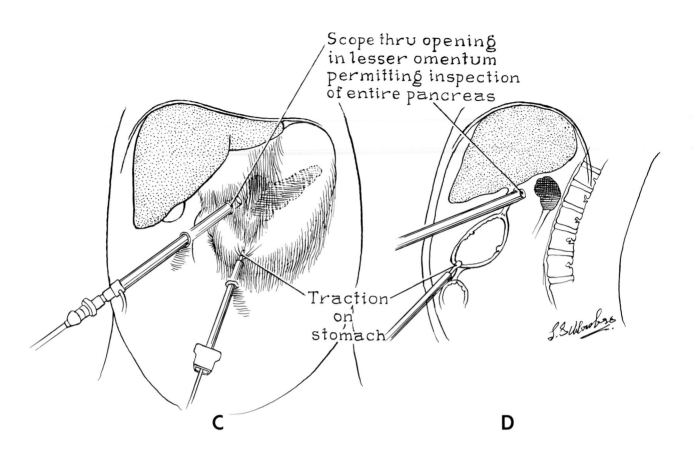

Scope thru opening
in lesser omentum
permitting inspection
of entire pancreas

Traction
on
stomach

C   D

Once the procedure is completed, the CO_2 is allowed to escape, and the skin wounds are closed with subcuticular absorbable sutures. Postoperative care is routine, with normal activity and diet being resumed promptly. The complication rate for this and other diagnostic laparoscopic procedures has been remarkably low. A review of the English literature revealed a complication rate of 1% and a mortality rate of 0.05%.[15]

Results

It has been our practice to use laparoscopy to help stage pancreatic cancer because of its unique capacity to detect small peritoneal metastatic disease. We do not think that direct visualization of the pancreatic tumor is necessary since a CT scan or ultrasonogram has already been obtained in the great majority of cases. Furthermore, the tumor can be biopsied percutaneously in most cases and perhaps should not be attempted in patients with potentially resectable tumors (see later discussion).

We evaluated the role of laparoscopy in pancreatic cancer staging in a series of 72 patients with this disease.[6] The staging protocol included CT, MRI, laparoscopy, and angiography. If a biopsy-confirmed metastasis was found, this sequence was ended, and the patients underwent appropriate palliative treatment. Although laparoscopy could not be performed in all patients because of adhesions from prior surgery, its contribution to accurate staging was significant, demonstrating peritoneal or superficial small liver metastases in 22 of 23 cases (96% accuracy) and correctly excluding them in 24 of 24 cases (overall accuracy of 98%). Typically these metastases were 1 to 3 mm nodules and were not detected by CT or MRI.

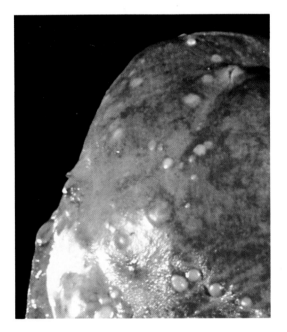

Superficial metastatic nodules on surface of liver were missed on CT scan.

The combination of CT, laparoscopy, and angiography (MRI was no better than CT alone) was effective in assessing resectability for pancreatic cancer. If any one of the three tests was positive, the tumor was unresectable 96% of the time (51 of 53 cases); if all three were negative, the resectability rate was 78% (15 of 19 cases).

Small liver and peritoneal metastases were found in 36% of patients with pancreatic tumors. Other authors report a rate between 40% and 73%.[13,16,17] This higher frequency is likely related to the fact that these investigators did not preselect their study population based on a negative CT scan as we did. Our results as well as theirs show that these malignant deposits are more frequent in cancer of the pancreatic body and tail (65%) than in cancer of the pancreatic head (27%).

We evaluated the cytologic study of peritoneal washings obtained during laparoscopy or at the time of surgery when laparoscopy was not carried out in 40 consecutive patients with pancreatic adenocarcinoma.[18] All patients were considered to have potentially resectable cancers on the basis of a CT scan showing no metastasis or vascular encasement. The presence of unequivocal malignant cells, either in the smears or in the tissue sections prepared from centrifuged blocks, was considered a positive study and occurred in 12 cases (30%).

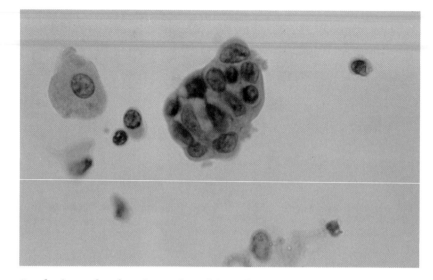

Cytologic study of peritoneal washings shows cluster of carcinomatous cells and macrophage laden with bile (left).

Of the patients with cancer of the pancreatic head with positive cytologic findings, only 1 of 10 underwent resection, whereas 13 of 25 with a negative study had resections. In addition, survival was significantly better in patients with negative cytologic findings, although this was most likely related to the rate of resectability.

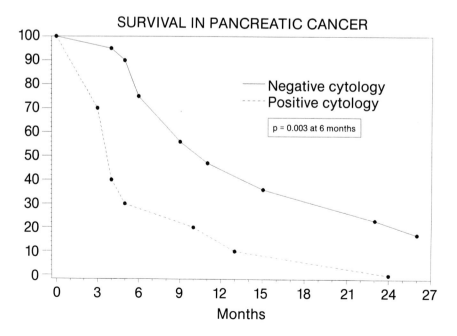

Two other findings of the study deserve comment. One is that positivity for malignant cells did not depend on the presence of visible peritoneal or liver metastasis (in fact, of six patients with liver metastases, none had positive cytologic results, and only one of the 12 patients with positive cytologic results had a visible omental implant) nor the presence of ascites (66% of positive studies were found in patients without ascites, and malignant cells were found in only 50% of those with ascites). This strengthens the point that the information gained by laparoscopy and by peritoneal cytologic examination is complementary. The other finding is that positive cytologic results were significantly increased in patients who had undergone per-cutaneous needle biopsy earlier compared to those who had not (75% vs. 19%). This is consistent with observations made by other investigators of rapid intra-abdominal spread and implantation after tumor manipulation and biopsy[19,20] and cautions against the use of preoperative biopsy in potentially resectable patients.

In summary, we believe that laparoscopy with cytologic examination of peritoneal washings significantly contributes to preoperative staging in pancreatic cancer. This procedure, together with CT and ultrasonography, can be easily carried out in the primary institution of care in most cases, allowing for effective triage and referral of only potentially resectable cases to more specialized institutions.

GASTRIC CANCER

The use of laparoscopy to assess the presence of peritoneal or liver metastasis in gastric carcinoma has been reported by several authors.[21-24] The two largest studies are by Chissov et al.,[21] who found evidence of dissemination in 22% of 625 patients, and Possik et al.,[22] who evaluated 360 patients and found peritoneal and liver metastases in 37% and in 18%, respectively. These numbers certainly suggest that the use of laparoscopy is justifiable in terms of detecting metastatic disease; however, it is not clear how subsequent therapy was influenced.

Surgery in gastric carcinoma has two main purposes—resection for cure and palliation of symptoms, mainly obstruction and bleeding. In contrast to pancreatic cancer, palliative gastrectomy is a well-established form of treatment[25,26] and is usually not limited by the presence of intraperitoneal metastatic spread. The main factor determining resectability, other than the general health status of the patient, is posterior fixation of the stomach to the retroperitoneum, especially at the celiac axis. Unfortunately laparoscopy does not yield reliable information in this regard. Thus foreknowledge of hepatic or peritoneal spread will not preclude laparotomy in many patients.

Recent reports concerning endoscopic laser ablation could change this picture.[27,28] Fleischer and Sivak[27] successfully managed to palliate the symptoms of 22 of 25 patients presenting with malignant obstruction of the gastric cardia. If this form of palliative treatment becomes more widespread, the information gained by laparoscopy would become more critical and would effectively contribute to the selection of patients to undergo curative surgery.

ESOPHAGEAL CANCER

A few studies are available on the use of laparoscopy for staging esophageal cancer.[23,29,30] Dagnini et al.[30] studied 369 patients with cancer of the esophagus or cardia. They found that in 14% of patients cancer had spread to the liver, peritoneum, omentum, stomach wall, or lymph nodes, precluding curative resection, and that in another 10% local spread had occurred and could be removed en bloc with the primary tumor. Metastases that had been missed at laparoscopy were found in 4.4% of 250 patients who subsequently underwent a laparotomy. The probability of finding subdiaphragmatic metastasis from cancers in the upper third of the esophagus was minimal but increased progressively in frequency with tumors of the middle and lower third of the esophagus and the cardia. Additionally, the authors noted that unsuspected cirrhosis was found at laparoscopy in 14.3% of cases and that the severity of portal hypertension precluded surgery in half of these. Concomitant primary hepatocarcinoma was found in three patients. Dagnini et al. concluded that CT and ultrasonography were primarily of use for staging esophageal cancer above the diaphragm and that laparoscopy was superior for infradiaphragmatic evaluation. It has been estimated that only 58% of patients with esophageal cancer are candidates for resection[30,31] and that only 39% have truly resectable cancer.[31] As with pancreatic cancer, the risks of operation are substantial and the chance of cure small. On the other hand, palliation of symptoms can be achieved by intubation or endoluminal laser therapy,[28] decreasing the need to perform surgery for this purpose. It is desirable to define the patients who are most likely to benefit from surgery, and laparoscopy could play a significant role in this process.

Recent developments in neoadjuvant (preoperative) chemotherapy and radiotherapy in this disease seem to have improved the poor outcome of these patients considerably.[32,33] A method such as laparoscopy to assess the presence of intra-abdominal metastases prior to surgery or to monitor for distant recurrence during follow-up may thus have a greater role.

LIVER AND GALLBLADDER CANCER

Two decades ago laparoscopy frequently was used to establish and to histologically confirm the diagnosis of hepatocarcinoma.[34-36] Its use increased the yield of hepatic biopsy to 70% as compared to 39% for blind biopsy and 52% for two blind biopsies.[34] The availability of CT and ultrasonography have largely superseded laparoscopy for this purpose; however, it can still be of value when small scattered lesions, fatty infiltration, or cirrhosis is present, in which case guidance of the biopsy needle with the aforementioned methods can be difficult. For purposes of staging, laparoscopy is of limited benefit in liver cancer. Extrahepatic metastases are generally hematogenous, with the lungs being the most frequently affected site. Diaphragmatic, pelvic, and peritoneal metastases, which could potentially be detected by laparoscopy and missed by other methods, only occur in 10%, 6%, and 4% of patients, respectively.[37] Attachment of an ultrasonic probe to the tip of the laparoscope has been used, although the extent to which this can increase the recognition of small or otherwise undetectable tumors has not yet been evaluated.[38,39]

Diagnosis of gallbladder malignancy can be difficult preoperatively, and after surgical exploration only about 10% of patients are found to have resectable cancers.[40] By allowing direct visualization of the tumor, obtaining tissue for diagnosis, and evaluating for possible metastatic spread, laparoscopy can prevent unnecessary surgery in many of these patients.[41,42]

CONCLUSION

Intra-abdominal metastases can be detected by a variety of scanning techniques, including ultrasonography, CT, MRI, and radionuclide scintigraphy. The sensitivity of these techniques varies widely, depending on the site and, more critically, on the size of the tumor implant, with metastases <2 cm frequently being missed.[43,44] Laparoscopy has the capacity to detect and permit biopsy of lesions over a wide range of sizes and locations, including the typical 1 to 2 mm nodules that are seen in peritoneal seeding,[6,22,45] that cannot be detected by any means other than laparotomy. It does have the limitation of surveying only surfaces, and deep-seated tumor deposits in organs such as the liver or in the retroperitoneal tissues or lymph nodes are likely to be missed, even when large. However, it would be unusual to perform laparoscopy without a prior ultrasound or CT scan. The intention is not to use laparoscopy as a substitute for these procedures but rather to complement them.

In our opinion the role of laparoscopy in gastrointestinal cancers is to aid in the staging process with the purpose of applying different therapeutic options. If the goal is to explore all cancers to see what can be accomplished surgically and to do it, then there is clearly no need for laparoscopy. If, however, the goal is to avoid operations that will have no therapeutic benefit and to select nonoperative alternatives that may do as well, information pertinent to those considerations must be obtained before deciding to open the abdomen. Thus the legitimate purpose of laparoscopy is to make strategic planning more accurate and meaningful, and the actual value of the procedure will be directly proportional to the likelihood of finding liver or peritoneal metastases of the cancer in question.

The prevalence of peritoneal and liver implants in pancreatic cancer (36% to 73%) makes foreknowledge of their existence highly desirable, except in cases where duodenal obstruction will mandate surgery. In gastric cancer the prevalence of these implants seems to be equally high; however, until now, having this information preoperatively has not been as critical because palliative gastrectomy was required for many incurable patients. In the case of esophageal cancer the overall frequency of metastatic deposits is smaller (about 15%), and this, coupled with a lower incidence rate (approximately one third that of pancreatic cancer), questions the real benefit of practicing laparoscopy in this setting.

Laparoscopy for diagnosing gastrointestinal cancers is rare in the United States, compared to its use in other parts of the world. In this era of cost containment, laparoscopy can optimize resources by avoiding unnecessary operations and prolonged hospital stays.

REFERENCES

1. Reynolds TB, Cowan RE. Peritoneoscopy. In Wright R, Alberti KG, Karran S, et al, eds. Liver and Biliary Disease. Philadelphia: WB Saunders, 1979.
2. Cortesi N, Zambarda E, Manenti A, Gibertini G, Gotuzzo L, Malagoli M. Laparoscopy in routine and emergency surgery: Experience with 1720 cases. Am J Surg 137:647, 1979.
3. Veronesi U, Spinelli P, Bonadonna G, et al. Laparoscopy and laparotomy in staging Hodgkin's and non-Hodgkin's lymphoma. AJR 127:501, 1976.
4. Barth RA, Jeffrey RB Jr, Moss AA, et al. A comparison study of computed tomography and laparoscopy in the staging of abdominal neoplasms. Dig Dis Sci 26:253, 1981.
5. Warshaw AL, Tepper JE, Shipley WU. Laparoscopy in the staging and planning of therapy for pancreatic cancer. Am J Surg 151:76, 1986.
6. Warshaw AL, Zhuo-Yun Gu, Wittenberg J, et al. Preoperative staging and assessment of resectability of pancreatic cancer. Arch Surg 125:230, 1990.
7. National Cancer Institute. Cancer Statistics Review 1973-1987 (SEER Program). Bethesda, Md.: The Institute, 1990.
8. Crist DW, Sitzmann JV, Cameron JL. Improved hospital morbidity, mortality, and survival after the Whipple procedure. Ann Surg 206:358, 1987.

9. Tsuchiya R, Noda T, Harada N, et al. Collective review of small carcinomas of the pancreas. Ann Surg 203:77, 1986.
10. Gudjonsson B. Cancer of the pancreas: 50 years of surgery. Cancer 60:2284, 1987.
11. Warshaw AL, Swanson RS. Pancreatic cancer in 1988: Possibilities and probabilities. Ann Surg 208:541, 1988.
12. Meyer-Burg J. The inspection, palpation and biopsy for the pancreas. Endoscopy 4:99, 1972.
13. Ishida H. Peritoneoscopy and pancreas biopsies in the diagnosis of pancreatic diseases. Gastrointest Endosc 29:211, 1983.
14. Cuschieri A, Hall AW, Clark J. Value of laparoscopy in the diagnosis and management of pancreatic carcinoma. Gut 19:672, 1978.
15. Mintz M. Risks and prophylaxis in laparoscopy: A survey of 100,000 cases. J Reprod Med 18:269, 1977.
16. Cuschieri A. Laparoscopy for pancreatic cancer: Does it benefit the patient? Eur J Surg Oncol 14:41, 1988.
17. Ivanov S, Keranov S. Laparoscopic assessment of the operability of pancreatic cancer. Khirurgiia (Sofiia) 42:12, 1989.
18. Warshaw AL. Implications of peritoneal cytology for staging of early pancreatic cancer. Am J Surg (in press).
19. Weiss SM, Skibber JM, Mohiuddin M, et al. Rapid intra-abdominal spread of pancreatic cancer. Arch Surg 120:415, 1985.
20. Martin JK Jr, Goellner JR. Abdominal fluid cytology in patients with gastrointestinal malignant lesions. Mayo Clin Proc 61:467, 1986.
21. Chissov VI, Maksimov IA, Vinogradov AL, et al. Laparoscopy in the diagnosis of gastric carcinoma spread. Khirurgiia (Mosk) 11:13, 1981.
22. Possik RA, Franco EL, Pires DR, et al. Sensitivity, specificity, and predictive value of laparoscopy for the staging of gastric cancer and for the detection of liver metastases. Cancer 58:1, 1986.
23. Shandall A, Johnson C. Laparoscopy or scanning in oesophageal and gastric carcinoma? Br J Surg 72:449, 1985.
24. Gross E, Bancewicz J, Ingram G. Assessment of gastric cancer by laparoscopy. Br Med J 288:1577, 1984.
25. Boddie AW, McBride CM, Balch CM. Gastric cancer. Am J Surg 157:595, 1989.
26. Adam YG, Efron G. Trends and controversies in the management of carcinoma of the stomach. Surg Gynecol Obstet 169:371, 1989.
27. Fleischer D, Sivak MV Jr. Endoscopic Nd:YAG laser therapy as palliation for esophagogastric cancer. Gastroenterology 89:827, 1985.
28. Suzuki H, Miho O, Watanabe M, et al. Endoscopic laser therapy in the curative and palliative treatment of upper gastrointestinal cancer. West J Med 13:158, 1989.
29. Sotnikov VN, Ermolov AS, Litvinof VI. The diagnosis of intra-abdominal metastases of esophageal cancer by means of laparoscopy. Vopr Onkol 35, 1973.
30. Dagnini G, Caldironi W, Martin G, et al. Laparoscopy in abdominal staging of esophageal carcinoma. Gastrointest Endosc 32:400, 1986.
31. Earlam R, Cunha-Melo JR. Oesophagel squamous cell carcinoma. A critical review of surgery. Br J Surg 67:381, 1980.
32. Orringer MB, Forastiere AA, Perez-Tamayo C, et al. Chemotherapy and radiation therapy before transhiatal esophagectomy for esophageal carcinoma. Ann Thorac Surg 49:348, 1990.
33. Kelsen D. Neoadjuvant therapy of esophageal cancer. Can J Surg 32:410, 1989.
34. Boyce WH. Laparoscopy. In Schiff L, Schiff ER, eds. Diseases of the Liver, 6th ed. Philadelphia, JB Lippincott, 1987.
35. Vilardell F. The value of laparoscopy in the diagnosis of primary cancer of the liver. Endoscopy 9:20, 1977.
36. Etienne JP, Chaput JC, Feydy P, et al. La laparoscopie dans le cancer primitif du foie du l'adulte. Ann Gastroenterol Hepatol (Paris) 49:53, 1973.
37. Nakashima T, Okuda K, Kojiro M, et al. Pathology of hepatocellular carcinoma in Japan: 232 consecutive cases autopsied in 10 years. Cancer 51:867, 1983.
38. Okita K. Kodma T, Oda M, et al. Laparoscopic ultrasonography. Diagnosis of liver and pancreatic cancer. Scand J Gastroenterol (Suppl) 94:91, 1984.
39. Fornari F, Civardi G, Cavanna L, et al. Laparoscopic ultrasonography in the study of liver diseases. Preliminary results. Surg Endosc 3:33, 1989.

40. Orloff MJ, Robinson GT. Tumors of the gallbladder. In Berk JE, Haubrick WS, Kalser MH, et al., eds. Bockus Gastroenterology, 4th ed. vol. 6. Philadelphia: WB Saunders, 1985.

41. Bhargava DK, Sarin S, Verma K, et al. Laparoscopy in carcinoma of the gallbladder. Gastrointest Endosc 29:21, 1983.

42. De Dios-Vega JF, Hita-Pérez J, Muro-González J, et al. Valor de la laparoscopía en el diagnóstico del cáncer de vesícula biliar. Rev Esp Enferm Apar Dig 41:867, 1973.

43. Smith TJ, Kemeny MM, Sugarbaker PH, et al. A prospective study of hepatic imaging in the detection of metastatic disease. Ann Surg 195:486, 1982.

44. Wittenberg J, Ferruci JT Jr, Warshaw AL. Contribution of computed tomography to patients with pancreatic adenocarcinoma. World J Surg 8:831, 1984.

45. Warshaw AL, Zhuo-Yun Gu. Laparoscopy for preoperative staging of foregut malignancies: Esophageal, gastric and pancreatic cancer. In Donahue PE, ed. Problems in General Surgery. Surgical Endoscopy. Philadelphia: JB Lippincott (in press).

CHAPTER 7

Therapeutic Options for Gallstone Disease

Keith D. Lillemoe, M.D.
Henry A. Pitt, M.D.

The treatment of gallstones has undergone dramatic changes in the past 5 years. Until recently cholecystectomy was the only accepted and effective therapy for symptomatic cholelithiasis. As a result, over 500,000 cholecystectomies were performed annually in the late 1980s. The overall contribution of the treatment of gallstones to annual U.S. health care costs is over 85 billion dollars, which represents 2.5% of the country's total health care expenditure.[1] Disability during convalescence further increases the high costs of traditional cholecystectomy.

The cost and disability associated with open surgical cholecystectomy as well as technologic developments and a better understanding of the biochemistry of gallstone dissolution have led to the introduction of a number of new treatment options. These techniques include dissolution with oral bile acids, extracorporeal shock wave lithotripsy, and percutaneous dissolution or ablation of gallstones. These treatments all share the common feature of preserving the gallbladder as a site for future gallstone recurrence, thus limiting their long-term effectiveness. In response to these new treatments for gallstones, laparoscopic cholecystectomy was introduced to the surgical community. This procedure has the potential for reducing hospital stay and postoperative disability while eliminating the potential for gallstone recurrence. We will review the current status of these newer treatment options for gallstones and define the role of these modalities and laparoscopic cholecystectomy in patient management.

SYMPTOMATIC VS. ASYMPTOMATIC GALLSTONES

Gallstones are common in the western world. An estimated 20 million people in the United States (10% of the adult population) have gallstones, and 1 million new cases are diagnosed each year. Gallstones are more common in females; however, the prevalence increases with age in both sexes. With this high prevalence, many asymptomatic patients with gallstones will be detected incidentally. The role of cholecystectomy in patients with asymptomatic or "silent" gallstones has been debated for years. A similar debate now exists concerning the role of less invasive procedures. The issues of cost, risks or side effects, and long-term results must be compared with the risk of symptoms or complications from gallstones developing in asymptomatic patients.

The spectrum of symptoms associated with gallstones is quite varied. Biliary colic is the most significant symptom of cholelithiasis. The pain—a steady, severe pain in the epigastrium or right upper quadrant—is often triggered by ingestion of a large meal and lasts 30 minutes to a few hours. The pathogenesis of these symptoms is a gallstone lodged in the cystic duct and, if prolonged, may progress to acute cholecystitis. Repeated episodes of biliary colic may lead to chronic cholecystitis with fibrosis and scarring of the gallbladder.

A number of nonspecific symptoms can also be associated with gallstones. Many patients have a chronic history of vague abdominal discomfort and dyspepsia without pain. Patients may complain of increased flatulence, eructations, or perhaps heartburn. Finally, in some patients a complication will mark the initial presentation of gallstones. Acute cholecystitis is the initial mode of presentation in up to 20% of patients.[2] Less than 10% of patients will present with other complications such as common bile duct obstruction, with or without cholangitis, or gallstone pancreatitis.

The type of symptoms patients with gallstones experience has been analyzed with respect to their long-term relief. A recent study by Gilliland and Traverso[3] provides not only important information for predicting success following cholecystectomy and other nonsurgical techniques but also modern standards for comparison of techniques. Over 670 patients undergoing elective cholecystectomy between 1982 and 1987 were analyzed with respect to their symptoms (Table 7-1). Biliary colic was the primary symptom in 91% of the patients. Dyspepsia, fatty food intolerance, flatulence, and other nonspecific symptoms occurred in 5% of patients. Atypical pain in variable locations was present in 4% of patients. Long-term

Table 7-1. Relief of Symptoms in Patients Undergoing Elective Cholecystectomy*

Symptoms	Patients (%)	Long-Term Relief of Symptoms (%)
Biliary colic	91	88
Dyspepsia and nonspecific complaints	5	75†
Atypical pain	4	91

*Modified from Gilliland TM, Traverso W. Modern standards for comparison of cholecystectomy with alternative treatments for symptomatic cholelithiasis with emphasis on long-term relief of symptoms. Surg Gynecol Obstet 170:329-344, 1990. By permission.
†$p < 0.01$ vs. biliary colic and atypical pain.

follow-up (mean 45 months) showed that 88% of patients were free of symptoms following cholecystectomy. Patients with biliary colic or atypical pain were more likely to have symptoms relieved than patients with nonspecific symptoms. In all patients, regardless of their presenting complaint, dyspepsia was the most prominent residual symptom. The authors concluded that cholecystectomy is a definitive operation that is highly selective in long-term relief of symptoms, especially biliary colic.

There is little doubt that patients with symptomatic gallstones should undergo treatment. In a series from Sweden, 150 patients with symptomatic gallstones refused cholecystectomy. The incidence of patients requiring urgent operations for serious complications of biliary tract disease within 2 years in this group was 27%.[4] In a series reported by McSherry et al.[5] in New York, 267 patients with symptomatic gallstones did not undergo cholecystectomy. Follow-up (mean 83 months) revealed that symptoms intensified in 48% of patients, whereas only 1 patient became asymptomatic.

The role of cholecystectomy or nonsurgical treatment of asymptomatic gallstones is less clear. The predominant issue remains the potential development of symptoms or complications of gallstones. Multiple natural history studies have been reported with variable results. The most frequently quoted natural history study is that of Gracie and Ransohoff[6] in which 123 faculty members at the University of Michigan (110 men, 13 women) were found to have asymptomatic gallstones on a screening oral cholecystogram. Only 18% of these patients became symptomatic during the follow-up period of 15 years. Moreover, operative morbidity or mortality did not increase in those patients who eventually required cholecystectomy. The authors concluded that "prophylactic cholecystectomy" for silent gallstones was not advisable. This study has been criticized because the population was primarily white males and over one fourth of the group underwent prophylactic cholecystectomy an average of 2 to 3 years after stone detection.

Recently McSherry et al.[5] used information from a large health maintenance organization to follow 135 patients with asymptomatic gallstones for a mean of almost 5 years. Only 10% of this group of patients, who represented a cross section of middle income Americans, developed symptoms of cholelithiasis. Of the 14 patients developing symptoms, however, five patients had complications of either acute cholecystitis or choledocholithiasis. Only 7.4% of the total group underwent biliary tract surgery for symptoms with no operative mortality and minimal morbidity. The median time interval between diagnosis and operation was 25 months. During the same interval, 18.5% of the asymptomatic patients died of nonbiliary tract diseases.

Similar results in 139 patients with gallstones, found incidentally during abdominal ultrasound examination for other indications, were recently reported from Duke University.[7] Only 11% of patients developed biliary symptoms over a 5-year follow-up period. Nine patients underwent cholecystectomy; three of these operations were incidental to other abdominal procedures and two were emergency operations for complications of gallstones. These patients, however, were older, and suspected malignancy or vascular disease was the primary reason for ultrasound examination. This point is emphasized by the fact that 40% of the patients died during the follow-up period. These results would also support a conservative approach to the management of asymptomatic gallstones, especially in the elderly.

Although most series seem to support a conservative approach in patients with asymptomatic gallstones, questions persist regarding the management of patients who have coexisting conditions such as diabetes or those who require laparotomy for another indication. In patients with diabetes mellitus the need for emergency surgery for complications is associated with increased operative morbidity and mortality.[8-10] In the elective setting, however, diabetes does not increase the operative risk.[8,9,11] As a result, many surgeons support the use of cholecystectomy in patients with diabetes regardless of their symptoms. Similar recommendations have been made for patients who are about to undergo renal or cardiac transplantation. Prophylactic cholecystectomy prior to instituting immunosuppression may be of some value in these patients. Similarly, patients with asymptomatic stones who are undergoing a laparotomy for another indication may benefit from an "incidental" cholecystectomy. Recent studies have indicated that as many as 50% of patients with asymptomatic cholelithiasis undergoing aortic reconstructive surgery will develop biliary symptoms later.[12-14] Cholecystectomy in this setting does not increase operative risk.

In conclusion, nondiabetic patients with asymptomatic gallstones can often be managed expectantly without risk of increased complications or death from gallstone disease or biliary tract surgery. Issues such as overall costs and quality of life, however, have not been addressed in most of the studies to date. If a highly effective, low-cost therapy became available, then treatment of asymptomatic patients in younger age groups may prove beneficial. Of the available treatments, laparoscopic cholecystectomy may best fulfill these criteria. More data on the true risks of this procedure are needed, however, before this conclusion can be drawn.

ORAL DISSOLUTION

The idea of treating gallstones with orally administered bile acids was suggested over a century ago. It was not until reports appeared from the Mayo Clinic[15] in the early 1970s, however, that the modern era of medical dissolution was entered. The normal human bile acid chenodeoxycholic acid (CDCA) was the first drug demonstrated to effectively dissolve gallstones on a large scale. The mechanism of action of CDCA is a decrease in cholesterol saturation of bile through two steps. First, the administration of exogenous bile acids expands the circulating bile salt pool and thus decreases endogenous bile acid biosynthesis. In addition, and probably more important, CDCA inhibits the hepatic enzyme hydroxymethylglutaryl coenzyme A reductase, thus decreasing cholesterol secretion into bile. The resulting desaturated bile draws cholesterol molecules on the surface of the gallstone to the unsaturated micelles and therefore into solution. This mechanism clearly indicates that CDCA is only effective in patients with cholesterol gallstones.

Encouraging results led to the use of CDCA in a multicenter trial throughout the United States in the early 1980s. This National Cooperative Gallstone Study was a randomized, double-blind prospective trial assigning 916 patients to one of three treatment groups: (1) low-dose CDCA (375 mg/day), (2) high-dose CDCA (750 mg/day), or (3) placebo.[16] The results of this trial were disappointing. In only 8% of all the patients receiving CDCA did the gallstones dissolve over a 2-year period, and the rate of cholecystectomy remained the same. Patients in the high-dose CDCA group (Table 7-2) experienced better results, with complete dissolution in 14% of patients and partial dissolution in 27% of patients (defined as a >50% decrease in gallstone size). These results were significantly poorer than those reported in previously published nonrandomized trials. This disparity was most likely the result of poor patient compliance due to side effects and also inclusion of patients with pigment gallstones. The best results were seen in women below their ideal body weight, with stones <1.7 cm in size, and with normal serum cholesterol levels. Success in these patients, however, still only approached 40%.

In addition to the limited efficacy, side effects experienced by patients in the cooperative study were high.[16] Significant, but reversible, liver injury was observed in 3% of patients taking high-dose CDCA. Eight percent of the patients reported diarrhea. These side effects were dose dependent. The diarrhea is caused by a direct secretory effect on the colon, whereas the conversion of CDCA by enteric flora to lithocholic acid, a known hepatotoxin, results in liver injury. A final side effect observed with CDCA was increased serum cholesterol and low-density lipoprotein (LDL) levels.

The overall poor results and side effects associated with CDCA led to a search for other bile acids that could dissolve gallstones. In the mid-1970s reports from Japan suggested that ursodeoxycholic acid (UDCA), the predominant bile acid in the bear, could dissolve gallstones at a faster rate than CDCA and with fewer side effects. UDCA appears to work by a different

Table 7-2. Results of the National Cooperative Gallstone Study: Efficacy of CDCA*

Group	No. of Patients	Partial Dissolution (%)	Complete Dissolution (%)
Placebo	305	10	1
CDCA, 375 mg/day	306	18	5
CDCA, 750 mg/day	306	27	14

*Modified, with permission, from Schoenfield LJ, Lachin JM, the Steering Committee, the National Cooperative Gallstone Study Group. Chenodiol (chenodeoxycholic acid) for dissolution of gallstones: The National Cooperative Gallstone Study: A controlled trial of efficacy and safety. Ann Intern Med 95:257-282, 1981.

mechanism than CDCA. UDCA does not suppress either cholesterol or bile acid biosynthesis, but rather it decreases intestinal absorption of cholesterol. The different methods of action of CDCA and UDCA have provided the rationale for administration of both drugs in combination.

The results of numerous prospective randomized studies comparing the effects of UDCA and CDCA have been reported[17-19] (Table 7-3). In addition, comparisons of UDCA and CDCA are now available. The conclusion is that UDCA is associated with more rapid dissolution than CDCA at lower comparable dosages. However, CDCA has the ability to "catch up" in time, and eventually the dissolution rates are nearly equal. The side effects of CDCA, including hepatotoxicity, diarrhea, and increased cholesterol and LDL levels, however, continue to be seen only with CDCA at the higher doses.

Improved results with combined CDCA and UDCA have been ascribed to their different mechanisms of action. Combination therapy also provides cost savings without increased side effects.[20] The cost of oral bile acid therapy is an especially relevant issue. The yearly cost of UDCA therapy ranges from $1200 to $2200, depending on the dosage. CDCA is somewhat cheaper. This cost, in addition to the expense of follow-up physician visits, gallbladder imaging, and blood tests, must be included in cost analyses of oral dissolution in comparison to elective cholecystectomy.

Table 7-3. Comparison of the Efficacy of UDCA and CDCA in Gallstone Dissolution

Study	Drug	Dose	No. of Patients	Success Rate* (%)
Barbera et al.[17]	UDCA	5 mg/kg/day	34	88
	UDCA	10 mg/kg/day	36	81
	CDCA	7 mg/kg/day	70	51
	CDCA	15 mg/kg/day	71	79
Bateson, Hill, and Bouchier[18]	UDCA	500 mg/day	13	38
	UDCA	1000 mg/day	24	42
	CDCA	750 mg/day	41	22
	CDCA	1000 mg/day	33	58
Fromm et al.[19]	UDCA	7-8 mg/kg/day	58	72
	UDCA	14-15 mg/kg/day	52	78
	CDCA	7-8 mg/kg/day	55	57
	CDCA	14-15 mg/kg/day	58	78

*Combined complete and partial dissolution.

The most significant drawback with respect to oral dissolution is the recurrence of gallstones. Numerous studies have documented a 10% recurrence per year in the 5 years after cessation of oral bile acid therapy with either CDCA or UDCA.[21-24] In many cases, however, recurrent stones are asymptomatic. Fortunately, reinstitution of oral bile acid therapy successfully manages recurrent stones in most series. Low-dose maintenance therapy has been suggested as a possible solution to the problem of recurrent stones. A recent report from Italy has shown that low-dose UDCA significantly reduces the frequency of gallstone recurrence.[24] This effect, however, was limited to younger patients. In patients older than 50 years no beneficial effect was noted with maintenance therapy.

In summary, oral dissolution with bile acids—primarily UDCA or combined UDCA and CDCA—can be used successfully to treat gallstones. The rate of success can be maximized by patient selection. The ideal patient has multiple, small floating gallstones that are radiolucent on an abdominal radiograph and is not obese (i.e., weight > 140% ideal body weight). Furthermore, gallbladder function should be documented on an oral cholecystogram. Unfortunately only a small number of patients with gallstones fit these criteria. When such criteria were applied to the patient population at the Johns Hopkins Hospital, only 20% of the patients with symptomatic gallstones were considered good candidates.[25]

ELIGIBILITY FOR NONOPERATIVE THERAPY

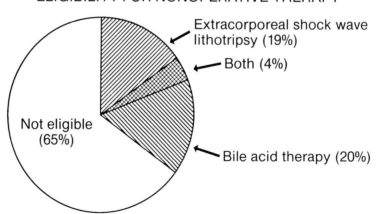

From Magnuson TH, Lillemoe KD, Pitt HA. How many Americans will be eligible for biliary lithotripsy? Arch Surg 124:1195-1200, 1989. Copyright 1989, American Medical Association.

A recommendation for oral dissolution thus should be made only in those patients meeting these favorable criteria who are increased surgical risks or have an overwhelming preference for nonsurgical therapy. If oral bile acid dissolution is elected, patients must expect a gradual recurrence of stones with the likelihood of lifelong therapy and increased costs.

EXTRACORPOREAL SHOCK WAVE LITHOTRIPSY

Extracorporeal shock wave lithotripsy (ESWL) for the treatment of gall-stones is a direct extension of the principles and techniques used in the treatment of kidney stones. Recognition of the destructive effect of shock waves stemmed from an investigation by the Dornier Corporation of Germany of the causes of pitting on the outer shell of its spacecraft and supersonic airplanes. Studies revealed that when aircrafts flying at high speeds collided with raindrops, shock waves were produced that created stresses within the material structure of the aircraft. Dornier researchers subsequently recognized that shock waves could exert a destructive effect on brittle solids but yet would pass harmlessly through organic tissue. Soon the ability to focus the shock wave to a fixed point led to in vitro experiments on the fragmentations of kidney stones. In 1980 the world's first kidney stone lithotripsy was performed. The tremendous success of urolithiasis has led to its extension to the treatment of gallstones.

Shock waves are high-intensity sound waves created when the velocity of a pressure front exceeds the speed of sound. All lithotriptors generate shock waves under water and focus the waves at a distance from the generator using a semielliptical reflector. Shock waves are initiated by four basic generating devices: (1) spark gap, (2) electromagnetic, (3) piezoelectric, and (4) microexplosive (Table 7-4). Shock waves can propagate through living tissue because of its high water content. However, the body must be adequately coupled to the lithotriptor, which requires the patient to be in contact with the water medium as the shock wave propagates. Direct contact with the water medium may be accomplished by placing the patient directly into a water bath or having the patient lie on a flexible

Table 7-4. Lithotriptor Models Available for Gallstone ESWL

Shock Wave Generator	Manufacturer	Imaging
Spark gap	Dornier	Ultrasound
	Medstone	Ultrasound + fluoroscopy
	Technomed	Ultrasound
	Northgate	Ultrasound
	Direx	Ultrasound + fluoroscopy
Piezoelectric	Wolf	Ultrasound
	EDAP	Ultrasound
	Diasonics	Ultrasound + fluoroscopy
	Storz	Ultrasound + fluoroscopy
Electromagnetic	Siemens	Ultrasound + fluoroscopy

membrane, which in turn is in contact with the water medium. Either ultrasonography or fluoroscopy can be used to visualize the gallstone for focusing the shock waves. However, since most gallstones are radiolucent, ultrasonography is the preferred method.

Gallstone disintegration is believed to result from collapse of cavitation bubbles in bile surrounding the gallstone when the pulse is generated. The energy required for fragmentation is proportional to the stone mass, with stone composition being less important. Thus shock wave lithotripsy can just as easily fragment calcified pigment gallstones as cholesterol stones, a principle easily predicted in that most kidney stones successfully treated are also calcified. To facilitate the dissolution of these stone fragments, litholitic therapy with oral bile acids is recommended.

The first report of gallstone lithotripsy described the experience with patients at the Klinikum Grosshardern in Munich, Federal Republic of Germany, using the Dornier spark-gap lithotriptor.[26] Since that initial report, numerous analyses have appeared in which all the various models of shock wave generators were used.[27-31] The Munich experience remains one of the largest and most successful. The most recent update of their experience is a follow-up of the first 175 patients.[27] All patients received oral bile acid therapy with a combination of CDCA and UDCA beginning 12 days before treatment and continuing for 3 months after stone disappearance. Fragmentation was achieved in all patients. Follow-up ultrasound examination revealed that 63% of patients were stone free at 4 to 8 months, 78% were stone free at 12 months, and 91% were stone free at 12 to 18 months (Table 7-5). Retreatment was necessary in 5.1% of patients. Results were significantly better in patients with solitary stones <20 mm in maximal diameter. Similar results have been reported in numerous other centers with all forms of shock wave generators (Table 7-6).

In the early series, ESWL treatments were performed under general anesthesia. However, experience has now shown that most patients tolerate the procedure well with intravenous analgesics alone. No analgesia is required using some models of lithotriptor (piezoelectric). In almost all series, outpatient treatment is routine, especially when general anesthesia is avoided.

Side effects of gallstone ESWL are generally minor, and significant complications are rare (Table 7-7).[27-31] Biliary colic occurs in one fourth to one third of patients after ESWL with the passage of stone fragments. Symptoms may occur for up to 1 year after the initial treatment. Transient microhematuria is observed in 10% to 20% of patients, but gross hematuria is seen in less than 5%. Cutaneous petechiae occur in about 15% of patients. Gallstone pancreatitis occurs in 1% to 3% of patients but usually can be managed conservatively. Acute cholecystitis due to cystic duct obstruction is seen in 1% to 2% of patients, but cholecystectomy generally is required in only 1% of cases. Deaths have been reported after ESWL, but few can be directly related to the lithotripsy procedure.

Table 7-5. Stone Clearance Following ESWL*

Follow-Up (mo)	Solitary Gallstone (%)	Two or Three Gallstones (%)	All Patients (90)
0-2	34	12	30
2-4	54	17	48
4-8	68	29	63
8-12	84	40	78
12-18	96	67	91
18-24	100	75	93

*Modified from Sackmann M, Delius M, Sauerbruch T, Holl J, Weber W, Ippisch E, Hagelauer U, Wess O, Hepp W, Brendel W, Paumgartner G. Shock-wave lithotripsy of gallbladder stones: The first 175 patients. N Engl J Med 318:393-397, 1988. Reprinted by permission.

Table 7-6. Results of ESWL for Gallstones

Machine	Type	No. of Patients	Oral Bile Acids	Retreatment (%)	Fragmentation (%)	Stone Free (%)	Follow-Up (mo)
Dornier[27]	Spark gap	173	CDCA & UDCA	5	100	63	4-8
						91	12-18
Medstone[28]	Spark gap	223	UDCA	13	95	51	6
Lithostar[29]	Electromagnetic	126	None	39	98	29	5
Pizolith[30]	Piezoelectric	75	CDCA & UDCA	50	98	53	4-6
Technomed[31]	Spark gap	135	CDCA & UDCA	46	76	63	12

Table 7-7. Complications of Gallstone ESWL

Machine	Biliary Colic (%)	Hematuria (%)	Pancreatitis (%)	Cholecystitis (%)
Dornier[27]	35	3	1	1
Medstone[28]	58	8	1	3
Lithostar[29]	—	3	1	7
Pizolith[30]	32	11	1	0
Technomed[31]	23	3	1	6

The key to successful treatment of gallstones with ESWL lies in proper selection of patients. Selection criteria for the treatment of gallstones with ESWL have generally been derived from the initial experience in West Germany. These criteria were based on theoretical considerations and have already been modified in many series with possible expansion of inclusion criteria as clinical data accumulate.

INCLUSION AND EXCLUSION CRITERIA
FOR GALLSTONE ESWL

Inclusion Criteria

Symptomatic gallstones
Functioning (visualized) gallbladder on oral cholecystogram or radionuclide
  study
Three gallstones or less with diameters no greater than 30 mm
Noncalcified gallstones (except rim or nidus <3 mm)
No cysts, aneurysms, or lung in the shock wave path
Ability to localize gallstone by ultrasonography

Exclusion Criteria

History of acute cholecystitis, cholangitis, pancreatitis, or bile duct obstruction
Known choledocholithiasis
Coagulopathy or anticoagulant therapy
Pregnancy
Allergy to radiographic contrast media
Active liver disease
Presence of a pacemaker or significant arrhythmia

The initial criteria for patient selection is symptomatic gallstones, preferably with a history of biliary colic. To date, the treatment has not been recommended for patients with asymptomatic gallstones. The stone must also be visualized on ultrasound examination. Although absolute size and number of stones vary among protocols, patients generally have four stones or less with stone sizes of between 5 and 30 mm. For stone fragments to pass out of the gallbladder, a patent cystic duct must be demonstrated by either oral cholecystography or nuclear scintigraphic scanning. Heavily calcified or pigment stones are excluded with radiolucent stones, whereas those with only a minimal rim of calcification are accepted. A number of absolute exclusion criteria have also been well defined.

These rigid criteria clearly limit the usefulness of ESWL for gallstone treatment. When accepted inclusion and exclusion criteria were applied to 100 consecutive patients undergoing cholecystectomy at the Johns Hopkins

Hospital, only 19% of patients were considered candidates for ESWL[25] (see p. 122). Moreover, if selection is based on those patients with the best chance of success (solitary stone <20 mm in diameter), only 12% of patients would be expected to be eligible for ESWL.

The exclusion of patients with calcified stones has been primarily based on failure of these stones to respond to adjuvant oral bile acid therapy. A prospective trial of ESWL in patients with calcified stones is now in progress. A recent progress report has been published concerning 38 patients with calcified stones who have been treated thus far.[32] However, in only 60% of these patients was fragmentation successful (all fragments <3 mm) despite an average of four treatment sessions and the administration of over 13,400 shock waves. Of the 18 patients with fragments <3 mm, only 3 were stone free after adequate follow-up (18 weeks). Comparison with patients with cholesterol stones treated at the same center showed that patients with calcified stones (1) required 50% more shock waves for fragmentation, (2) cleared fragments more slowly, and (3) had a higher frequency of acute pancreatitis (5% vs. 2%) and transient hematuria (8% vs. 3%).

The role of adjuvant oral bile acid therapy has recently been addressed by a prospective multicenter trial in the United States.[33] The Dornier spark-gap lithotriptor was used to treat 600 randomized patients. UDCA (10 mg/kg/day) was given to 49.3% of the patients, with the remainder receiving placebo. Follow-up data are available at 6 months for 511 patients, but data were reported for all 600 patients who entered the study with an intent to treat (Table 7-8). In this study, fragmentation was achieved in 95% of patients. Among all 600 patients, only 14.8% were stone free at 6 months.

Table 7-8. Results of Dornier National Biliary Lithotripsy Study*

| Group | Success at 6 Months | |
	All Patients (%)	Solitary Stone <20 mm (%)
UDCA	20.6†	35‡
Placebo	9.2	18

*Modified from Schoenfield LJ and the investigators of the Dornier National Biliary Lithotripsy Study. The role of bile acids in extracorporeal shock wave lithotripsy of gallbladder stones. Gastroenterology 98:392-396, 1990.
†$p < 0.0001$ vs. placebo.
‡$p < 0.01$ vs. placebo.

The treatment success for UDCA was 20.6% vs. only 9.2% for the placebo group ($p < 0.001$). The best results were again seen in patients with noncalcified solitary stones <20 mm in diameter who received UDCA (a stone-free rate of 35%).

The results of this study appear to be worse than previous reports using the Dornier model. Three factors have been cited to explain this discrepancy. First, the total stone volume was greater in the U.S. series in that up to three stones, each with a diameter of up to 30 mm, may have been included. Second, the U.S. series employed that Dornier MPL-9000 lithotriptor as opposed to earlier reports from Munich in which a prototype model requiring a water bath and general anesthesia was used. The energy provided by the two units is not directly comparable, and it is likely that less energy was delivered to the gallstones in the U.S. series. Finally, a combination of CDCA and UDCA was given in the Munich series. As discussed earlier, combination therapy appears to improve gallstone dissolution.

Side effects in the U.S. series were also greater than those from the previous Dornier reports. At least one episode of biliary colic was reported in 73% of patients. Abdominal wall tenderness was a complaint in 46% and transient hematuria in 42%. The incidence of acute pancreatitis (1.5%) was comparable to other reports, but 2.3% of patients in the U.S. series required cholecystectomy within the 6-month follow-up period for either intractable biliary colic or other complications of gallstone disease. Patients receiving UDCA also had a slightly higher incidence of diarrhea than patients receiving placebo (33% vs. 25%, $p < 0.04$).

This study strongly suggests that oral bile acid therapy is crucial for the success of ESWL. The explanation for this finding is the known action of bile acids on the surface of existing gallstones. Fragmentation of gallstone increases the surface area and thus increases the success of stone dissolution. This study also provides an explanation for the lack of success observed with calcified and noncholesterol gallstones. Clearly, fragmentation without dissolution leads to ineffective stone clearance.

The similarity between ESWL and oral bile acid therapy alone is the potential for stone recurrence. Both techniques, of course, leave the gallbladder in situ with the potential risk for recurrent gallstones. Numerous reports have documented that the gallstone recurrence rate after successful oral bile acid dissolution is approximately 10% per year.[21-24] Initial reports of gallstone recurrence following ESWL are now also appearing and seem to be similar. In the Munich experience 58 of the first 60 patients became stone free after ESWL and were followed up for 1 year after discontinuing adjuvant oral bile acid therapy.[34] The rate of gallstone recurrence was 9% within 1 year but only 15% at 2 years. In contrast to stone recurrence after oral dissolution, five of six patients had biliary colic. Recurrent stones were successfully managed with the administration of bile acids in four of the six patients. Repeat ESWL has not yet been necessary.

The clinical experience with ESWL suggests that this technique is safe and well tolerated. Patients do not require general anesthesia and are treated on an outpatient basis, thus minimizing hospital costs and immediate procedure-related risks. Biliary colic is a common symptom after treatment, but severe adverse complications such as cholecystitis and pancreatitis are uncommon.

The role of ESWL is limited by the number of patients in which excellent results can be expected and the potential for gallstone recurrence with the necessity of reinstitution of oral bile acid therapy or possible repeat ESWL. These possibilities limit the cost effectiveness of ESWL despite its apparent early advantages when compared to traditional cholecystectomy. Using a computer model, Bass et al.[35] at Johns Hopkins have analyzed mortality projections, quality of life, and cost effectiveness of ESWL vs. cholecystectomy in the treatment of symptomatic gallstones. Their estimates suggest minimal differences in mortality projections or quality of life for all patients, regardless of sex, age, or stone characteristics. However, cost projections suggest that at 5-year follow-up the average cumulative charge for ESWL treatment will exceed that for surgical treatment by over $1700 for a 45-year-old woman with the most favorable ESWL criteria (single stone <2 cm). Moreover, in a 45-year-old woman with two or three stones (a less favorable patient with respect to ESWL results), cumulative charges for lithotripsy at 5 years would exceed surgical charges by almost $3000. One must note that these figures were based on cost figures for traditional cholecystectomy, including several days of hospitalization. Certainly outpatient or single-day hospitalization following laparoscopic cholecystectomy would provide an even greater cost advantage for cholecystectomy. These results as well as the limited proportion of gallstone patients who are good candidates for ESWL would appear to limit the widespread usefulness of this procedure.

PERCUTANEOUS DISSOLUTION AND GALLSTONE ABLATION

Advancements in the field of invasive biliary radiology over the past decade have opened an entirely new arena of gallstone treatment. Recognition that the gallbladder can be easily and safely cannulated has paved the way for installation of contact solvents or actual mechanical ablation of gallstones with extraction of fragments. Present experience with these techniques is limited, and long-term follow-up is not available.

The continuing interest in gallstone dissolution by the Mayo Clinic led to the discovery that the gasoline additive methyl-*tert*-butyl ether (MTBE) rapidly dissolved cholesterol gallstones in vitro.[36] MTBE, which is liquid at body temperature, was subsequently demonstrated to dissolve human gallstones implanted in a canine gallbladder using percutaneous transhepatic gallbladder catheterization.[37]

Collaboration with interventional radiologists has culminated in a simple, rapid technique of transhepatically placing a pigtail catheter into a patient's gallbladder.

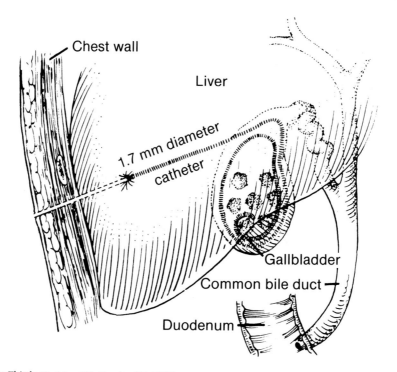

Chest wall

Liver

1.7 mm diameter catheter

Gallbladder

Common bile duct

Duodenum

From Thistle JL, May GR, Bender CE, Williams HJ, LeRoy AJ, Nelson PE, Peins CJ, Petersen BT, McCullough JE. Dissolution of cholesterol gallbladder stones by methyl *tert*-butyl ether administered by percutaneous transhepatic catheter. N Engl J Med 320:633-638, 1989. Reprinted by permission.

Gallstone dissolution occurs within hours of MTBE infusion into the gallbladder. MTBE, however, must be extracted to avoid excessive overflow of the solvent from the gallbladder. To accomplish this, the Mayo Clinic group has developed an oscillating pump that transfers a defined volume into and out of the gallbladder. This volume is chosen based on the volume of contrast material required to fill the gallbladder on initial fluoroscopic examination. Further technical advancements have made it possible to monitor intraluminal gallbladder pressure.[38] A miniprocessor then controls the solvent infusion rate to keep the intraluminal pressure below the "escape pressure."

The largest group of patients treated with MTBE was reported in 1989 by Thistle et al.[39] at the Mayo Clinic. Of 75 patients with symptomatic cholesterol gallstones treated, 72 had complete (or ≥95%) dissolution of all stones. Twenty-one patients were clear of stones immediately after treatment. Of the remaining 51 with residual debris, 15 were stone free at 6 to 35 months of follow-up, and only seven patients have had persistent symptoms. Only 6 of the 75 patients have undergone cholecystectomy during a 6- to 42-month follow-up. Similar results have also been reported at a number of other centers.[38,40,41]

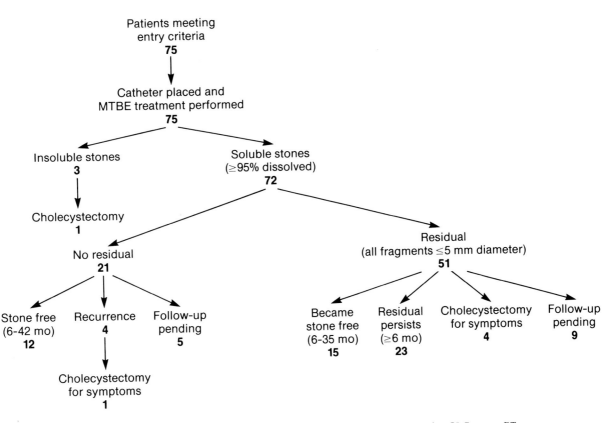

From Thistle JL, May GR, Bender CE, Williams HJ, LeRoy AJ, Nelson PE, Peins CJ, Petersen BT, McCullough JE. Dissolution of cholesterol gallbladder stones by methyl *tert*-butyl ether administered by percutaneous transhepatic catheter. N Engl J Med 320:633-638, 1989. Reprinted by permission.

As with ESWL and oral dissolution, patients undergoing MTBE treatment must meet certain inclusion criteria. Patency of the cystic duct must be confirmed on an oral cholecystogram. At the Mayo Clinic CT was used to detect gallstone calcification.[39] Significant calcification will decrease the efficacy of MTBE since it is purely a cholesterol solvent. Obvious exclusion criteria include coagulopathy, pregnancy, and common bile duct obstruction. The number and size of cholesterol stones do not affect eligibility; however, the added stone burden lengthens the time necessary for dissolution to occur.

The total treatment time for all patients averaged 12.5 hours (range 3.8 to 30.8 hours). Two or three sessions of several hours each were usually required. Patients were fasted prior to the sessions but were given low-fat meals on the evenings of treatment. In the initial series, UDCA was given for 6 to 12 months to aid in fragment clearance. Currently a randomized trial addressing the role of UDCA is under way.

Most patients received parenteral analgesics on the day of the initial procedure. Twenty-three of 75 patients experienced nausea with or without vomiting. An overflow of MTBE can be associated with mild transient sedation and can often be detected by the presence of MTBE on the patient's breath. Other potential risks include those related to gallbladder puncture and the effect of MTBE if accidentally infused into the hepatic parenchyma, intravascularly, or with excessive overflow into the duodenum. Although not harmful to the gallbladder mucosa, hemorrhagic ulcerative duodenitis can occur with overflow from the gallbladder. Long-term follow-up is available following successful MTBE therapy in 21 patients cleared of all stone debris. In 4 of these 21 patients, stones had recurred at 6- to 16-month follow-up. One patient eventually had a cholecystectomy. Thus a recurrent stone rate similar to that documented after successful oral dissolution can be expected.

The role of MTBE in the overall management of gallstone disease is likely to be limited. Although the technique is applicable to most patients with cholesterol gallstones regardless of stone size or number, expertise and diligence in treatment are necessary to avoid complications. Thus it is likely that gallstone dissolution with MTBE will remain limited to specialized centers dedicated to the technique. Moreover, when compared to laparoscopic cholecystectomy, MTBE therapy is unlikely to be cost effective. The major advantage of MTBE is the avoidance of general anesthesia, which makes it efficacious for extremely high-risk patients.

Ablation or extraction of gallstones is a similar technique in which percutaneous gallbladder cannulation is required, but experience is also quite limited. Several methods have been reported for fragmentation of gallstones, including mechanical fragmentation, electrohydraulic lithotripsy, and laser fragmentation.[42-44] Small stones and fragments are then removed with radiologic baskets. However, these procedures are complex and technically demanding, which makes for a steep learning curve.

A recent report from the University of Pennsylvania is typical of this early experience.[42] Percutaneous cholecystolithotomy was performed in 20 consecutive patients. The procedures were performed with intravenous sedation and epidural anesthesia. The gallbladder was punctured directly (not transhepatically), aspirated with a small needle, and a short 5 Fr catheter was inserted over a guidewire. An anchoring device provided traction to fix the gallbladder against the abdominal wall to prevent bile leakage. A second cholecystostomy tract was then erected with the same technique. This tract was then dilated with 14 to 24 Fr catheters for insertion of a cholecystostomy cannula. Small stones were flushed out with saline irrigation, medium-size stones were removed with a basket, and large stones were fragmented with a catheter electrohydraulic lithotriptor. Gallbladder endoscopy was then performed to check for and remove remaining fragments. A second session on the next day was necessary in one third of the patients. The sessions varied between 1 and 2 hours.

After stone extraction the patients were observed for 24 hours. The cholecystostomy cannula was exchanged for a Foley or similar catheter, which was left in place for external drainage. After 4 to 5 days the catheter was closed. Cholecystography and final gallbladder endoscopy were repeated before removal of the final catheter 4 to 6 weeks after the initial procedure.

Of the 20 patients treated, 17 had successful stone extraction of all gallstones during a 3- to 5-day hospital stay. Both pigment and cholesterol stones were successfully managed. The three patients who were treatment failures all had cholecystectomies. Complications, mostly minor, occurred in eight patients. Furthermore, of the 17 patients thought to be free of fragments after the procedure, residual stones were found in three patients on follow-up ultrasonography. The remaining patients were stone free at a follow-up period of 1 year or less.

This technique appears to be another effective nonsurgical alternative for the treatment of gallstones. It represents the only nonoperative alternative for pigment or calcified stones and is not limited by stone size or number. The major advantage over cholecystectomy is avoidance of general anesthesia. However, epidural anesthesia may have definite risks.

Several disadvantages of the technique are again obvious. First, no method is presently available to reliably ablate the gallbladder mucosa or cystic duct; thus the potential for gallstone recurrence still remains.[45] Second, the length of hospital stay and most likely total hospital and professional charges exceed that of laparoscopic cholecystectomy and perhaps even traditional cholecystectomy. The patients are further inconvenienced by an externally draining cholecystostomy tube for 4 to 6 weeks. Finally, as with the use of MTBE, the technical skill and expertise required for this procedure will probably limit its widespread use.

A final method of gallstone treatment that employs similar principles is endoscopic removal of gallbladder stones. This technique, which is still in the developmental stage, involves the introduction of a "daughter scope" into the common bile duct after routine endoscopic retrograde cholangiography and sphincterotomy. The daughter scope is then advanced through the cystic duct directly into the gallbladder for stone extraction or dissolution. Although no large series of patients have been reported, this technique seems unlikely to offer any advantage over percutaneous techniques.

TRADITIONAL CHOLECYSTECTOMY

The first cholecystectomy was performed more than 100 years ago. Over the last century tremendous progress has been made in the surgical treatment of calculous biliary tract disease. Traditional cholecystectomy is the gold standard by which the numerous new nonoperative techniques for gallstone management as well as laparoscopic cholecystectomy must be compared.

A number of factors must be considered when comparing the multitude of options for treatment of gallstones. First, and most important, is procedure-related mortality and morbidity. Second, the overall efficacy of the technique must be considered. Third, cost considerations, both short- and long-term, are becoming increasingly important factors in health care. Finally, factors such as patient inconvenience, disability, and quality of life are also extremely important.

Published data with respect to the safety of cholecystectomy are abundant. One of the largest series reported in this country was from the New York Hospital; over 14,200 patients were operated on for nonmalignant biliary tract disease from 1932 to 1984.[46] Cholecystectomy alone was performed in 10,749 patients with an operative mortality over the entire period of 0.6%. This series includes patients with both acute and chronic cholecystitis. The operative mortality for chronic cholecystitis, which would include most patients considered for nonsurgical techniques, was 0.4% in almost 9000 patients. Cholecystectomy for acute cholecystitis increased operative mortality to 1.2%. In the time period from 1978 to 1984, however, the operative mortality was only 0.2%. The most frequent cause of death was cardiovascular complications followed by disorders of the hepatobiliary system. Cirrhosis contributed to the majority of these deaths. Extrahepatic, intra-abdominal, pulmonary, and renal problems and infection were less frequent causes of death.

Evidence supporting the low operative mortality for traditional cholecystectomy is available from numerous other sources[3,47-51] (Table 7-9). Moreover, two series with a combined total of 1451 patients undergoing elective cholecystectomy have recently been published that report no mortality.[3,51] Critics of cholecystectomy point to increased operative mortality in elderly patients with coexisting medical conditions. Indeed, in an earlier report from the New York Hospital the operative mortality did increase with increasing age.[52] Operative mortality was 0.3% in patients under 50 years of age, 1.6% between the ages of 50 and 64 years, and 4.9% over age 65 years. However, these figures include all biliary tract operations for benign disease. If one looks only at those patients over age 50 undergoing operation for chronic cholecystitis, the operative mortality was only 0.9%. Death was most commonly due to cardiovascular complications in this age group.

Operative morbidity is also quite low following cholecystectomy. In a number of elective cholecystectomy series the morbidity has been less than 5%.[3,49-51] Complications following cholecystectomy can be either medical, anesthetic related, or procedure related. In the recent report by Gilli-

Table 7-9. Operative Mortality Following Traditional Cholecystectomy

Author	Year	Number	Operative Mortality (%)
Meyer, Capos, and Mihlepunkt[47]	1967	680	0.7
DeMarco, Nance, and Cohn[48]	1968	394	0.8
Gallbladder Survey Committee[49]	1970	28,621	1.5
Pickelman and Gonzalez[50]	1986	269	0.4
Ganey et al.[51]	1986	801	0.0
McSherry[46]	1989	10,749	0.6
Gilliland and Traverso[3]	1990	650	0.0

land and Traverso[3] total morbidity was 4.5%, whereas procedure-related morbidity was 2.2%. One might expect that procedure-related morbidity would be similar regardless of age, whereas anesthetic and other medical complications might be increased in older patients. The most feared procedure-related morbidity is a bile duct injury resulting in a biliary fistula or stricture. Numerous series have documented the current incidence of bile duct injury to be one case per 500 to 1000 cholecystectomies.[53-55]

The efficacy of cholecystectomy has been difficult to determine. Clearly, when compared to nonoperative techniques, cholecystectomy offers the advantage of removing the gallbladder and thus eliminating the chance of recurrent gallbladder stones. Yet some patients frequently do have persistent symptoms following cholecystectomy. In many cases persistent symptoms are found not to be related to gallstones at all but attributable to some other cause. Most patients with gallstones present with biliary colic. Biliary colic in its classic form is seldom due to causes other than gallstones. As reported by Gilliland and Traverso,[3] 88% of patients presenting with biliary colic were free of all symptoms at the time of long-term follow-up. Dyspepsia, flatulence, fatty food intolerance, or indigestion are nonspecific symptoms that may be indicative of a number of upper gastrointestinal disorders. Cholecystectomy relieved symptoms in 75% of patients who presented with these complaints. Thus an effort should be made to rule out other conditions before cholecystectomy is performed. Dyspepsia was the most common symptom following cholecystectomy regardless of the presenting complaint.

The postcholecystectomy syndrome is a generic term used frequently by critics of cholecystectomy for any and all complaints of patients who have had this procedure. However, this term should be reserved only for those patients experiencing severe episodes of upper abdominal pain similar to those preceding cholecystectomy. The incidence of this syndrome may be as high as 5% and can be attributable to a number of specific causes:
1. Common duct stones
2. Cystic duct remnant
3. Retained gallbladder
4. Bile duct stricture
5. Sphincter of Oddi stenosis
6. Sphincter of Oddi dysfunction

Stenosing papillitis and biliary dyskinesia are two potential causes of postcholecystectomy pain that remain controversial. These diagnoses can be established with manometric measurements of the sphincter of Oddi with treatment directed at lowering sphincter pressure. Endoscopic sphincterotomy has been recommended to treat many of the conditions causing the postcholecystectomy syndrome. However, a relatively high incidence of failure in some series has made many experts skeptical of the diagnosis.

Cost considerations are a major driving force behind the introduction of nonsurgical approaches to the treatment of gallstones. Outpatient measures such as oral bile acid therapy or ESWL have a markedly reduced "upfront" cost as compared to cholecystectomy. Yet, when long-term costs of oral bile acid therapy for the initial course of up to 2 years plus the treatment of recurrent stones is considered, the differences are less impressive. Add to that the cost of lifelong follow-up with physician visits, ultrasound examinations, and laboratory testing, the upfront cost for most patients undergoing elective cholecystectomy seems small. Although no randomized or comparative studies exist, a computer model comparing ESWL and surgery would favor cholecystectomy for most patients.[35]

In recent years the costs of cholecystectomy have been reduced significantly. Most patients are now admitted on the day of surgery and discharged on the second or third postoperative day. Laparoscopic cholecystectomy as an outpatient or a single overnight procedure will obviously further reduce these costs. Finally, the issues of patient inconvenience, disability, and quality of life must be considered. A traditional cholecystectomy, regardless of the type or length of the incision, is painful. Regional blocks may help in some cases for a few hours, but most patients need postoperative analgesics. Elimination of the routine use of nasogastric tubes and wound drains has led to some alleviation of postoperative discomfort. Disability following cholecystectomy is impossible to predict and clearly is based on the individual patient's motivation, pain threshold, type of work, and the desire to return to normal life. However, postoperative disability following traditional cholecystectomy obviously is greater than for most nonoperative techniques.

The final issue is quality of life and has not been addressed for cholecystectomy alone or in comparison to nonoperative techniques. How does one compare general anesthesia, a laparotomy, a 3-day hospital stay, and 3 weeks off work to taking pills twice a day for the rest of one's life or undergoing repeated ESWL or the various percutaneous therapies? This issue was again addressed in the Johns Hopkins computer model comparing ESWL and cholecystectomy.[35] In this report ESWL was favored over cholecystectomy only in patients with a single stone (best treated by ESWL). However, in young patients with multiple stones (higher failure and recurrence rates), the quality of life was actually judged to be better with traditional cholecystectomy.

LAPAROSCOPIC CHOLECYSTECTOMY

A similar stepwise comparison of laparoscopic cholecystectomy must be made with traditional cholecystectomy and nonoperative techniques. At present only scattered reports of the results of laparoscopic cholecystectomy are available from pioneers in the field. Although these reports suggest that operative morbidity and mortality are low and comparable to traditional cholecystectomy, more time will be necessary to determine whether these same results can be obtained by general surgeons throughout the world.

If comparisons of morbidity and mortality are excluded because of lack of data, laparoscopic cholecystectomy would appear to be the ideal procedure. It provides all of the advantages of cholecystectomy (relief of symptoms and removal of the gallbladder) with the advantages of nonoperative techniques (minimal pain and disability, low cost, outpatient or short hospital stay, and patient acceptance). Despite these potential advantages, the success of laparoscopic cholecystectomy will be judged ultimately by its postoperative morbidity and mortality.

In theory, the operative mortality of laparoscopic cholecystectomy should be the same as that for traditional cholecystectomy. Although the mortality rate is presently very low (Table 7-9), a small number of patients will continue to have perioperative cardiovascular problems and pulmonary emboli that preclude a zero mortality rate. Other potential problems such as bowel perforation at cannula insertion, the incidence of bile duct injury, and the long-term fate of retained intraperitoneal gallstones may affect the eventual role of laparoscopic cholecystectomy. However, to date, these problems have been very uncommon and should not limit the application of this new technique.

The relative and absolute contraindications to laparoscopic cholecystectomy, discussed in subsequent chapters, remain a matter of debate. Patients with coexisting problems such as pregnancy, severe bleeding disorders, peritonitis, and cholangitis represent only a very small percentage of all patients who are having traditional cholecystectomies. Other problems such as acute cholecystitis, gallstone pancreatitis, advanced liver disease, and prior upper abdominal surgery are only relative contraindications, and many patients with these problems have successfully undergone laparoscopic cholecystectomy.

Initial data from several institutions suggest that laparoscopic cholecystectomy can be completed successfully in more than 95% of patients. Analysis of patients referred to Johns Hopkins for laparoscopic cholecystectomy suggests that 82% met established criteria for the procedure. In this analysis a significant percentage of patients with relative contraindications were able to have their gallbladder removed laparoscopically. This analysis suggests that 80% to 85% or more of patients with symptomatic cholecystitis and cholelithiasis may be eligible for laparoscopic cholecystectomy.

REFERENCES

1. Bilhartz LE. Southwestern Internal Medicine Conference. Cholesterol gallstone disease: The current status of nonsurgical therapy. Am J Med Sci 296:45-56, 1988.
2. Hermann RE. The spectrum of biliary stone disease. Am J Surg 158:171-173, 1989.
3. Gilliland TM, Traverso W. Modern standards for comparison of cholecystectomy with alternative treatments for symptomatic cholelithiasis with emphasis on long-term relief of symptoms. Surg Gynecol Obstet 170:329-344, 1990.
4. Wenckert A, Robertson B. The natural course of gallstone disease: Eleven-year review of 781 nonoperated cases. Gastroenterology 50:376-381, 1966.
5. McSherry CK, Ferstenberg H, Calhoun F, Lahman E, Virshup M. The natural history of diagnosed gallstone disease in symptomatic and asymptomatic patients. Ann Surg 202:59-63, 1985.
6. Gracie WA, Ransohoff DF. The natural history of silent gallstones: The innocent gallstone is not a myth. N Engl J Med 307:798-800, 1982.
7. Cucchiaro G, Rossitch JC. Clinical significance of ultrasonographically detected coincidental gallstones. Dig Dis Sci 35:417-421, 1990.
8. Turill FL, McCarron MM, Mikkelsen WP. Gallstones and diabetes: An ominous association. Am J Surg 102:184-190, 1961.
9. Sandler RS, Maule WF, Baltus ME. Factors associated with postoperative complications in diabetes after biliary tract surgery. Gastroenterology 91:245-246, 1986.
10. Ransohoff DF, Miller GL, Forsythe SB, Hermann RE. Outcome of acute cholecystitis in patients with diabetes mellitus. Ann Intern Med 106:829-832, 1987.
11. Goldstein ME, Schein CJ. The significance of biliary tract disease in the diabetic—Its unique features. Am J Gastroenterol 39:630-634, 1963.
12. Thompson JS, Philben VJ, Hodgson PE. Operative management of incidental cholelithiasis. Am J Surg 148:821-824, 1984.
13. Ouriel K, Ricotta JJ, Adams JT, DeWuse JA. Management of cholelithiasis in patients with abdominal aortic aneurysm. Ann Surg 198:717-719, 1983.
14. String ST. Cholelithiasis and aortic reconstruction. J Vasc Surg 1:664-669, 1984.
15. Danzinger RG, Hofmann AF, Schoenfield LJ, Thistle JL. Dissolution of cholesterol gallstones by chenodeoxycholic acid. N Engl J Med 286:1-8, 1972.
16. Schoenfield LJ, Lachin JM, the Steering Committee, the National Cooperative Gallstone Study Group. Chenodiol (chenodeoxycholic acid) for dissolution of gallstones: The National Cooperative Gallstone Study: A controlled trial of efficacy and safety. Ann Intern Med 95:257-282, 1981.
17. Barbera L, Roda E, Mazzela G, et al. Efficacy of UDCA versus CDCA in cholesterol gallstone patients: A double-blind trial. In Fungalli et al, eds. Drugs Effecting Lipid Metabolism. Amsterdam: Elsevier, 1980.
18. Bateson MC, Hill A, Bouchier IAD. Analysis of response to ursodeoxycholic acid for gallstone dissolution. Digestion 20:358-364, 1980.
19. Fromm H, Roat JW, Gonzales V, Sarva RP, Farivar S. Comparative efficacy and side effects of ursodeoxycholic and chenodeoxycholic acids in dissolving gallstones: A double-blind controlled study. Gastroenterology 85:1257-1264, 1983.

20. Podda M, Zuin M, Battezzati PM, Ghezzi C, de Fazio C, Dioguardi ML. Efficacy and safety of a combination of chenodeoxycholic acid and ursodeoxycholic acid for gallstone dissolution: A comparison with ursodeoxycholic acid alone. Gastroenterology 96:222-229, 1989.

21. Ruppin DC, Dowling RH. Is recurrence inevitable after gallstone dissolution by bile acid treatment? Lancet 1:181-185, 1982.

22. Marks JV, Lan SO. The Steering Committee and The National Cooperative Gallstone Study Group. Low dose chenodiol to prevent gallstone recurrence after dissolution therapy. Ann Intern Med 100:376-381, 1984.

23. O'Donnell LDJ, Heaton KW. Recurrence and re-recurrence of gallstones after medical dissolution: A long-term follow-up. Gut 29:655-658, 1988.

24. Villanova N, Bazzoli F, Taroni F, Frabboni R, Mazzela G, Festi D, Barbera L, Roda E. Gallstone recurrence after successful oral bile acid treatment: A 12-year follow-up study and evaluation of long-term postdissolution treatment. Gastroenterology 97:726-731, 1989.

25. Magnuson TH, Lillemoe KD, Pitt HA. How many Americans will be eligible for biliary lithotripsy? Arch Surg 124:1195-1200, 1989.

26. Neubrand M, Sauerbruch T, Stellaard F, Paumgartner G. In vitro gallstone dissolution after fragmentation with shock waves. Digestion 34:51-54, 1986.

27. Sackmann M, Delius M, Sauerbruch T, Holl J, Weber W, Ippisch E, Hagelauer U, Wess O, Hepp W, Brendel W, Paumgartner G. Shock-wave lithotripsy of gallbladder stones: The first 175 patients. N Engl J Med 318:393-397, 1988.

28. Burnett D, Ertan A, Jones R, O'Leary JP, Mackie R, Robinson JE, Salen G, Stahlgren L, Van Thiel DH, Vassy L, Greenberger N, Hofmann AF. Use of external shock-wave lithotripsy and adjuvant ursodiol for treatment of radiolucent gallstones. Dig Dis Sci 34:1011-1014, 1989.

29. Rawat B, Fache JS, Malone DE, et al. Biliary lithotripsy without oral chemolitholysis: The Vancouver experience. In Burhenne HJ, Paumgartner G, Ferrucci JT, eds. Biliary Lithotripsy, vol II. Chicago: Year Book, 1990, pp 111-122.

30. Ell C, Kerzel W, Schneider HT, et al. Piezoelectric lithotripsy of gallbladder stones: The Erlangen experience. In Burhenne HJ, Paumgartner G, Ferrucci JT, eds. Biliary Lithotripsy, vol II. Chicago: Year Book, 1990, pp 93-109.

31. Ponchon T, Barkun AN, Pujol B, Mestar JL, Lambert R. Gallstone disappearance after extracorporeal lithotripsy and oral bile acid dissolution. Gastroenterology 97:457-463, 1989.

32. Rawat B, Burhenne HJ. Extracorporeal shock wave lithotripsy of calcified gallstones: Work in progress. Radiology 175:667-670, 1990.

33. Schoenfield LJ and the investigators of the Dornier National Biliary Lithotripsy Study. The role of bile acids in extracorporeal shock wave lithotripsy of gallbladder stones. Gastroenterology 98:A261, 1990.

34. Sackmann M, Ippisch E, Sauerbruch T, Holl J, Brendel W, Paumgartner G. Early gallstone recurrence rate after successful shock-wave therapy. Gastroenterology 98:392-396, 1990.

35. Bass E, Steinberg E, Pitt HA, et al. Cost effectiveness of extracorporeal shock wave lithotripsy versus surgery for gallstones (submitted for publication).

36. Allen MJ, Borody TJ, Thistle JL. In vitro dissolution of cholesterol gallstones: A study of factors influencing rate and a comparison of solvents. Gastroenterology 89:1097-1103, 1985.

37. Allen MJ, Borody TJ, Bugliosi TF, May GR, LaRusso NF, Thistle JL. Cholelitholysis using methyl tertiary butyl ether. Gastroenterology 88:122-125, 1985.

38. Zakko SF, Hofmann AF, Schteingart C, vonSonnenberg E, Wheeler HO. Percutaneous gallbladder stone dissolution using a microprocessor assisted solvent transfer (MAST) system [abstract]. Gastroenterology 92:1794, 1987.

39. Thistle JL, May GR, Bender CE, Williams HJ, LeRoy AJ, Nelson PE, Peine CJ, Peterson BT, McCullough JE. Dissolution of cholesterol gallbladder stones by methyl *tert*-butyl ether administered by percutaneous transhepatic catheter. N Engl J Med 320:633-638, 1989.

40. Hellstern A, Leuschner M, Fischer H, Lazarovici D, Guldutung S, Kurtz W, Leuschner U. Perkutan-transhepatische Lyse von Gallenblasensteinen mit methyl-tert-butyl-äther. Dtsch Med Wochenschr 113:506-510, 1988.

41. vonSonnenberg E, Casola G, Zakko SF. Gallbladder and bile duct stones: Percutaneous therapy with primary MTBE dissolution and mechanical methods. Radiology 169:505-509, 1988.

42. Cope C, Burke DR, Meranze SG. Percutaneous extraction of gallstones in 20 patients. Radiology 176:19-24, 1990.

43. Picus D, Marx MV, Hicks ME, Lang EV, Edmundowicz SA. Percutaneous cholecystolithotomy: Preliminary experience and technical considerations. Radiology 173:487-491, 1989.
44. Hruby W, Stackl W, Urban M, Armbruster C, Marberger M. Percutaneous endoscopic cholecystolithotripsy: Work in progress. Radiology 173:477-479, 1989.
45. Gibney RG, Chow K, So CB, Rowley VA, Cooperberg PL, Burhenne HJ. Gallstone recurrence after cholecystolithotomy. AJR 153:287-289, 1989.
46. McSherry CK. Cholecystectomy: The gold standard. Am J Surg 158:174-178, 1989.
47. Meyer KA, Capos JN, Mihlepunkt AI. Personal experience with 1261 cases of acute and chronic cholecystitis and cholelithiasis. Surgery 61:661-668, 1967.
48. DeMarco A, Nance F, Cohn I Jr. Chronic cholecystitis: Experience in a large charity institution. Surgery 63:750-756, 1968.
49. Gallbladder Survey Committee. 28,621 cholecystectomies in Ohio. Am J Surg 119:714-717, 1970.
50. Pickleman J, Gonzalez R. Improving results of cholecystectomy. Arch Surg 121:930-934, 1986.
51. Ganey JB, Johnson PA Jr, Prillaman PE, McSwain GR. Cholecystectomy: Clinical experience with a large series. Am J Surg 151:352-357, 1986.
52. McSherry CK, Glen F. The incidence and causes of death following surgery for nonmalignant biliary tract disease. Ann Surg 191:271-275, 1980.
53. Andrén-Sandbera A, Alinder G, Bengmark S. Accidental lesions of the common bile duct at cholecystectomy: Pre- and perioperative factors of importance. Ann Surg 201:328-332, 1985.
54. Andrén-Sandbera A, Johansson S, Bengmark S. Accidental lesions of the common bile duct: II. Results of treatment. Ann Surg 201:452-455, 1985.
55. Madsen CM, Sörenson HR, Truelsen I. The frequency of bile duct injuries illustrated by a Danish county survey. Acta Chir Scand 119:110-111, 1960.

Laparoscopic Guided Cholecystectomy With Electrocautery Dissection

Karl A. Zucker, M.D.

PATIENT SELECTION

The preoperative evaluation of candidates for laparoscopic guided cholecystectomy differs little from that of patients undergoing traditional open cholecystectomy. A careful history and physical examination are performed to exclude the possibility of other gastrointestinal diseases that may mimic biliary colic, such as peptic ulcer disease or reflux esophagitis. At the University of Maryland Medical Center we continue to perform cholecystectomy only on patients with symptomatic gallbladder disease except for individuals with diabetes or those who may be required to spend long periods away from medical facilities (i.e., military personnel). In addition, it is important to elicit any information suggestive of choledocholithiasis, such as a history of pancreatitis or jaundice. Since we cannot routinely extract common bile duct stones with laparoscopic surgical techniques at this time, all attempts are made to screen for such patients before surgery. In addition to the routine blood work such as a coagulation panel, complete blood count, and serum electrolytes, we obtain a serum amylase and a liver function panel containing one or more hepatic transaminases and alkaline phosphatase. We have found the most cost-effective imaging study of the biliary tract to be a high-quality abdominal ultrasonogram, which can document the presence of gallstones as well as intra- or extra-hepatic bile duct dilatation that may suggest the presence of choledocholithiasis. The number and size of the gallstones do not affect the patient's eligibility for laparoscopic surgery. We have removed gallbladders containing stones as large as 4.0 cm without major difficulty. Similarly, information such as gallbladder wall thickening and surrounding fluid has not proved useful in predicting how successful laparoscopic cholecystectomy will be. If there is a history of atypical pain or previous peptic ulcer disease, we perform flexible esophagogastroduodenoscopy.

If choledocholithiasis is not suggested by the history, sonographic results, or blood work, additional diagnostic studies are not ordered. In patients with suspected common bile duct stones a preoperative endoscopic retrograde cholangiopancreatogram (ERCP) is advised. If the ERCP demonstrates choledocholithiasis, endoscopic sphincterotomy and stone extraction are attempted prior to laparoscopic surgery. In most centers that are experienced in biliary endoscopy, common bile duct stones are successfully treated in over 90% of patients.[1] If common bile duct stones cannot be removed via the endoscopic approach, the patient may require an open laparotomy and common bile duct exploration.

In contrast to other, nonoperative approaches to gallbladder disease, there are relatively few absolute and relative contraindications to laparoscopic guided cholecystectomy. At any time during laparoscopic cholecystectomy the surgeon can, if necessary, elect to convert the procedure to an open laparotomy. Situations that may render the laparoscopic approach difficult or impossible include extensive adhesions from prior surgery or recurrent attacks of cholecystitis, unusual vascular or ductal anomalies, unsuspected pathologic findings, acute inflammation distorting the normal tissue planes, excessive bleeding, and inability to safely identify the ductal and vascular anatomy. To cover this eventuality, the surgeon must properly inform the patient of this option and obtain an informed consent for both laparoscopic and open procedures. Thus the patient will not interpret conversion to a laparotomy as a complication of laparoscopic surgery. We have developed a special addendum to our standard operative consent that emphasizes this point as well as the innovative nature of this new procedure.

University of Maryland Medical System
University of Maryland Hospital

LAPAROSCOPIC CHOLECYSTECTOMY

Consent For Surgery: Addendum

Laparoscopic cholecystectomy is a surgical procedure which involves complete removal of the gallbladder through a half-inch incision near the navel. A laparoscope, which consists of a long, narrow tube with a light at one end and a miniature video camera attached to the other end, is inserted into the abdomen and allows the surgeon and his assistants to visualize the gallbladder. In addition, two to three smaller incisions (approximately 1/4 inch) are made in the upper abdomen through which various operating instruments are inserted. These instruments are used to separate the gallbladder from its surrounding attachments.

This procedure was first performed in 1987 in Europe and in 1988 in the United States. A laparoscopic cholecystectomy program was initiated at the University of Maryland Medical System in October of 1989. Experience with this new approach to cholecystectomy is rapidly increasing, but is still limited. Potential complications are similar to those of standard gallbladder surgery and include, but are not limited to: bleeding, infection or abscess formation, injury to the bile ducts, leaving stones behind in the main bile duct, infection of the incision sites, or perforation of the large or small bowel. It is unknown at this time whether the complication rate from this new approach will be the same as that of open cholecystectomy.

I understand and agree that the surgeon may decide to stop the laparoscopic procedure at his discretion and proceed with standard, open removal of the gallbladder. The surgeon will make this decision during the operative procedure based on a number of different factors such as the ability to safely identify important blood vessels and bile ducts, the presence of extensive adhesions (scar tissue), unusual gallbladder anatomy, the presence of other intraabdominal disease, and bleeding. An x-ray of the bile ducts connected to the gallbladder may be performed during the operation if deemed necessary by the surgeon.

I hereby acknowledge that I have read the above information and understand the potential risks of laparoscopic cholecystectomy and open cholecystectomy. The current experience with laparoscopic cholecystectomy at the University of Maryland Medical System has been clearly explained to me by Dr._____ and I give consent to undergo laparoscopic cholecystectomy, and, if deemed appropriate intraoperatively, open cholecystectomy.

_____   _____
Witness   Patient or Legal Guardian

_____
Date

Currently, the only absolute and relative contraindications to laparoscopic cholecystectomy are as follows:

Absolute Contraindications	Relative Contraindications
Pregnancy	Acute cholecystitis
Acute cholangitis	Prior upper abdominal surgery
Septic peritonitis	Minor bleeding disorders
Severe bleeding disorders	Untreated choledocholithiasis
	Known abdominal malignancy
	Advanced liver disease
	Inability to tolerate general anesthesia

Since the effects of pneumoperitoneum on the developing fetus are unknown, laparoscopic surgery should not be attempted in pregnant women. Patients with acute cholangitis generally have an obstructed ductal system that cannot be readily cleared via the laparoscope. In such patients the common bile duct should be drained by open surgery, endoscopic techniques, or under percutaneous radiologic guidance, depending on the expertise available and the patient's condition. Patients with abdominal sepsis or generalized peritonitis often will have some sort of abdominal catastrophe that may or may not be limited to the biliary tract. Under such circumstances we perform a formal surgical exploration. We also exclude patients with major bleeding disorders. Although a number of techniques for ensuring hemostasis during laparoscopic surgery are available, they are less effective in the face of major blood loss. Thus patients with uncorrectable coagulopathies should undergo an open procedure since the surgeon will be better equipped to control major hemorrhage during an open laparotomy.

Patients with one or more of the relative contraindications should be evaluated on a case-by-case basis. The experience of the operative team is perhaps the most important factor. Many patients we would not consider candidates early in our experience will now routinely undergo laparoscopic surgery. The most commonly encountered relative contraindications include acute cholecystitis and patients with prior upper abdominal surgery. The inflammation and edema that accompany acute cholecystitis often distort the normal tissue planes surrounding the gallbladder and cystic duct. We currently tell such patients that we will attempt laparoscopic guided cholecystectomy but inform them that the possibility of converting the procedure to an open laparotomy is increased. Individuals with prior abdominal surgery, inflammatory bowel disease, or known abdominal malignancy may also pose a challenge to the surgeon since extensive inflammatory or malignant adhesions may preclude safe dissection around the porta hepatis and increase the possibility of injury during insertion of the insufflation needle and trocar. Laparoscopic guided cholecystectomy also may prove to be technically difficult in patients with advanced liver disease (i.e., cirrhosis). The diseased liver may be enlarged and immobile, making exposure of the cystic and common bile ducts difficult. In addition, coagulopathy may be associated with liver disease. Patients who are not considered candidates for open laparotomy due to coexisting medical illness or poor prognosis should not routinely be considered candidates for laparoscopic guided cholecystectomy. Under such circumstances this less invasive procedure is not necessarily safer since conversion to an open laparotomy is always a possibility.

At the University of Maryland we do not consider morbid obesity an absolute or relative contraindication to laparoscopic guided cholecystectomy. Although insufflation and trocar insertion may prove more difficult because of abdominal wall adipose tissue, the actual operative procedure often is no more difficult than in thinner individuals. Exposure may be somewhat compromised by fat in the omentum and transverse colon mesentery; however, this generally is not a major limiting factor. It is advisable for the inexperienced laparoscopic surgeon to avoid operating on such patients; however, there does not appear to be any specific contraindication to laparoscopic surgery. In fact, these patients recover remarkably well following laparoscopic guided cholecystectomy as compared to the open procedure. The majority of patients are able to ambulate and return home the following morning. Wound infections, pneumonia, prolonged ileus, and pulmonary emboli appear to be much less of a problem with laparoscopic surgery.

TECHNIQUE

Patients are generally admitted on the morning of the procedure. Laparoscopic guided cholecystectomy is performed under rigid sterile conditions in a fully equipped operating room (see Chapter 2). Patients are prepared for both a laparoscopic procedure and an open cholecystectomy. Either general anesthesia or a combination of regional anesthetics and local anesthesia may be used successfully (see Chapter 4). We do not recommend attempting this procedure under regional anesthesia until the surgeon becomes experienced at laparoscopic guided cholecystectomy. It is usually necessary to employ less insufflation pressure for the pneumoperitoneum, which may limit exposure of the porta hepatis. To facilitate laparoscopic exposure in the upper and lower abdomen and minimize risk of injury in this area, a urinary catheter and nasogastric tube are used to decompress the bladder and stomach. Pneumoperitoneum is necessary to visualize the abdominal cavity with the laparoscope. CO_2 is the gas most commonly used because it is relatively innocuous to the patient and will not support combustion, an important consideration during electrocautery or laser dissection of tissues. Insufflation of the abdominal cavity may be accomplished percutaneously using an insufflation (Veress) needle or under direct visualization (open laparoscopy or the Hasson technique). We routinely use the percutaneous method because it has proved to be a safe technique in properly selected patients and can be performed quickly. If patients have had a prior surgical incision near the umbilicus or if there are other reasons to suspect underlying adhesions, we will perform the open procedure (see Chapter 5).

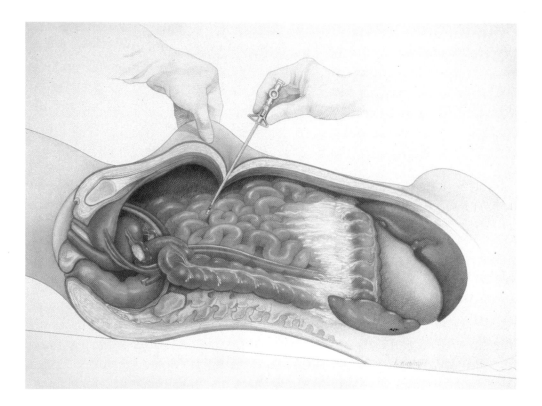

To establish pneumoperitoneum, the patient is initially placed in a 10- to 20-degree reverse Trendelenburg position. The insufflation needle is inserted through a small skin incision in the folds just above or below the umbilicus. To avoid injury to the underlying aorta or vena cava, the needle is angled slightly toward the pelvis.

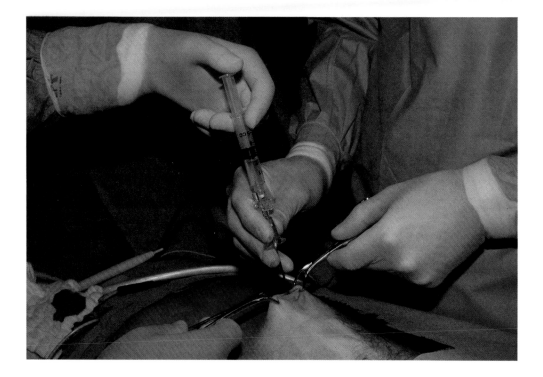

The Trendelenburg position allows the intestines to fall cephalad, thus minimizing the risk of needle injury as it is directed toward the pelvis. Because the thinnest portion of the anterior abdominal wall is at the umbilicus, the surgeon is able to feel the needle pass through the fascia and peritoneum. Raising the abdominal wall gently with a pair of penetrating towel clamps or by hand will provide countertraction of the abdominal fascia. This may assist the surgeon in determining when the needle passes through the fascial layer and into the peritoneal cavity. Several maneuvers have been described in an attempt to ensure proper placement of the insufflation needle. The simplest procedure is to draw back with a small syringe attached to the needle.

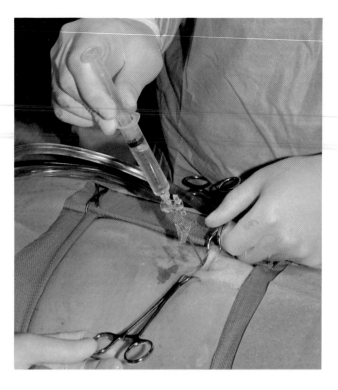

Aspiration of blood, urine, or intestinal contents indicates improper placement of the needle. The so-called drop test is performed by placing a drop of saline solution within the open lumen (the hub) of the insufflation needle. As the needle enters the peritoneal cavity, the relative negative intra-abdominal pressure pulls the fluid through the needle.

Electronic high-flow insufflators are now capable of direct intra-abdominal pressure readings through the insufflation needle and are also used to confirm proper positioning of the needle (see Chapter 2).

Gas flow is initiated at 1 to 2 L/min. If the tip of the insufflation needle is within the free intraperitoneal space, the intra-abdominal pressure should be 8 to 10 mm Hg. This amount of pressure is the result of resistance to the flow of CO_2 through the small bore of the needle. Higher pressures suggest that the needle has been improperly positioned into a relatively closed space such as within the subcutaneous tissues, preperitoneal fat, or intestinal lumen or buried in the omentum. After proper needle placement is confirmed, gas flow may be increased. However, we continue to insufflate at 1 to 2 L/min to minimize the amount of postoperative shoulder pain. This discomfort is believed to be referred pain from the diaphragm. This may occur as a result of rapid stretching or direct irritation from the CO_2. Slow insufflation at the beginning of the procedure will reduce this complaint. Once the abdomen is fully distended, high-flow insufflation is used to maintain pneumoperitoneum. As the abdominal cavity distends, the surgeon should percuss all four quadrants to ensure symmetric insufflation. The insufflation instrument should be set at a maximum pressure of 14 to 15 mm Hg. When the intra-abdominal pressure reaches this level, gas flow should stop. Pressures higher than this may result in a gas embolus from CO_2 being forced through an exposed blood vessel during the operative dissection.[2] Most electronic insufflators are equipped with an alarm mechanism that informs the operating room team if the intra-abdominal pressure exceeds the desired amount. This can occur if one of the members of the surgical team accidently leans against the abdominal wall or may be caused by the gas plume that is used in some types of surgical lasers (see Chapter 3). The abdomen is filled with 3 to 4 L of CO_2; when pneumoperitoneum is established, the insufflation needle is removed.

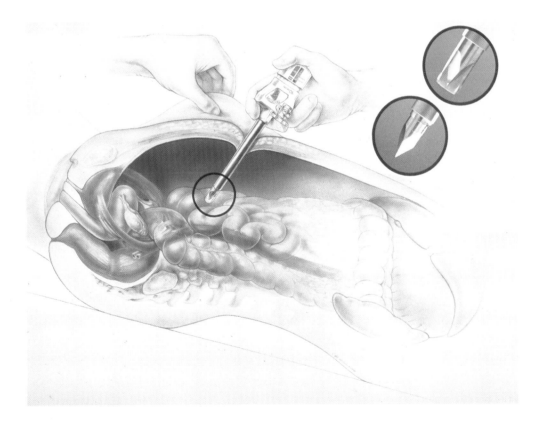

The skin incision is enlarged, and a 10 or 11 mm (depending on the instrumentation set being used) trocar and sheath are inserted, aiming slightly toward the pelvis.

Both reusable metal trocars and sheaths as well as plastic or fiberglass disposable units are now available (see Chapter 2). We prefer the disposable trocars (SurgiPort; United States Surgical Corporation, Norwalk, Conn.) because they have a number of features that are useful in laparoscopic biliary tract surgery. First, the disposable sheaths are completely radiolucent, which is important if the surgeon wants to perform laparoscopic cholangiography. The reusable instruments are radiopaque and may obscure the x-ray image.

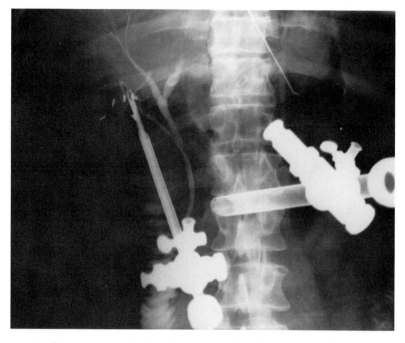

Radiopaque sheath blocks view of distal common bile duct on laparoscopic cholangiogram.

Also, the disposable instruments are always sharp and thus minimize the amount of force necessary to penetrate the fascia and peritoneum.[3] Excessive force during insertion of the trocar may result in an uncontrolled entry into the abdominal cavity with subsequent injury to underlying tissue. Another advantage of the disposable trocars is their locking safety shield. This shield withdraws during fascia penetration, exposing the sharp tip. After entry into the free peritoneal space, the safety shield rapidly retracts over the sharp trocar tip and prevents the trocar from lacerating underlying bowel or vascular structures. However, for the safety shield to retract back over the sharp trocar, the instrument must first be exposed to the free peritoneal space. Therefore the disposable devices will not prevent an injury if bowel is fixed to the underlying abdominal wall.

An operating (10 mm) laparoscope with attached camera is then inserted through the umbilical sheath to confirm intraperitoneal placement. Either a forward- (zero degree) viewing or side-viewing (30- to 45-degree fixed-angle) laparoscope may be used. The angled instrument is actually more useful because the assistant can manipulate the laparoscope to look directly up at the anterior abdominal wall as well as around a distended transverse colon or duodenum. Unfortunately the angled laparoscope requires a great deal more skill to operate. The assistant must orient not only the attached camera but also the angle of the viewing lens. However, once these skills are achieved, the surgical team often will prefer the greater versatility offered by the side-viewing laparoscope.

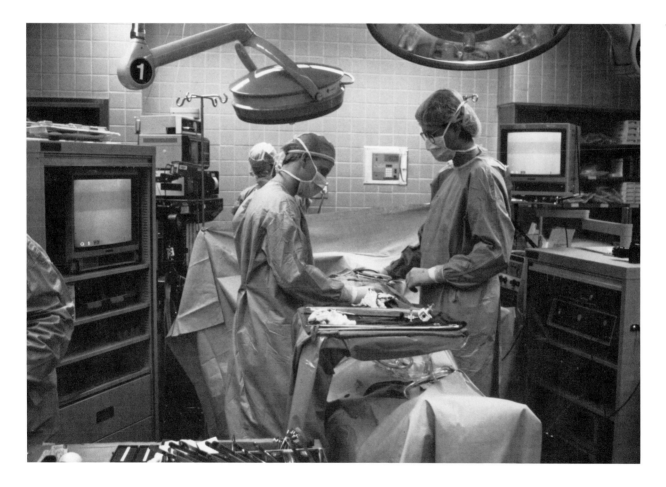

Positioning of the surgeon and the first assistant is left to each individual's choice. We prefer to have the surgeon stand at the patient's left side with the assistant directly across the operating room table. Video monitors are then situated to allow all the members of the surgical team to visualize the procedure.

Generally we use two professional-grade monitors with a resolution greater than 500 lines per inch. Accessory electronic equipment is organized on sturdy carts, which allow the surgical team to monitor these instruments. The insufflation instrument also should be in the surgeon's direct view to allow for continuous monitoring of the gas flow rate and insufflation pressure.

After the umbilical sheath is properly placed, the patient is moved to a 30-degree reverse Trendelenburg position. This allows the transverse colon and small bowel to fall inferiorly and away from the gallbladder. Tilting the patient slightly to the left may further help expose the gallbladder and the cystic duct. Three additional skin incisions are made for the placement of accessory trocars and sheaths. One incision (5.0 mm) is placed two fingerbreadths below the right midcostal margin, and a second small puncture site (5.0 mm) is made over the right midaxillary line. The fourth trocar site is placed one third the distance between the xiphoid and umbilicus and just to the right of the midline. This incision is made to accommodate a larger (10 or 11 mm) trocar and sheath.

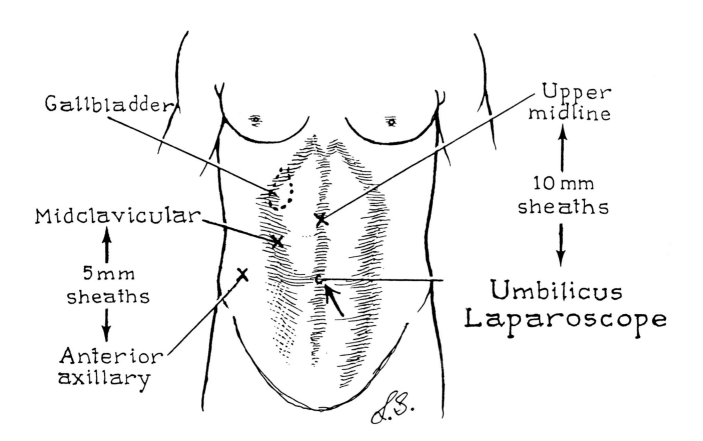

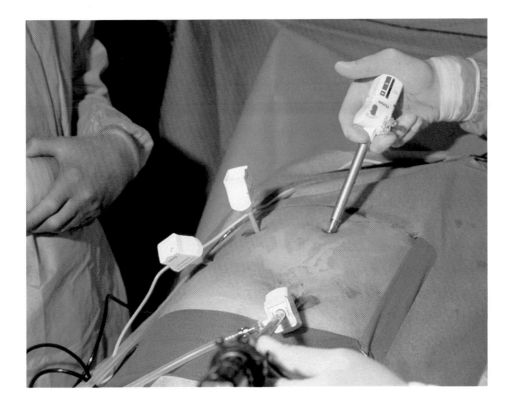

These accessory trocars and sheaths are inserted into the abdominal cavity under direct laparoscopic vision to preclude any injury to the abdominal organs.

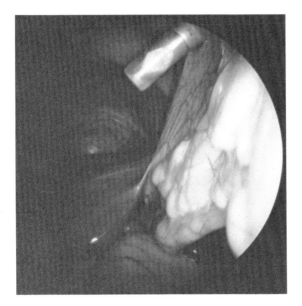

The epigastric trocar is positioned just to the right of the patient's falciform ligament.

If indicated, the surgeon may elect to insert a fifth trocar and sheath, with the portal placed in the left midcostal region or midway between the umbilical and epigastric sites. This may be necessary if additional grasping or retracting instruments are needed. The additional skin incision and trocar insertion do not result in added discomfort or scarring and would seem to be preferable to aborting the laparoscopic procedure in favor of a laparotomy.

These accessory sheaths or portals are used to insert the various laparoscopic surgical instruments.

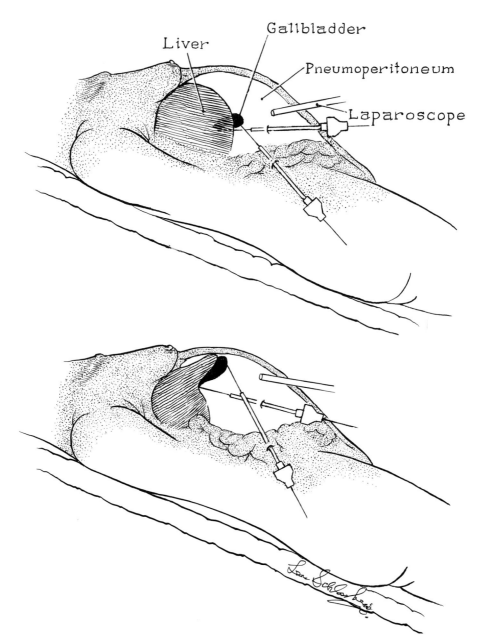

Blunt atraumatic or alligator forceps are inserted through the 5.0 mm sheaths and used to expose the gallbladder and porta hepatis. The anterior axillary forceps is placed on the dome of the gallbladder and used to push the right lobe of the liver toward the diaphragm.

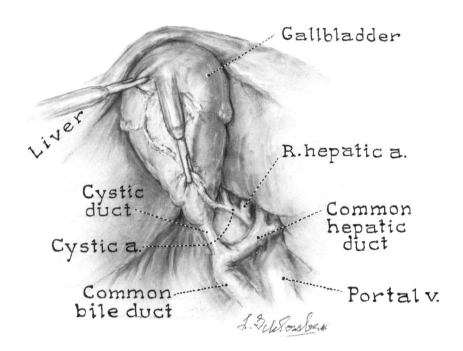

The midclavicular instrument is applied near the neck of the gallbladder and further exposes the cystic and common bile duct.

This maneuver draws the cystic and common bile duct out of the hepato-duodenal ligament. It is important to recognize that the cephalad traction of the gallbladder fundus and neck may distort the normal anatomy and position of the cystic duct and common bile duct junction. Such distortion could precipitate inadvertent injury.

Excessive force applied to these forceps may also result in a tear or avulsion off the gallbladder wall, which may lead to bile or stones escaping into the peritoneal cavity. A small opening may be easily and quickly controlled by simply repositioning the grasping forceps to occlude the opening.

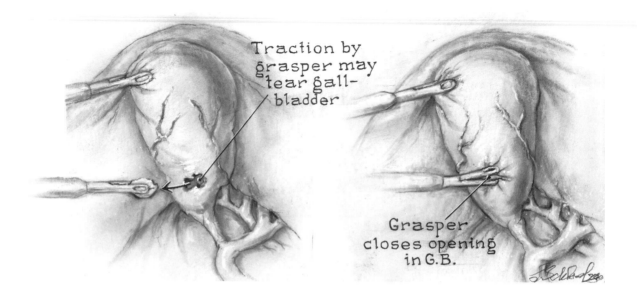

Larger defects generally require the application of a laparoscopic suture (EndoLoop; Ethicon, Inc., Sommerville, N.J.). This pretied suture (slip or fisherman's knot) is made of either plain or chromic catgut.

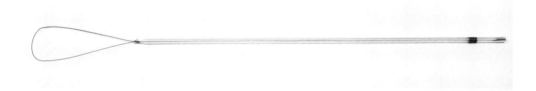

The gallbladder is allowed to partially collapse and then a grasping forceps is used to tent the wall outward for application of the EndoLoop.

The forceps is placed through the loop of the suture prior to grasping the gallbladder wall. The knot is then secured by tightening the knot with the incorporated plastic guide.

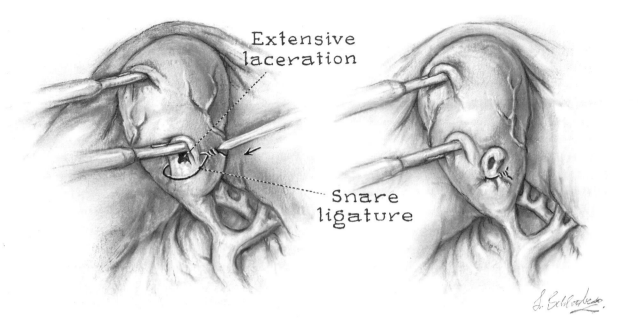

Extensive laceration

Snare ligature

Dissection of the cystic duct and artery is carried out almost entirely from the midline accessory sheath. These structures are freed from the surrounding tissue by using blunt dissection with straight or curved forceps (Maryland dissector; American Surgical Instruments, Pompano, Fla.). Dissection always begins along the gallbladder and proceeds toward the cystic and common bile duct junction.

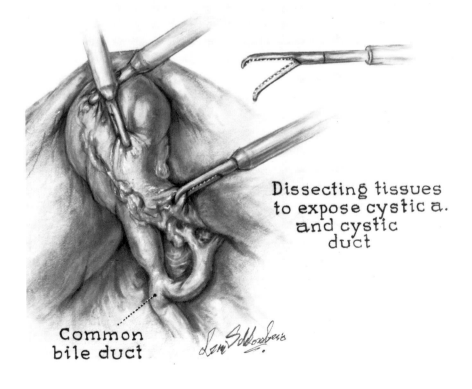

Dissecting tissues to expose cystic a. and cystic duct

Common bile duct

Careful incision of the peritoneal reflection over the cystic and common bile duct with a laparoscopic scissors facilitates this dissection. Retrograde dissection of the gallbladder and cystic duct is not advised with laparoscopic surgery. If the gallbladder is detached from the liver before the cystic and common bile ducts are completely visualized, the surgeon can no longer use this as a retraction aid. In addition, even a small amount of blood or bile resulting from prior dissection near the gallbladder fundus may make identification of the cystic and common bile duct junction difficult. The entire length of the cystic duct is exposed, with special attention directed at the junction with the common bile duct.

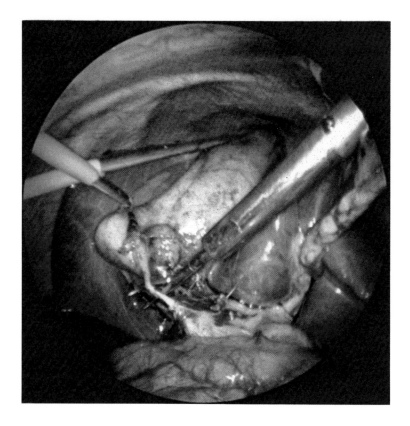

The entire length of the cystic duct and its junction with the common bile duct has been freed from the surrounding tissue.

The cystic artery is dissected free from the surrounding tissues before the cystic duct is divided.

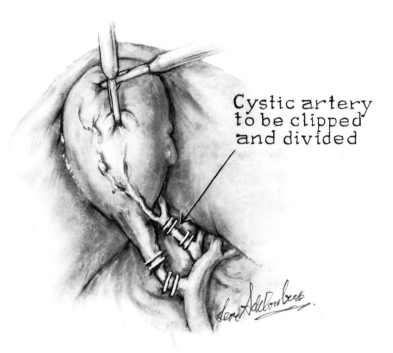

Cystic artery to be clipped and divided

Note the exposure and ligation of the cystic artery before bifurcation of the anterior and posterior branches.

It is important for the surgeon to recognize that the cystic artery divides into an anterior and posterior branch at variable locations near the gallbladder wall. The lack of depth perception as well as the fact that the view from the laparoscope is from caudad to cephalad may result in exposure of only the anterior branch of the cystic artery. The posterior branch is later encountered during dissection of the gallbladder off the liver bed and may then bleed profusely. Although this can be easily controlled by applying surgical clips or sutures, proper identification and ligation of the cystic artery proximal to the anterior and posterior branching will eliminate this problem. If the cystic artery is inadvertently injured or divided, the intact cystic duct will prevent retraction of the proximal artery into the hepatoduodenal ligament. Occasionally the cystic artery will lie directly posterior to the cystic duct and cannot be safely exposed until after the duct is divided.

Following exposure of the cystic duct, the surgeon may elect to perform a laparoscopic cholangiogram (see Chapter 10). We obtain a cholangiogram in almost every patient undergoing laparoscopic cholecystectomy to exclude the presence of common bile duct stones and to gather as much information as possible regarding the ductal anatomy. We also believe it is important for surgical residents at our institution to become proficient in performing laparoscopic cholangiography. However, I do not advocate that cholangiography be done routinely in all patients undergoing laparoscopic cholecystectomy. Surgeons should follow the same indications as for open cholecystectomy. I do believe it is essential that any surgeon performing this procedure have the expertise and equipment available for laparoscopic cholangiography. With the development of specialized cholangiogram clamps such as the Olsen cholangiography fixation clamp (Karl Storz Endoscopy, Culver City, Calif.), this procedure has been greatly simplified.

The surgeon has the same options for ligating the cystic duct and artery during laparoscopic cholecystectomy as in the open procedure. Surgical clips, free ties, and suture ligatures are available. In the vast majority of our cases we use titanium surgical clips to control both the cystic duct and artery. Both reusable and disposable laparoscopic clip appliers are now available. The reusable instruments hold only one clip and therefore must be withdrawn from the abdomen each time it is loaded. Although these clip appliers work very well, they can add as much as 15 to 20 minutes to the surgical procedure. Often as many as eight clips or more are used, and each time one is used the surgeon and camera operator must reorient the laparoscope and the instruments. In addition, these clips often fall off the end of the applicator as it is being inserted through the sheath. Therefore we prefer a multi-fire, spring-loaded clip applier (EndoClip; United States Surgical Corporation, Norwalk, Conn.).

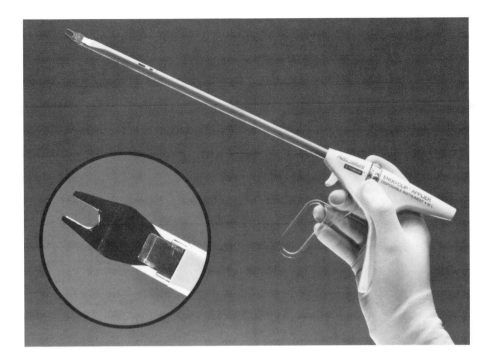

This instrument holds over 20 titanium clips 9.0 mm in length. The clip applicator is inserted through the upper midline sheath, and under direct vision two clips are applied proximally and distally on both the duct and the artery.

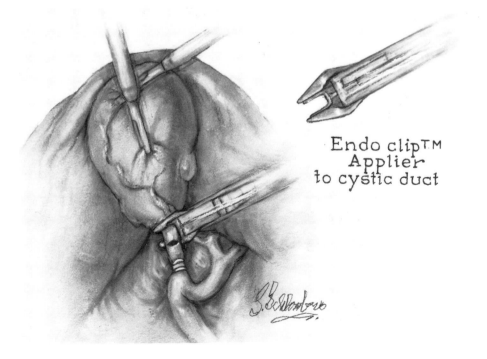

Endo clip™
Applier
to cystic duct

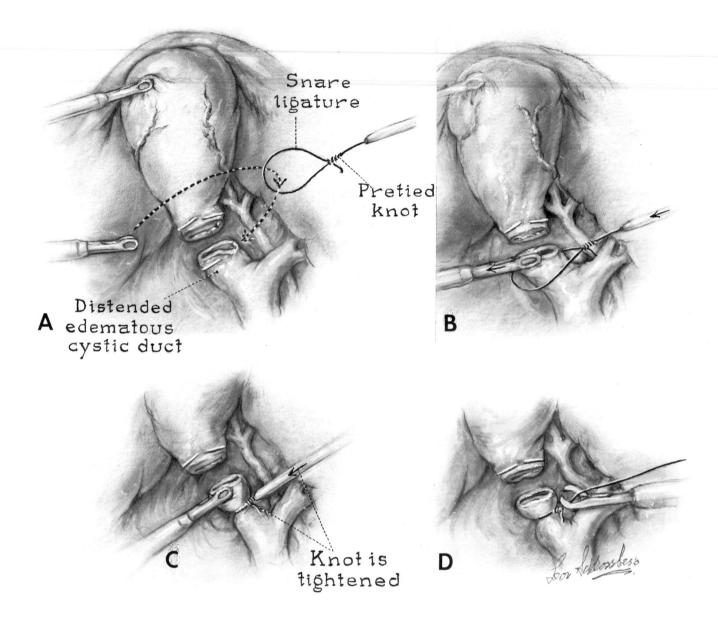

Snare ligature

Pretied knot

A Distended edematous cystic duct

B

C Knot is tightened

D

If the cystic duct or artery appears inflamed or edematous, we may also elect to apply pretied laparoscopic sutures (EndoLoop) so that the clips will not become loose or fall off if the edema resolves soon after the surgical procedure. Therefore, under these circumstances, we will apply a single clip on each side of the structure (to prevent leakage of bile or small stones), divide it, and then apply the EndoLoop.

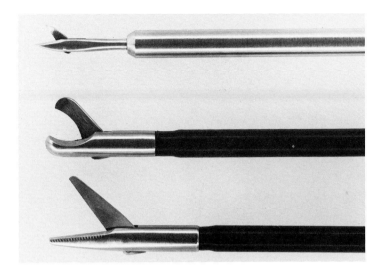

A variety of laparoscopic scissors, designed as either curved, hooked, or straight, are currently available.

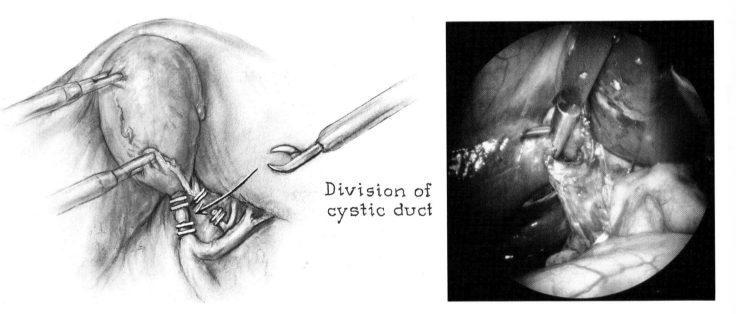

Division of cystic duct

The lack of depth perception afforded by the imaging equipment may create problems when the straight or curved instruments are used. As the surgeon opens the jaws of the scissors to encompass the duct or artery, the location of the tips of the instrument may be misleading. Because of this, adjacent tissues may also be divided or torn. With the hook scissors the surgeon places the duct or artery within the curved jaws and lifts the tissue out of the operative field and away from surrounding tissues.

Existing laparoscopic scissors are only 5.0 mm in diameter, which may lead to difficulty in dividing some tissues. In addition, the scissors are almost impossible to keep sharp. Fortunately a larger (10 mm) set of scissors has recently been introduced by American Surgical Instruments. After dividing the cystic duct and artery we continue with meticulous blunt dissection until the neck of the gallbladder is free from the liver edge. This minimizes the risk of injury to adjacent ductal structures such as the right hepatic duct or major blood vessels.

The gallbladder may be dissected from the liver bed using either monopolar electrocautery or laser dissection. We have used both modalities and find them equally effective. We now exclusively use electrocautery to avoid the increased cost of the laser (instrument purchase, maintenance, additional personnel, disposable fibers, cables, tips, etc.). A number of electrocautery instruments may be used for this dissection. We have found the spatula and hook cautery instruments to be the most useful.

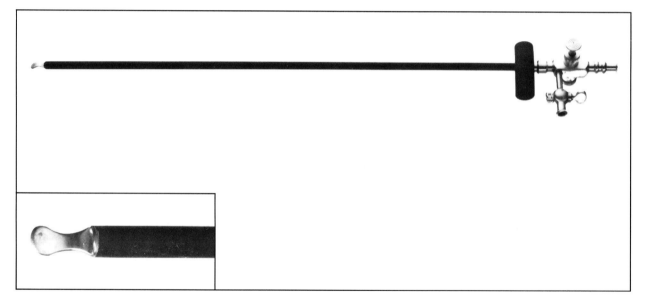

Monopolar spatula cautery

The broad tip of the spatula allows the surgeon to have tactile sensation and to bluntly dissect with this device as well. We use a pure, monopolar coagulation current set at approximately 30 to 35 watts. The spatula instrument was originally designed with two channels to allow the surgeon to irrigate and suction with the same instrument. Although the small size of these channels (each is less than 2.0 mm) does not make this practical, it does result in an effective smoke evacuation device. One of the channels may be left open to room air, and because of the increased pressure within the abdominal cavity, this results in a controlled air leak. Since the internal opening is adjacent to the cautery tip, the smoke escapes through this lumen, and there is no accumulation of cautery-induced smoke to obstruct the surgeon's view of the operative field. The high-flow electronic insufflator easily replaces the lost CO_2. The dissection begins near the mobilized gallbladder neck and proceeds superiorly along the medial and lateral attachments to the liver bed. The midclavicular forceps is placed just proximal to the cystic duct clips and is used to retract the gallbladder neck cephalad and anterior.

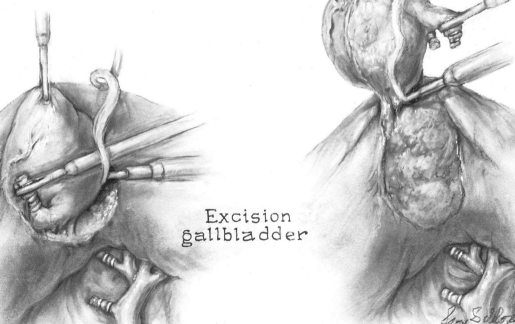

Excision
gallbladder

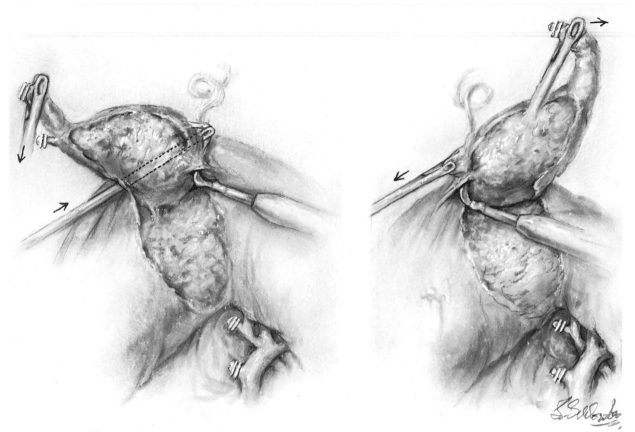

Right twist   Left twist

It is important to keep the gallbladder on tension so that the cautery instrument can effectively dissect tissue. By manipulating the 5.0 mm lateral grasping forceps, the assistant can maintain tension and also expose the medial and lateral surfaces of the gallbladder.

The so-called right twist is performed by advancing the anterior axillary forceps toward the midline and pulling the midclavicular forceps laterally. This maneuver exposes the medial attachments of the gallbladder to the liver.

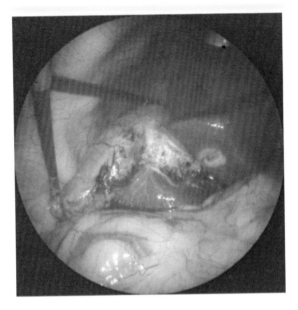

Reversing the direction of the forceps accomplishes the left twist. This allows the surgeon to dissect the lateral surface of the gallbladder. If the dissection remains in the proper plane of tissue between the gallbladder and the liver, there is minimal coagulation injury to the underlying tissue. Partial electrocautery dissection of the gallbladder from the liver bed is shown.

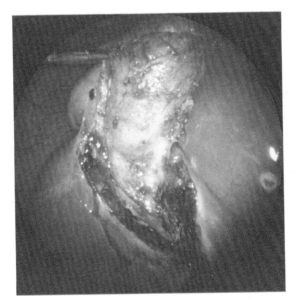

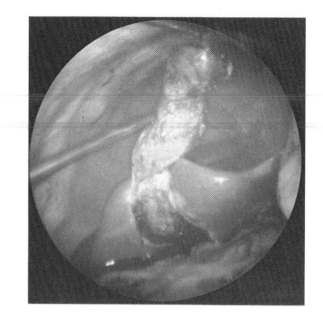

Before the gallbladder is completely detached, we irrigate the operative field with saline solution and examine the liver bed for possible sites of bleeding or bile leak.

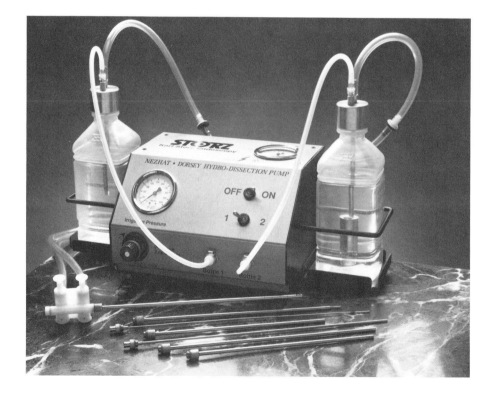

This laparoscopic irrigation/aspiration instrument is gas driven and has two saline reservoirs.

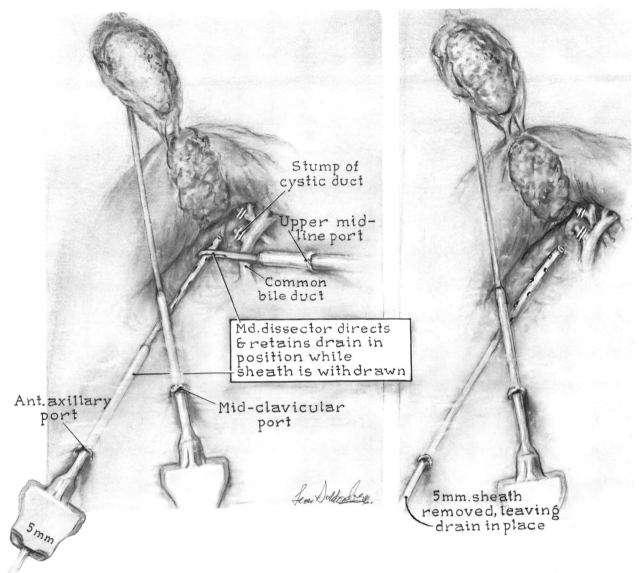

We also reexamine the clips or sutures applied to the distal end of the cystic duct and the proximal cystic artery to confirm continued placement. We do not routinely drain the site after open or laparoscopic guided cholecystectomies; however, a small drainage catheter may be inserted if clinically indicated. A closed suction drain is placed through the lateral sheath and into the abdominal cavity.

A grasping forceps or dissector is inserted through the upper midline sheath and is used to direct the drainage catheter into place and hold it in position as the sheath is removed. The drain is then secured to the skin.

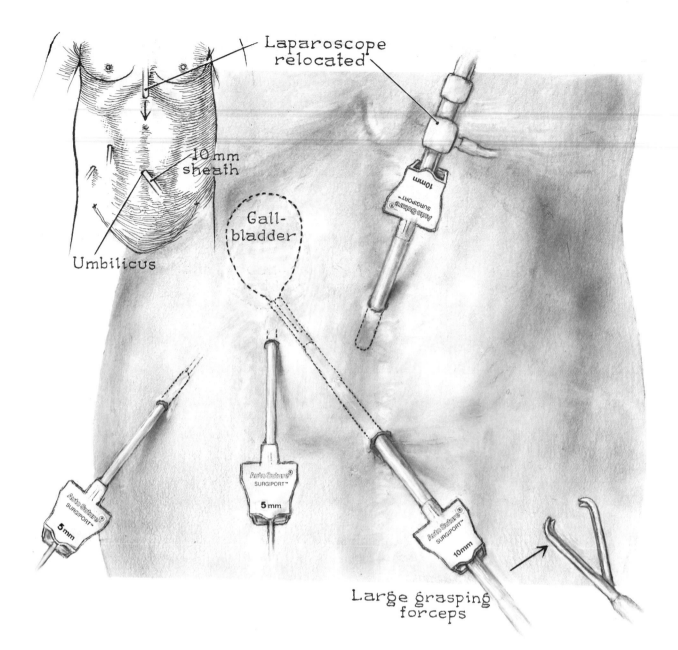

The gallbladder is routinely removed from the abdominal cavity through the umbilical incision. The laparoscope and camera are moved to the upper midline sheath, and a large grasping forceps is placed on the gall-bladder neck under direct visualization.

Positioning of the clamp is important to prevent the escape of bile or stones from the transected portion of the cystic duct during gallbladder extraction. We advise using a 10 or 11 mm toothed grasping instrument for extracting the gallbladder.

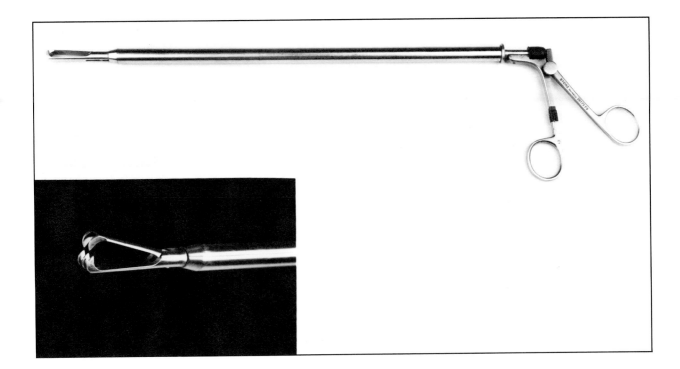

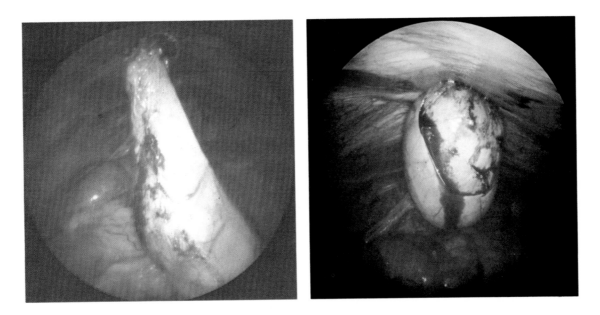

Smaller and/or less traumatic instruments may not secure the gallbladder adequately, and it may become dislodged and be lost within the loops of bowel as the surgeon attempts to manipulate the gallbladder through the umbilical fascial opening. A number of surgeons have then been forced to perform a lower midline laparotomy to retrieve the gallbladder. The large grasping forceps is shown secured to the neck of the gallbladder as it is pulled partially into the umbilical sheath.

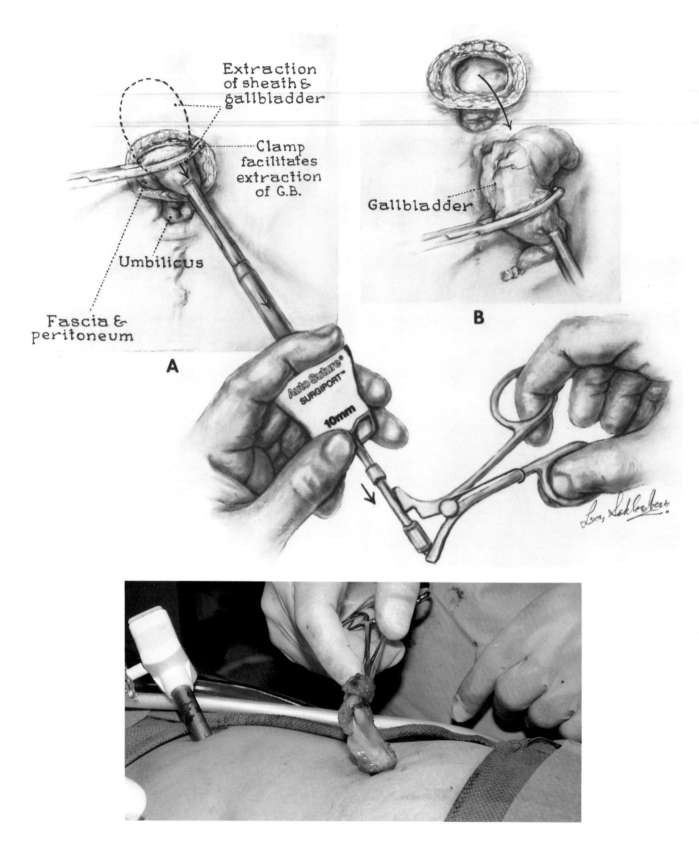

The entire sheath and gallbladder neck are withdrawn to just above the skin incision, and a Kelly or Kocher clamp is used to secure the tip of the gallbladder and manipulate it further from the abdominal cavity.

Gallbladder partially with-drawn—too large to pass thru incision

Tip of gallbladder excised

Stones & fluid aspirated from specimen

Collapsed gallbladder withdrawn

Often the gallbladder is distended with bile or multiple stones and will not pass easily through the 10 mm sheath. In these circumstances the gallbladder neck is grasped just above the fascial opening with two Kelly clamps and further manipulated out of the abdomen. The gallbladder neck is amputated, allowing the bile and small stones to be aspirated.

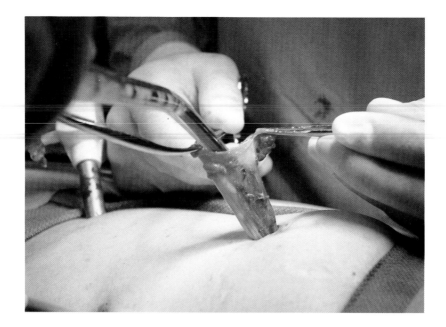

The wound is covered with sponges or towels, and a large suction catheter is used to remove small stones and bile. The collapsed gallbladder is then easily withdrawn from the abdomen.

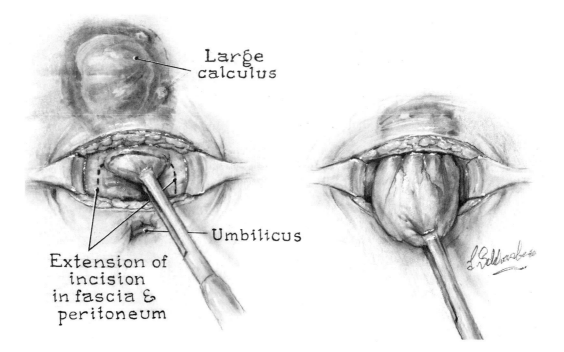

Occasionally the presence of very large stones (>1.0 cm) precludes removal through the standard umbilical fascial opening. In such cases the incision is extended as necessary around the folds of the navel and held open with a pair of right-angled retractors.

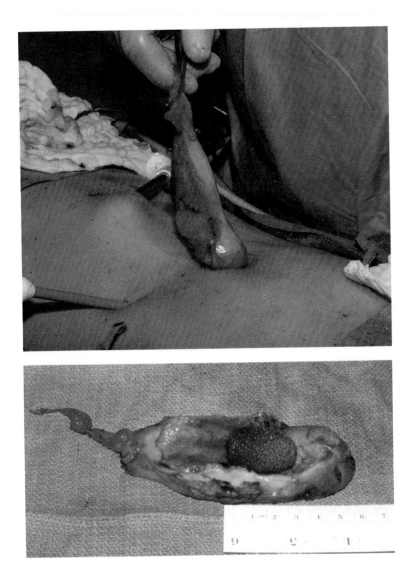

The gallbladder is then easily pulled through the enlarged incision.

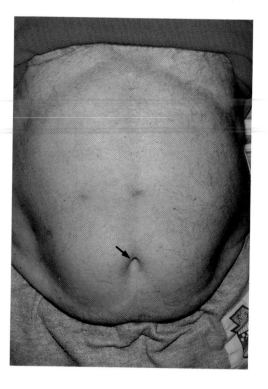

If the extended incision (arrow) continues circumferentially around the navel, the resulting scar will be almost invisible despite its greater length.

Longer incisions do not appear to cause any additional pain or discomfort than the smaller puncture wounds, and the majority of patients will still be able to return home within 24 hours of the procedure.

A single absorbable suture is used to close the umbilical and upper midline fascial openings. Occasionally the upper fascial incision cannot be easily closed in obese patients. We then prefer to leave the defect open rather than extend the skin incision. To date, no complications of interval ventral hernia formation at this location have been reported. A number of laparoscopic surgeons routinely leave this fascial defect open without ill effect. However, we always close the umbilical fascial opening because this site is much more prone to abdominal hernia. The smaller lateral puncture wounds do not require fascial closure. An absorbable subcuticular suture is used to approximate the skin over the larger midline puncture sites. The smaller lateral openings are approximated with Steri-Strips.

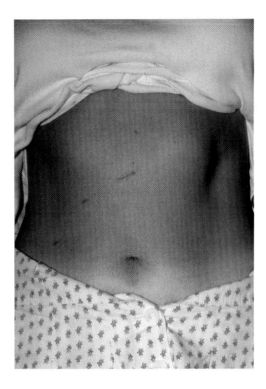

Minimal cosmetic disfigurement is seen 10 days following laparoscopic guided cholecystectomy.

POSTOPERATIVE CARE

The nasogastric tube and urinary catheter are normally removed before the patient leaves the recovery room. Approximately one fifth of our patients are discharged home the afternoon or evening of the procedure. Individuals who have urinary retention, prolonged nausea, or difficulty ambulating or those who live a great distance from the hospital are admitted. The majority of patients are sent home the next morning. We routinely administer a three-dose regimen of a broad-spectrum antibiotic, with the first dose infused 1 hour before the surgical procedure. Initially the operating team was unfamiliar with the various aspects of laparoscopic surgery, and breaks in sterile technique were not uncommon. Although such occurrences are now rare, we continue to administer this short course of antibiotics. To date, we have not encountered any intra-abdominal or superficial wound infections. In addition, we apply a transdermal scopolamine patch prior to the operative procedure. This compound has a duration of action of up to 3 days. It appears to greatly diminish the postoperative nausea resulting from the anesthetic agents and narcotic analgesics.

Postoperative pain is generally minimal, with only minor discomfort at the trocar insertion sites. A few patients complain of mild shoulder pain for up to a week after the procedure, which is believed to be the result of diaphragmatic stretching or irritation from the CO_2. This pain, usually described as an arthralgic-like pain, is easily controlled with oral analgesics and anti-inflammatory agents. Slow insufflation of CO_2 at the onset of the procedure and complete removal of the gas at the end of the procedure will significantly reduce this discomfort. Generally patients are able to assume moderate activity within 48 to 72 hours, and most return to normal activity within a week.

RESULTS

In 1988 Reddick and Olsen[4] reported the first extensive series of patients undergoing laparoscopic guided cholecystectomy in the English literature. They reported the results of their initial 25 patients undergoing laparoscopic surgery and compared them to a similar number of patients with "mini-cholecystectomy." Although this was early in their clinical experience, the advantages were clearly demonstrated. In early 1990 Dubois et al.[5] at the University of Paris reported on their first 36 patients who underwent laparoscopic biliary tract surgery. Their findings of diminished pain, shortened hospital stay, and a more rapid return to normal activity were similar to those of Reddick and Olsen.

Our clinical experience with laparoscopic guided cholecystectomy at the University of Maryland Medical Center began in September 1989.[6] Over 200 procedures were performed in the first year of our program. In only 10 individuals ($<5\%$) was it necessary to convert the laparoscopic operation to a standard laparotomy. Four patients were found to have extensive adhesions, which precluded a safe dissection of the gallbladder and cystic duct. The laparoscopic procedure was aborted in two individuals when unsuspected malignancies were found. Congenital anomalies of the biliary ductal system were identified in two patients, and to avoid a possible ductal injury, these patients underwent exploratory surgery. In addition, there was one cystic duct injury and one common bile duct injury that required laparotomy and repair. A more detailed discussion regarding complications associated with laparoscopic guided cholecystectomy and other laparoscopic procedures is found in Chapter 16. Four of the patients who required laparotomy were among the first 10 patients we treated with this procedure. As our operative experience has increased, the need for conversion to laparotomy has diminished. The ages of patients undergoing laparoscopic surgery at the University of Maryland Medical Center ranges from 16 to 94 years. Twelve patients were operated on for acute cholecystitis, with only one of these individuals requiring an open laparotomy because of inflammatory adhesions. Five patients were admitted for gallstone pancreatitis and underwent laparoscopic cholecystectomy during the same admission without major difficulty. A preoperative ERCP was obtained for each of these patients. In two patients common duct stones were identified and extracted following endoscopic sphincterotomy.

The only postoperative death that occurred was a 77-year-old man who had a myocardial infarction 4 days after an otherwise uneventful laparoscopic cholecystectomy. Although the timing of the death would suggest an association with the surgical procedure, we believe it was unrelated to the fact that the operation was performed under laparoscopic guidance. Most of the major postoperative complications seen after abdominal surgery, such as pneumonia, intra-abdominal or wound infections, urinary tract infections, deep venous thrombosis, or pulmonary emboli, were not seen in patients who underwent laparoscopic cholecystectomy. This is despite the fact that we have performed this procedure on a number of elderly and high-risk individuals.

In our first series of 200 patients who successfully underwent laparoscopic guided cholecystectomy, all but 12 were discharged within 24 hours of the operation. In these individuals a second day was required primarily because of prolonged nausea and vomiting associated with the procedure. Approximately 15% of our patients complained of mild to moderate shoulder pain following laparoscopic surgery, which delayed their recovery. However, this complaint has significantly diminished in the last 100 patients. This appears to be the result of using a much slower gas flow to initially establish pneumoperitoneum and a more concentrated effort at removing all the CO_2 from the abdominal cavity before closing the fascia and skin. Over 90% of our patients were able to return to normal activity within 5 to 7 days of the procedure. Approximately one third returned to their normal routine within 3 to 4 days of surgery.

Our experience with laparoscopic guided cholecystectomy is certainly not unique. A number of other institutions that have started laparoscopic surgical programs have reported similar experiences (Table 8-1). In addition to laparoscopic biliary tract surgery, clinical programs offering laparoscopic appendectomy, laparoscopic assisted bowel resection, laparoscopic pelvic lymphadenectomy, staging laparoscopy for various malignancies, and laparoscopic parietal cell vagotomy have been recently instituted.

Table 8-1. Experience with laparoscopic guided cholecystectomy at selected centers as of August 1, 1990

Surgeon(s)	Location	No. of Patients	Date of First Procedure
F. Dubois	Paris, France	700	June 1987
Reddick and Olsen	Nashville, Tenn.	500	Oct. 1988
Petelin	Kansas City, Mo.	300	Sept. 1989
Daly	Pittsburgh, Penn.	230	Oct. 1989
Corbitt	West Palm Beach, Fla.	225	Dec. 1989
Phillips and Carroll	Los Angeles, Calif.	225	Aug. 1989
Zucker and Bailey	Baltimore, Md.	200	Sept. 1989
Soper	St. Louis, Mo.	170	Nov. 1989
Saye, McKernnan, and Rives	Marrieta, Ga.	150	Oct. 1988
Fitzgibbons and Hinder	Omaha, Neb.	150	Oct. 1989

REFERENCES

1. Cotton PB, Williams CB. Duodenoscopic sphincterotomy. In Cotton PB, Williams CB, eds. Practical Gastrointestinal Endoscopy. Oxford, England: Blackwell, 1982, pp. 86-95.
2. DePlater RMH, Jones ISC. Non-fatal carbon dioxide embolism during laparoscopy. Anaesth Intensive Care 17:359-361, 1989.
3. Corson SL, Batzer SR, Gocial B, Naislin G. Measurement of the force necessary for laparoscopic trocar entry. J Reprod Med 34:282-284, 1989.
4. Reddick EJ, Olsen DO. Laparoscopic laser cholecystectomy: A comparison with mini-lap cholecystectomy. Surg Endosc 3:34-39, 1989.
5. Dubois F, Icard P, Berthelot G, Levard H. Coelioscopic cholecystectomy: Preliminary report of 36 cases. Ann Surg 211:60-62, 1990.
6. Zucker KA, Bailey RB, Gadacz TR, Imbembo AL. Laparoscopic guided cholecystectomy. Am J Surg 161:36-44, 1991.

Laparoscopic Laser Cholecystectomy

Eddie Joe Reddick, M.D.

Gynecologists for years have combined laser technology and laparoscopy to treat intra-abdominal pathologic conditions, but only recently have general surgeons embraced this minimal access approach for the treatment of gastrointestinal disease. Laparoscopic laser cholecystectomy was the first such minimally invasive procedure to gain wide acceptance by general surgeons in the United States.[1-3] Standard cholecystectomy has been the mainstay of treatment for gallstone disease for over a century. Neither the efficacy of this procedure nor its extremely low mortality rate has been questioned. However, the large abdominal incision associated with traditional open cholecystectomy resulted in considerable morbidity in terms of the prolonged hospital stay and recovery interval. In addition the patient is often left with an unsightly scar. Laparoscopic laser cholecystectomy provides all of the benefits of complete gallbladder removal without the cosmetic disfigurement, longer hospitalization, and loss of productivity associated with the traditional procedure.

Laparoscopic laser cholecystectomy was initially used selectively, but with greater operative experience surgeons soon learned the procedure could be performed on almost every patient with gallstone disease. Morbid obesity, multiple stones, large stones, choledocholithiasis, previous abdominal surgery, and acute cholecystitis are no longer considered absolute contraindications to laparoscopic laser cholecystectomy.[4]

PREOPERATIVE EDUCATION

The clinical diagnosis of gallbladder disease is usually made based on a history of right upper abdominal pain, fatty food intolerance, and nausea. Cholelithiasis is then confirmed by a radiographic study such as ultrasonography, oral cholecystography, or a nuclear scan. Occasionally a biliary drainage or stimulation test may be required to diagnose acalculous cholecystitis. Since general anesthesia is usually required, a preoperative laboratory screening test and electrocardiography are performed. Patients should be counseled concerning the possibility of a laparotomy. An open procedure will be required in approximately 3% because adhesions or acute infection will prohibit adequate visualization and safe dissection.[4] Complex common bile duct stones, abnormal ductal or vascular anatomy, as well as surgical misadventures may lead to conversion to open cholecystectomy. It is an unusual case, however, in which bleeding cannot be controlled laparoscopically; therefore most of these conversions to open cholecystectomy can be performed in a controlled fashion.

Many patients erroneously think that laparoscopic laser cholecystectomy is true "belly button" surgery. They must understand that four abdominal incisions will be made, resulting in four small scars.

INSTRUMENTATION
Lasers

The lasers most commonly used in general surgery are the KTP/YAG, argon, Nd:YAG, and CO_2. Each has its own advantages and disadvantages, but all can be used to perform laparoscopic laser cholecystectomy. The KTP 532/YAG laser has an internal configuration that utilizes YAG energy to stimulate the KTP crystal to form the 532 nm green light used for cutting and superficial coagulation. The KTP energy may be changed to YAG energy for deeper coagulation since the machine has both YAG and KTP crystals. Cutting as well as superficial and deep coagulation are accomplished with a single 6 μm quartz fiber, thereby decreasing the need for cautery or tip exchanges. The fiber is disposable but may be recleaned if the tip becomes damaged during a procedure. The fiber cuts on contact and gives a blend of cutting and coagulation if the beam is defocused. Color distortion is minimized by a video filter inserted into the video camera. The argon laser has properties similar to the KTP laser, but considerable color distortion occurs with the use of currently available filters.

With the standard fiber the Nd:YAG is strictly a coagulating laser; however, with the addition of contact scalpel tips it will dissect and cut easily. For added coagulation the cutting tip must be changed or removed so that the bare fiber can be used. Contact tips must be precisely placed on the tissue for adequate cutting and to decrease heat buildup, which will crack the tips. This can be difficult for the beginner learning to work in a two-dimensional video environment. A distinct advantage of the contact tip is lack of forward scatter, alleviating the need for a backstop. Recently sculptured fibers have been introduced for the Nd:YAG laser. These permit cutting and coagulation through the same fiber, although the cutting power does not seem as great as with contact tips and the coagulation seems more superficial than with a bare fiber.

The CO_2 laser has been used more sparingly than fiber lasers for laparoscopic laser cholecystectomy. The beam can cause a destructive tissue effect several centimeters beyond the target tissue, and it has less coagulating ability than the previously described fiber lasers. The energy is more difficult to deliver since it cannot be refracted down a flexible fiber. For these reasons, surgeons have been less enthusiastic about the CO_2 laser in laparoscopy.

Ancillary Equipment

Since visualization is paramount to performance of laparoscopic laser cholecystectomy, a high-resolution video system is essential (see Chapter 2). The dark color of the liver absorbs a large amount of light as the laparoscope and light source are directed toward the right upper quadrant. Therefore the camera aperture must be large enough to allow adequate light return but small enough to allow an adequate depth of field. An automatic iris is sometimes helpful since the camera may have different light requirements, depending on its distance from the gallbladder. Unfortunately some of these work poorly, and each camera must be evaluated on its individual merits. Monitors should be of high quality but easily maintained and adjustable by the operating room personnel. Some of the more sophisticated monitors have a control panel with far too much detail for the average assistant.

Insufflators should have a gas flow of 6 L/min or greater to maintain adequate pneumoperitoneum. Numerous instrument exchanges and evacuation of smoke will overwhelm the output of lesser machines. Recirculating devices are helpful but are sometimes a bulky addition to a procedure that already requires numerous tubes and wires.

Operating Instruments

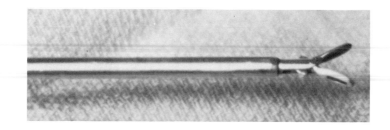

Since the gallbladder is vulnerable to tears during laparoscopic laser chole-cystectomy, dissecting and grasping instruments should be designed with atraumatic jaws, similar to those of a Kelly clamp or DeBakey forceps. The tips should be rounded to decrease the chances of puncturing the gallbladder during retraction.

Grasping forceps should have heavier jaws. Dissecting forceps should be finer and thinner to facilitate blunt removal of peritoneal attachments and adhesions. An angled instrument such as the Maryland dissector (American Surgical Instruments, Pompano, Fla.) may be beneficial in certain situations. All grasping instruments should be insulated to facilitate cauterization of small blood vessels or lymphatics. Cholangiography can be facilitated with the use of a cholangiogram clamp (see Chapter 10). The clamp permits placement of the cholangiogram catheter through the center of the instrument and into the cystic duct. The jaws of the clamp are placed across the entry site into the cystic duct to secure the catheter and prevent leakage of contrast material. A laparoscopic clip applier is essential to the procedure. Ligating the cystic duct and artery with sutures is time consuming and difficult. The applier will markedly expedite the operation.

OPERATING THEATER DESIGN

Laparoscopic laser cholecystectomy requires a vast amount of instrumentation, and the operating theater should be designed to keep the various devices out of the traffic pattern and permit visualization of equipment by operating room personnel.

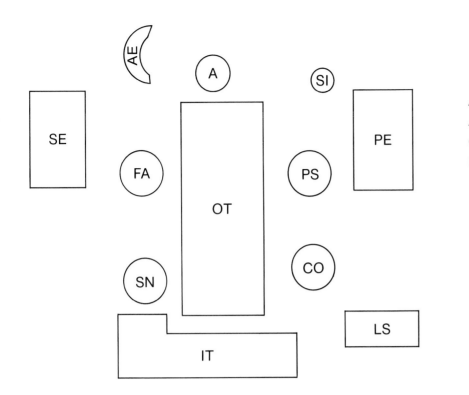

A – Anesthesiologist
AE – Anesthesia equipment
CO – Camera operator
FA – First assistant
IT – Instrument tray
LS – Surgical laser and laser
       safety officer
OT – Operating table
PE – Primary equipment cart
PS – Primary surgeon
SE – Secondary equipment cart
SI – Suction irrigation device
SN – Scrub nurse

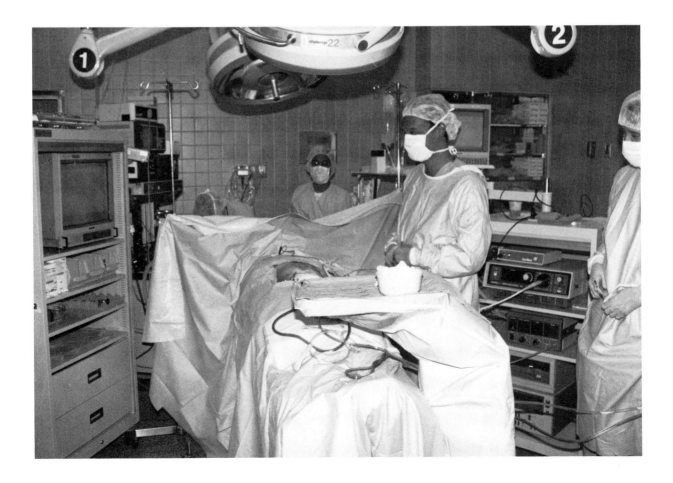

The laser should be placed against a wall away from the traffic pattern with the fiber elevated and brought to the operating table. If the fiber is left on the floor or brought across a frequently traveled area, it often gets broken. Specialized carts safely secure expensive and fragile video monitoring and insufflation equipment. These carts may also store accessory instruments such as the choledoscope, backup camera, laparoscopes, and sutures. The primary equipment cart is positioned so the larger video screen is in direct view of the surgeon and camera operator. Monitors should be placed at 45 degrees from the head of the table to facilitate viewing by the surgeon and his assistants. The surgeon and camera operator stand on the patient's left side. The first assistant and scrub technician stand on the opposite side.

The secondary equipment cart has a smaller video screen attached to a swivel arm that allows it to be positioned for the first assistant.

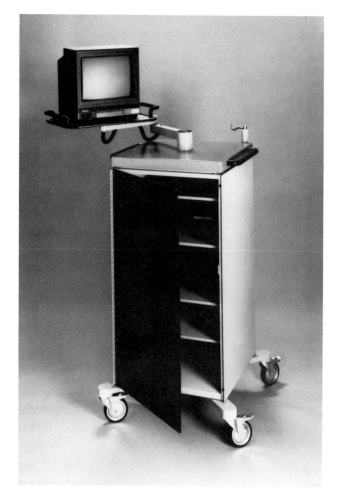

TECHNIQUE

Access to the abdominal cavity is gained by standard laparoscopic techniques. If the patient has not had previous abdominal operations, an insufflation needle is inserted through the umbilicus (see Chapter 8). If the patient has undergone lower abdominal surgery (hysterectomy, appendectomy, etc.), it may be safer to insert the insufflation needle through an upper abdominal site. A position in the midclavicular line, 2 cm below the right costal margin, is the site of choice. After pneumoperitoneum is obtained, a 5 mm trocar is placed through the same site, and a 5 mm laparoscope is used to examine the umbilical area for adhesions. If present, they may be dissected away or the umbilical trocar may be guided around the adhesions under direct vision. If a patient has had extensive abdominal surgery and has no obvious clear site for trocar insertion, an open laparoscopy (Hasson technique) may be utilized (see Chapter 5). This is performed by making a small cutdown in the infraumbilical area and exposing the peritoneum. The blunt Hasson trocar is inserted and fixed with sutures to the peritoneum and fascia, making a seal for insufflation.

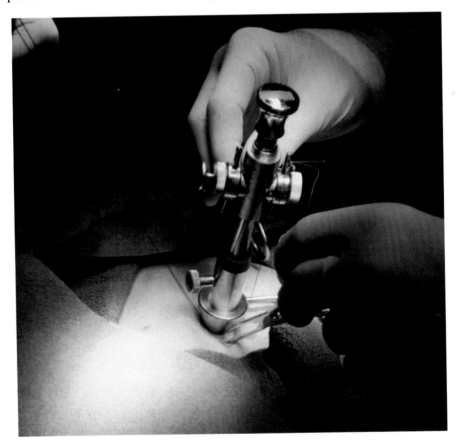

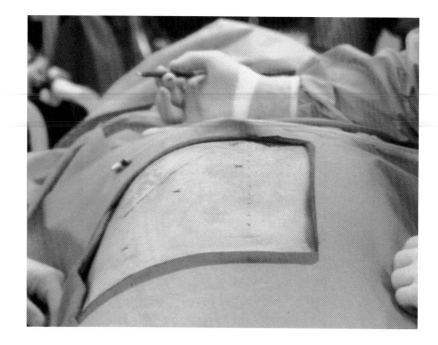

Accurate placement of trocars is essential for optimal retraction, visualization, and dissection angles. A 10 mm trocar placed in the folds of the umbilicus is used for placement of the laparoscope and attached video camera. A second 10 mm trocar placed 5 cm below the xiphoid in the midline is used for dissection and as an entry portal for the clip applicator. Five-millimeter trocars are placed 2 cm below the right costal margin in the midclavicular line and at the level of the umbilicus in the anterior axillary line. Both are utilized for retraction of the gallbladder and liver. The midclavicular trocar site is constant for all body types; however, the lateral trocar may be moved closer to the costal margin in obese patients and closer to the iliac crest in very thin patients. This will allow more maneuverability of the gallbladder fundus in these two extremes of habitus.

Retraction

The dome of the gallbladder is controlled with the lateral grasping forceps and pushed superiorly and laterally (toward the right shoulder). This places the gallbladder on stretch and elevates the liver, simulating the same movements used in traditional open cholecystectomy. The midclavicular forceps controls Hartmann's pouch and places tension on the cystic duct and artery. The gallbladder should be kept on stretch and Hartmann's pouch pulled away from the liver. This maneuver will most effectively expose the triangle of Calot. If Hartmann's pouch is pushed into the liver, the triangle will collapse, making safe dissection impossible. *Failure to follow this technique will make common bile duct injury more likely.*

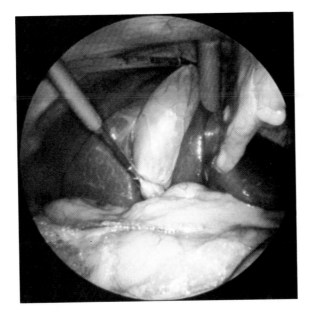

Dissection

Dissection is performed through the upper midline sheath and begins at the neck of the gallbladder and proceeds toward the common bile duct. The cystic duct is identified initially at the neck and then dissected posteriorly and laterally from the surrounding tissues until the cystic–common duct junction is visualized. The cystic artery can be safely dissected at this point, starting at the neck of the gallbladder and working toward the right hepatic artery. All dissection around the triangle of Calot is performed bluntly.

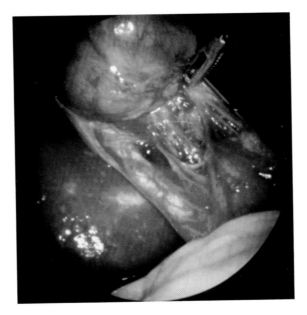

If any bleeding is encountered during the cystic artery dissection, appropriate control (cautery or clip) can be obtained since the other important structures have been identified. If possible the cystic artery should be clipped prior to dividing the cystic duct. Otherwise the proximal end of the vessel may retract into the hepatoduodenal ligament if the artery is torn following division of the cystic duct. Control of the bleeding artery will then be difficult. If the cystic duct remains intact, the surrounding tissues will prevent the torn vessel from retracting out of the operative field. Also, the artery should be clipped and left intact during cholangiography. Should the cystic duct be transected inadvertently, the artery will keep it tethered to the gallbladder and allow for better control.

Cholangiogram

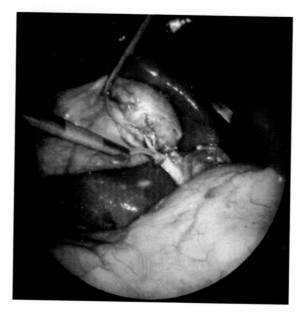

Numerous techniques have been devised for cholangiography and all work equally well (see Chapter 10). The gallbladder may be punctured, drained of bile, and injected with contrast material to obtain a cholecystocholangiogram. Occasionally, however, a cystic duct may be obstructed, prohibiting the flow of dye into the common bile duct. Direct cystic duct cholangiography may be performed by inserting a cholangiogram catheter through the lateral port and into the cystic duct.[5] An alternative method is to make a separate 14-gauge needle puncture through the anterior abdominal wall and pass a small catheter through the bore of the needle and into the cystic duct. The catheter may then be fixed in the cystic duct with a surgical clip or a cholangiogram clamp. Specialized balloon-tipped catheters have been designed (Reddick cystic duct catheter; Ideas for Medicine, Clearwater, Fla.) to remain secure in the cystic duct without specialized clamps or clips.

Radiolucent (disposable) sheaths do not interfere with cholangiography. If radiopaque sheaths are used, they must be positioned parallel to the spine to keep them from overlying the opacified common duct. The upper midline and midclavicular trocar sheaths are the most common offenders.

Laser Dissection

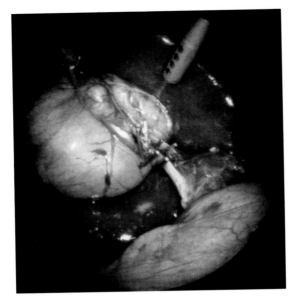

After cholangiography is completed and the catheter has been removed, the cystic duct is clipped. The laser fiber is introduced through a suction-irrigation catheter through the upper midline cannula. The duct and artery are then transected with the laser. When using the KTP, argon, CO_2, or YAG laser with a sculptured fiber, the duct and artery should be positioned so any forward scatter of the laser will be absorbed by the liver. This will result in only superficial injury to the liver capsule.

The gallbladder should be pulled laterally and the laser utilized to transect all the attachments to the liver. Most bleeding can be controlled by defocusing the laser (KTP) beam. Defocusing is accomplished by retracting the fiber 2 to 5 mm from the tissue, thereby decreasing the energy applied to the area and allowing coagulation. Minimal coagulation effect can be gained with the YAG laser with a cutting contact tip. Therefore cautery may have to be used more often with the YAG laser to ensure hemostasis.

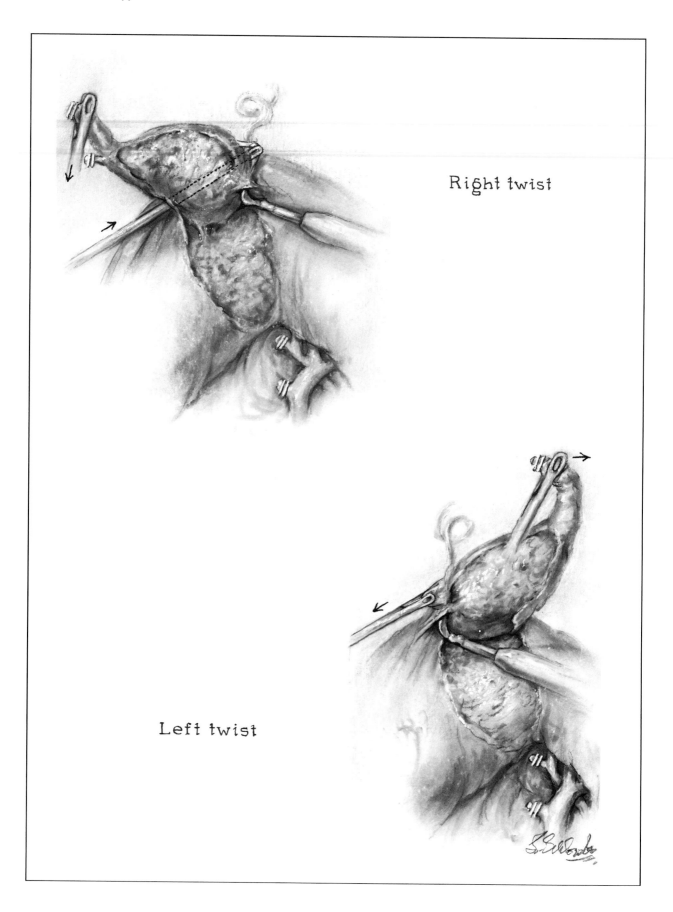

Right twist

Left twist

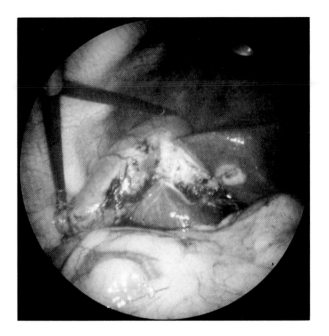

The dissection then continues, exposing the peritoneal attachments of the gallbladder on either side. This can be accomplished by manipulating the lateral and midclavicular grasping forceps, causing a twisting motion on the gallbladder. To expose the inferior peritoneal attachment, the midclavicular trocar is pushed medially and superiorly and the lateral trocar, holding the fundus of the gallbladder, is pulled inferiorly and laterally (left twist). The superior peritoneal attachment can be exposed using exactly opposite motions (i.e., the midclavicular trocar is pulled inferiorly and laterally, and the lateral trocar is pushed superiorly and medially [right twist]).

Should a perforation of the gallbladder occur, dissection should continue until enough gallbladder wall is freed from the liver bed to allow a grasping forceps to control the opening (see p. 159). A pretied suture (EndoLoop) is passed through the upper midline sheath and tied around the hole. Scissors are passed through a separate trocar to cut the suture.

Near the end of the dissection care should be taken to ensure hemostasis of the bed. After the gallbladder is completely removed from the liver bed, it becomes difficult to expose the bed to check for bleeding.

Once hemostasis is ensured, the gallbladder can be dissected free and the abdomen irrigated and suctioned dry. A solution of normal saline solution with heparin (5000 units/L) and antibiotics are used for irrigation. Heparin will decrease clot formation, thereby allowing easier aspiration of spilled blood.

Extraction of the Gallbladder

The gallbladder is most easily removed through the umbilical puncture site since only a single layer of fascia is present. The camera and laparoscope are removed from the umbilical trocar and placed through the upper midline sheath. The gallbladder is held over the liver near its neck with grasping forceps placed through the lateral sheath. A forceps is placed through the umbilical port to grasp the neck of the gallbladder. The neck of the gallbladder is pulled up into the umbilical sheath and the sheath pulled out of the abdominal cavity. This sometimes leaves a distended gallbladder bulb inside the abdominal cavity.

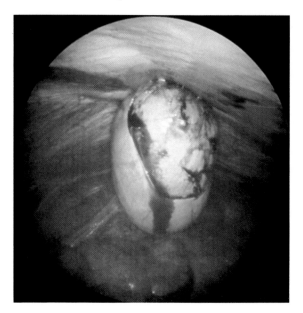

The neck of the gallbladder is extracted out of the abdominal cavity and just outside of the umbilicus. Gentle traction on the neck of the gallbladder will usually force the bile through the umbilical fascial opening, much like sand through an hourglass.

If the gallbladder will not come through the small fascial opening, the neck of the gallbladder can be opened and a small suction device placed through it to decompress the gallbladder.

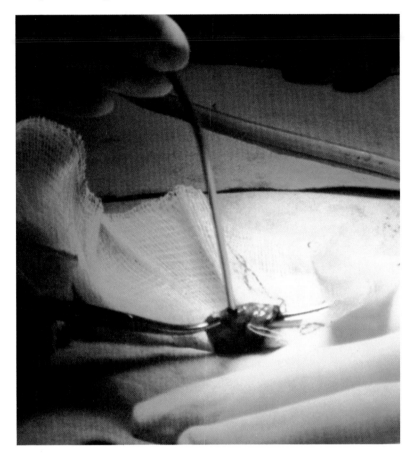

If stones prevent the gallbladder from coming through the fascial opening, they may be crushed or removed with a ring forceps placed through the neck of the gallbladder. If a stone is still too large to allow removal of the gallbladder, the fascial opening may be enlarged a millimeter at a time until the gallbladder and stone are delivered or the stone may be fractured with an ultrasonic device or pulsed-dye laser. The umbilical fascial defect is closed with a single figure-of-eight suture. Skin incisions are closed with subcuticular sutures and covered with plastic dressings.

POSTOPERATIVE CARE

Nearly half the patients undergoing laparoscopic laser cholecystectomy can have outpatient procedures[6]; those who must be hospitalized can return home within 24 hours. Nausea, urinary retention, and pain are the primary reasons for hospital admission. Nausea can be controlled with a 1.5 mg scopolamine patch placed behind the patient's ear at the termination of surgery. Pain may be decreased by the instillation of local anesthetics into the puncture sites. There is usually minimal discomfort, which may be alleviated by mild oral analgesics. Patients may complain of right shoulder and chest pain for 24 to 36 hours after surgery. This is self-limited and will resolve with only symptomatic treatment. Patients may have a clear liquid diet the day of surgery, followed by a regular diet the following morning. Ileus has been a problem only in an occasional older patient. Activities may be resumed without restrictions at the patient's discretion. Most patients may drive and resume other routine activities within 72 hours of surgery. All patients should be able to return to work within a week regardless of their occupation.

An office visit is scheduled 1 week after surgery to remove dressings and assess the patient's recovery. The patient may be discharged from care at that point.

SPECIAL PROBLEMS

Although most gallbladders are easily removed using the previously described technique, some pose special problems. The acute gallbladder or one with hydrops is sometimes so tense that grasping it becomes impossible. These gallbladders should be decompressed through the fundus by a laparoscopic needle passed through the lateral or midclavicular ports.

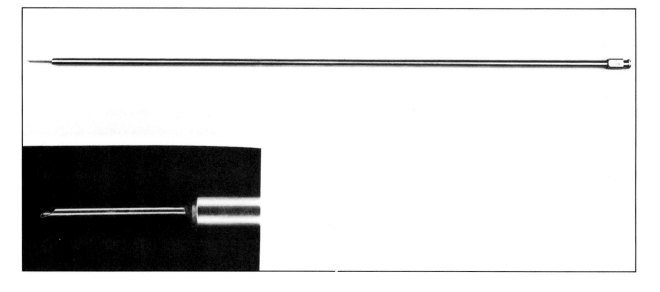

The hole in the fundus can be controlled easily with the lateral forceps grasping the gallbladder in that area. If the gallbladder wall is still too thick to hold securely, an instrument with small teeth may be used. Since this is a traumatic forceps, care should be taken to grasp only the serosa of the gallbladder to preclude tearing a hole in the gallbladder wall.

If the gallbladder becomes torn during the operation, a decision must be made whether to terminate the laparoscopic procedure. If the hole is small, it can be controlled with an EndoLoop as previously described. However, if the hole is large or the gallbladder is torn in half, it may become impossible to maintain traction on the gallbladder, which prohibits safe dissection. If this is the case, it may be preferable to abort the laparoscopic procedure and open the patient's abdomen.

Common bile duct stones may be found during cholangiography and force a decision concerning open common bile duct exploration. Although opening the patient's abdomen at this point is an acceptable alternative, I prefer to attempt removing the stones through a flexible (fiberoptic) chole-dochoscopy (see Chapter 10). A flexible ureteroscope with bidirectional control and a working channel can be inserted over a guidewire through the cystic duct and into the common bile duct. Stones can be removed with a Dormier basket or broken up with a pulsed-dye laser or electromechanical lithotriptor.[7] If these methods fail to clear the duct of stones, endoscopic retrograde cholangiopancreatography with papillotomy and stone removal may be performed the day following surgery. Selective use of chole-dochotomy through the laparoscope has been performed, but laparoscopic suturing of the common bile duct is tedious and should only be undertaken by surgeons skilled in suturing techniques.

CONCLUSION

Most patients with documented gallbladder disease can be considered candidates for laparoscopic laser cholecystectomy using the methods described herein. After mastering the technique of laparoscopic laser cholecystectomy, the laparoscopic surgeon should approach an open rate of 5% or less. The incidence of bile duct injuries should be no greater than that for open cholecystectomy. Since there are no large open incisions with subsequent tissue trauma and hypoxia, the incidence of wound infection should be markedly reduced over that for open cholecystectomy.

REFERENCES

1. Reddick E, Olsen D. Laparoscopic laser cholecystectomy: A comparison with mini-lap cholecystectomy. Surg Endosc 3:34-39, 1989.
2. Reddick EJ, Olsen D, Daniell J, Saye W, McKernan B, Miller W, Hoback M. Laparoscopic laser cholecystectomy. Laser Med Surg News Adv 7:38-40, 1989.
3. Reddick EJ, Baird D, Daniell J, Olsen D, Saye W. Laparoscopic laser cholecystectomy. Ann Chir Gynecol (in press).
4. Zucker KA, Bailey RW, Gadacz TR, Imbembo AL. Laparoscopic guided cholecystectomy. Am J Surg 161:36-44, 1991.
5. Reddick E, Alexander W, Bailey A, Baird D, Olsen D, Price N, Pruitt R. Laparoscopic laser cholecystectomy and choledocholithiasis. Surg Endosc (in press).
6. Reddick EJ, Olsen D. Outpatient laparoscopic laser cholecystectomy. Am J Surg (in press).
7. Perissat J, Collet D, Belliard R. Gallstones: Laparoscopic treatment—Cholecystectomy, cholecystotomy lithotripsy. Surg Endosc 4:1-5, 1990.

Laparoscopic Cholangiography and Management of Choledocholithiasis

Robert W. Bailey, M.D.
Karl A. Zucker, M.D.

Any new procedure such as laparoscopic guided cholecystectomy should achieve results that are as safe and effective as the traditional open procedure. The ability to perform intraoperative cholangiography during laparoscopic biliary tract surgery, therefore, is essential. In addition to determining the presence of choledocholithiasis, cholangiography has become an important adjuvant for evaluating the ductal anatomy during laparoscopic cholecystectomy. Common bile duct injuries are a well-known complication of biliary tract surgery and may occur more often during the learning phase when a surgeon first begins performing laparoscopic cholecystectomy.[1] Many of these injuries may be avoided if a cholangiogram is obtained. This is especially important in those patients with complicated biliary tract disease.

Unlike open cholecystectomy, common bile duct stones that are discovered during the preoperative evaluation or during laparoscopic cholangiography are usually not managed via a formal common bile duct exploration. Therefore it is important that surgeons performing laparoscopic biliary tract surgery be aware of the available alternatives in the treatment of choledocholithiasis. The operative techniques involved in performing laparoscopic cholangiography as well as currently available options in the management of common bile duct stones form the basis of this chapter.

PATIENT SELECTION

Prior to performing laparoscopic guided cholecystectomy an attempt should be made to screen patients for choledocholithiasis. The majority of patients with persistent common bile duct stones can be identified prior to surgery. Patients may give a history of abdominal pain distinctly different from their typical gallbladder symptoms. Occasionally such episodes will be associated with transient jaundice or dark-colored urine. Usually such patients have already sought medical attention, and a careful review of their previous medical records may reveal elevations in liver transaminases, alkaline phosphatase, or pancreatic enzymes (i.e., amylase or lipase). Choledocholithiasis is also suggested by the presence of intra- or extrahepatic ductal dilatation on the abdominal ultrasound or CT scan. If there is reason to suspect persistent common bile duct stones on the basis of the history, laboratory tests, or imaging studies, endoscopic retrograde cholangiopancreatography (ERCP) is advised. If choledocholithiasis is confirmed, endoscopic sphincterotomy and stone extraction are performed during the same procedure. In an experienced biliary endoscopy center, sphincterotomy and stone extraction should be successful in over 90% of patients.[2] ERCP and sphincterotomy may not be successful in certain situations: common bile duct stones >20 mm in diameter, the presence of impacted intrahepatic stones, prior gastric surgery such as a Billroth II gastrectomy, large duodenal diverticulum adjacent to the ampulla, distal common bile duct stenosis, and of course an inexperienced endoscopist.[2] All reasonable attempts are made to clear the common bile duct of stones prior to laparoscopic cholecystectomy since we cannot routinely extract these stones during laparoscopic surgery at the present time. In the near future, however, methods of exploring the biliary tract with the choledochoscope and other innovative approaches may be developed to the point that this will be possible.

LAPAROSCOPIC CHOLANGIOGRAPHY
Indications

When to perform intraoperative cholangiography continues to be a controversial issue. The primary purpose of this chapter is to provide insight into the technical aspects of laparoscopic cholangiography and not to debate the use of *selective* vs. *routine* intraoperative cholangiography. Although a strong case for selective cholangiography can be made on the basis of available clinical data,[3-5] laparoscopic cholecystectomy is a new procedure and clinical experience is limited. Indications for laparoscopic cholangiography cannot be compared directly to standards established for open cholecystectomy. Issues such as training, operative experience, and the need for precise definition of the ductal anatomy are important in determining the need for laparoscopic cholangiography. The latter may be especially true during the learning phase of this procedure.

Inherent limitations of laparoscopic surgery may result in surgeons depending more on the information gleaned from cholangiography than with open cholecystectomy. Although current video imaging systems allow for excellent visualization of the gallbladder and cystic ducts, many surgeons are reluctant to completely mobilize and identify the junction of the cystic and common bile duct. This is especially true in patients with acute or subacute cholecystitis. Inflammation near the common bile duct may make dissection tedious. If bleeding occurs in this region, it may prove difficult to control and may increase the risk of a ductal injury. In such circumstances the surgeon may prefer to dissect only the proximal cystic duct and gallbladder neck, relying on the cholangiogram to visualize the junction with the common bile duct. In many instances laparoscopic surgeons routinely prefer to limit dissection to the gallbladder neck area to avoid possible injury to the ductal or vascular structures. This approach often results in a longer cystic duct remnant than is normally left after open cholecystectomy, and stones may be left within the cystic duct stump that may later result in symptomatic choledocholithiasis.

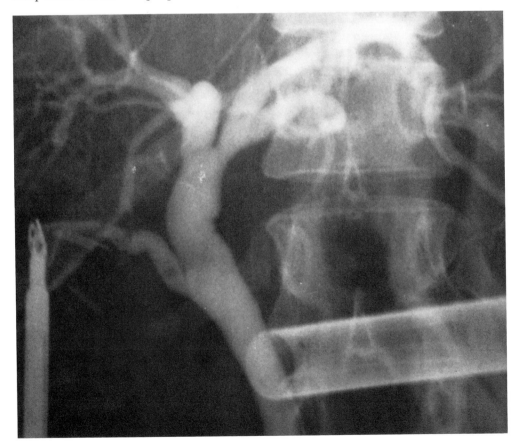

A high-quality cholangiogram should demonstrate a retained stone within the cystic duct stump and allow the surgeon to take appropriate action. Congenital anomalies of the biliary tract are also difficult to identify during laparoscopic surgery and may result in an increased incidence of ductal injuries (see Chapter 16). The distortion of the hepatic and common bile ducts occurring with cephalad retraction of the gallbladder and right lobe of the liver compound this problem (see Chapter 8). Routine cholangiography may help identify these anomalies and reduce the risk of injury.

Although cholangiography may not be indicated for every patient who has a cholecystectomy, it will eventually be required at some point. Unless the technique is practiced and mastered, it may not be possible to perform laparoscopic cholangiography when it is indicated. Furthermore, laparoscopic cholecystectomy is under intense scrutiny by the medical community, and demonstrating the feasibility of and indications for laparoscopic cholangiography is of important clinical value.

Technique

Cystic duct cholangiography is the most accepted method of intraoperative cholangiography. Although cholangiography via direct injection into the gallbladder or common bile duct is possible, this discussion will center on techniques involving cannulation of the cystic duct.

The components essential for the successful completion of laparoscopic cholangiography include (1) the ability to maintain exposure of the gallbladder and cystic duct during the procedure, (2) opening the cystic duct for access to the biliary tract, (3) a catheter for the injection of contrast material, (4) a method to introduce this catheter into the abdominal cavity, (5) a means to guide the catheter into the cystic duct, and (6) a method of securing the catheter within the cystic duct that also prevents extravasation of contrast material. A number of surgeons, having recognized the importance of performing cholangiography, have independently developed their own techniques for this procedure. These clinical investigators have shown that laparoscopic cholangiography can be performed with the same efficiency and quality as during open cholecystectomy. The instrumentation necessary to perform laparoscopic cholangiography will vary according to the specific technique employed. The most popular method requires the use of specially designed cholangiogram clamps (Olsen cholangiography fixation clamp; Karl Storz Endoscopy, Culver City, Calif.).

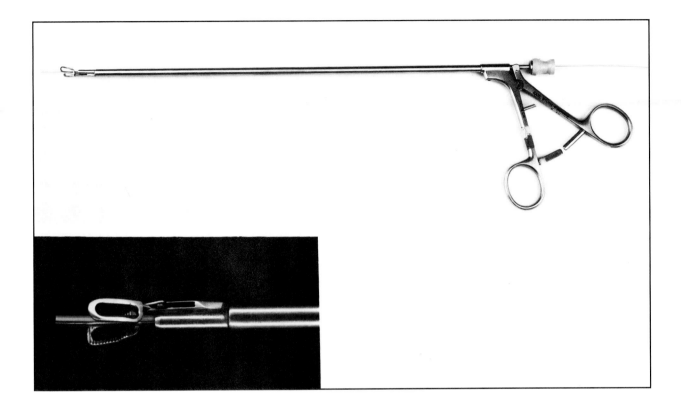

In the following discussion the general principles and techniques of laparoscopic cholangiography will be introduced. This is followed by a description of the more commonly used alternative methods that do not employ this type of instrument.

Method using specially designed cholangiogram clamps

An essential feature of laparoscopic cholangiography is the ability to maintain exposure of the gallbladder and cystic duct. During routine laparoscopic cholecystectomy, four portals of entry are made into the abdominal cavity. The right upper abdominal 5 mm portals are used to provide retraction of the gallbladder. The most lateral (anterior axillary) 5 mm instrument is used to retract the dome of the gallbladder cephalad and allows visualization of the fundus and neck of the gallbladder. Additional retraction on the neck of the gallbladder is usually required to provide proper exposure for dissection and eventual ligation of the cystic duct. Therefore partial or complete loss of exposure by removing either 5 mm grasping forceps during cholangiography will make insertion of the cystic duct catheter difficult. Although the midepigastric (10 mm) cannula may be used to introduce the cholangiogram catheter, the midline approach is awkward since the cystic duct is situated more lateral. In addition, if a specialized cholangiogram clamp is inserted from the midline, the radiopaque shaft of the instrument may impair visualization of the bile ducts. This problem is overcome by removing the midclavicular forceps from the neck of the gallbladder and placing it through the midepigastric portal.

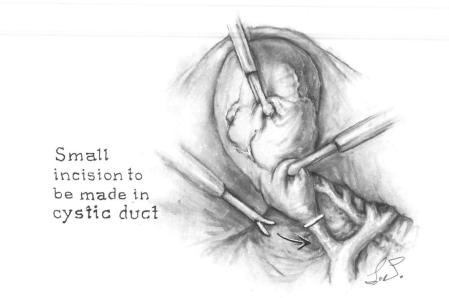

Small incision to be made in cystic duct

The forceps are then used for retraction at the same site. The midclavicular cannula is then available to introduce the instruments necessary to perform cholangiography. The lateral 5 mm grasping forceps, attached to the fundus of the gallbladder, is left in place. This maneuver will maintain exposure for opening the cystic duct and inserting the cholangiogram catheter.

Several different types of catheters have been used successfully for laparoscopic cholangiography. One obvious requirement is that the catheter be long enough to pass through the abdominal wall and reach the cystic duct. This distance is increased during laparoscopic surgery because of the pneumoperitoneum. For the most part, any catheter that is used for cystic duct cholangiography during open cholecystectomy may also be used for laparoscopic cholangiography. We routinely use a 24-inch plastic central venous access catheter (Intracath; Desert Medical Inc., Sandy, Utah). The tip of this catheter may be beveled slightly prior to insertion into the abdomen to facilitate its entry into the cystic duct. Another catheter commonly used during "open" cholangiography is the Taut catheter, which has a flange at one end (operative cholangiogram catheter; Taut Inc., Geneva, Ill.). This flange was designed to secure the catheter within the cystic duct during open cholecystectomy by tying a suture around the duct.

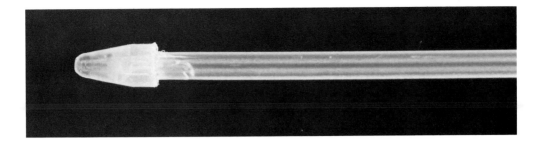

Since the Taut catheter is a very stiff device, care must be taken not to perforate the back wall of the cystic duct or common bile duct during insertion. The limited tactile sensation afforded by laparoscopic surgery makes this more of a concern than with open cholecystectomy. Another catheter, recently developed specifically for laparoscopic cholangiography, is 5 mm in diameter with a curved and tapered tip at one end (American Catheter Corporation, Danielson, Conn.). This larger catheter was designed to fit tightly within the cystic duct and therefore eliminate the need for a suture, surgical clip, or specially designed clamps.

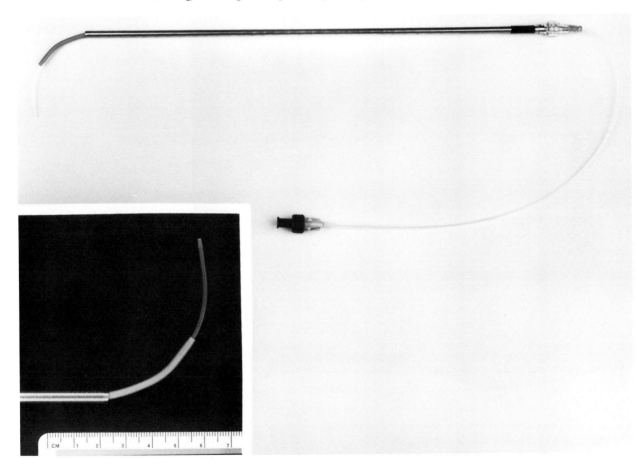

Experience with this device is still limited, and its ability to remain within the cystic duct without additional control is not known at this time. One potential disadvantage of this catheter is its larger size, which may limit its use when attempting to cannulate small-caliber cystic ducts (<5 mm diameter). Another option many laparoscopic surgeons prefer is guiding small ureteral catheters into the cystic duct. These catheters come in a variety of sizes and incorporate a tapered, flexible tip that minimizes the risk of ductal perforation. Additional catheters will undoubtedly be designed that offer distinct advantages over the current models.

An opening must be made in the cystic duct for insertion of the cholangiogram catheter. If the surgeon is confident of the anatomy near the proximal cystic duct, a single surgical clip may be placed where the cystic duct joins the gallbladder. This avoids leakage of bile or small stones after the duct is opened. Curved or straight microscissors are then inserted through the midclavicular cannula and directed toward the cystic duct. This must be done with caution as the tips of these scissors are extremely sharp.

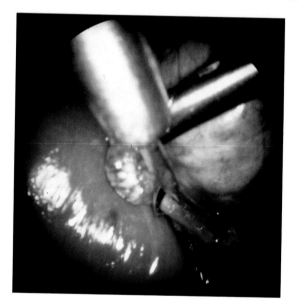

The microscissors are used to make a small opening into the cystic duct. Care must be taken to avoid complete transection of the duct. If this occurs, it is almost impossible to guide the catheter into the lumen of the cystic duct. After incising the cystic duct, the scissors are withdrawn from the cannula and replaced with the Olsen cholangiography fixation clamp, which has a central lumen and two atraumatic ring forceps at the distal tip. The cholangiogram catheter is introduced through the lumen of the instrument and then guided into the cystic duct by the ring forceps.

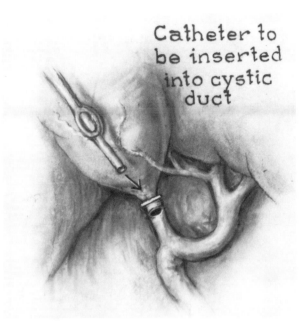

The same atraumatic forceps are then applied around the catheter as it enters the cystic duct. These forceps secure the catheter within the duct and prevent extravasation of contrast material.

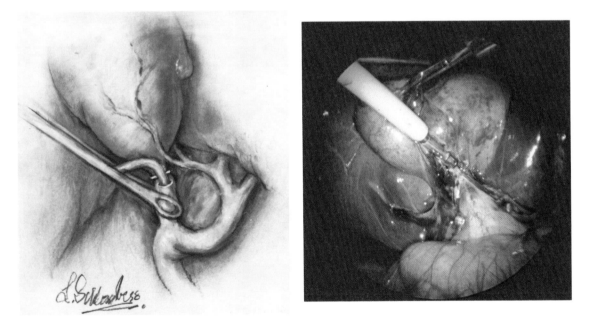

Use of this instrument eliminates the need for additional punctures or trocar placement to introduce the cholangiogram catheter. In addition, sutures or clips are not needed to hold the catheter in place, thereby saving the time it takes to apply and remove them. The cholangiogram clamp used to secure the duct must remain in the abdomen during x-ray exposure. If not held by the surgeon, this clamp tends to fall toward the patient's right side. This motion causes the distal tip of the clamp to move medially and override the common bile duct.

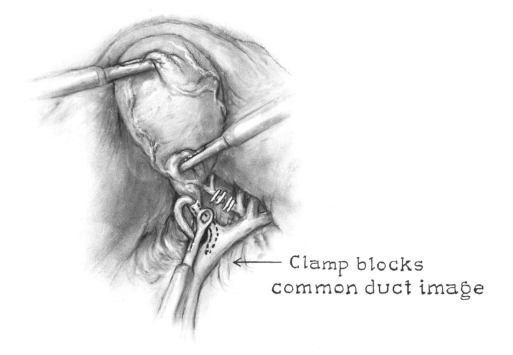

Clamp blocks
common duct image

This may result in the clamp partially obstructing the flow of contrast to the more proximal ducts as well as obscuring the radiographic visualization of the cystic and common bile duct junction. If the proximal sheath is tethered externally toward the midline with a suture, the distal tip of the clamp will remain lateral to the cystic and common bile duct junction.

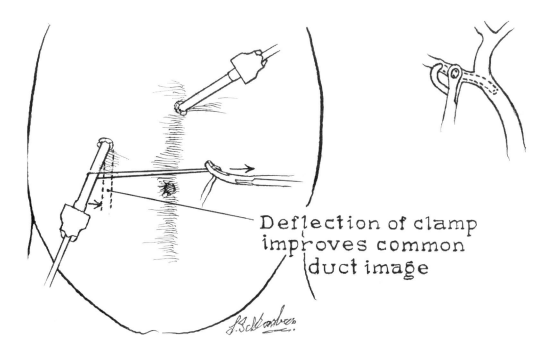

Deflection of clamp
improves common
duct image

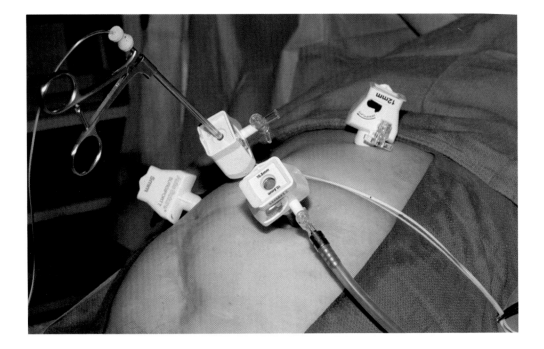

Once the cholangiogram catheter has been secured within the duct, several maneuvers may help avoid inadvertent removal of the catheter. If the grasping forceps on the neck of the gallbladder are not removed, they may interfere with radiographic visualization of the bile ducts. They should be removed in such a manner that the catheter is not accidentally dislodged. Release of the forceps from the fundus of the gallbladder results in the entire liver falling down to its normal anatomic location. This will, by definition, pull the common and cystic ducts inferiorly and posteriorly in the abdomen. Sudden release of the gallbladder may create excessive tension on the catheter, which is fixed in position by the cholangiogram clamp. The forceps should be backed slowly out of the sheath prior to release; at the same time the cystic duct clamp is advanced in the same direction the common bile and cystic ducts are moving. We routinely infuse 5 to 7 ml of contrast material into the catheter prior to removing the grasping forceps. In the event that the catheter is pulled from the cystic duct, this initial injection will usually provide sufficient contrast to visualize the common bile duct and document flow into the duodenum. If reusable radiopaque laparoscopic sheaths are used, they must be positioned away from the underlying bile ducts. However, this may prove difficult if four or more of these metal cannulas have been used. For this reason we routinely use radiolucent disposable cannulas (SurgiPort; United States Surgical Corporation, Norwalk, Conn.) if there is a possibility a cholangiogram must be obtained.

The laparoscope is subsequently removed from the abdomen and the patient moved from the reverse Trendelenburg to the supine position. Additional contrast material (5 to 7 ml) is infused through the catheter and a standard x-ray film obtained.

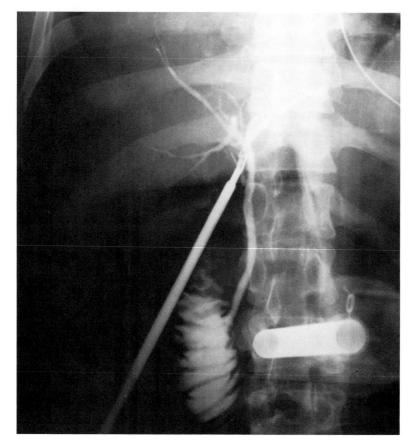

Occasionally the proximal hepatic duct and intrahepatic ducts may not adequately fill with contrast. Placing the patient in a slight head-down position facilitates filling of the upper tracts. While the surgeon waits for the radiograph to be developed, the patient is returned to the reverse Trendelenburg position, the laparoscope reinserted into the umbilical cannula, and traction on the fundus of the gallbladder reapplied. The operation then proceeds normally from this point with the remaining clips (or sutures) placed on the cystic duct and artery.

Alternative methods

There are a number of alternative techniques for introducing a catheter into the cystic duct. The cholangiogram catheter may be inserted through one of the laparoscopic sheaths using a suture introducer (with a diaphragm at one end to prevent air leak) or an aspiration needle.

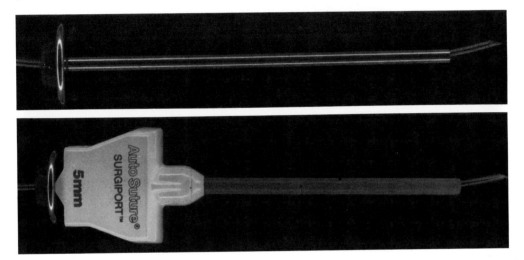

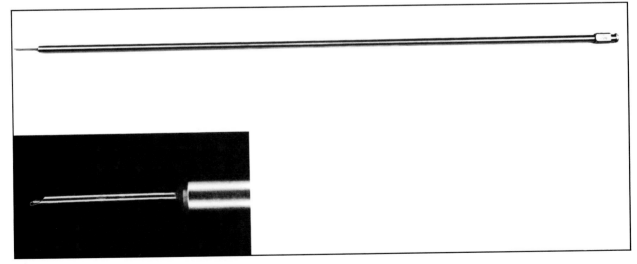

If the catheter is introduced by some means other than a cholangiogram clamp, it will need to be directed into the cystic duct with either a 5 mm grasping forceps or laparoscopic needle holder.

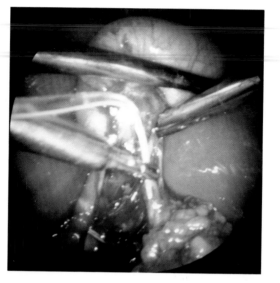

A catheter introduced by one of these methods must be secured within the cystic duct by either a surgical clip or suture. Although laparoscopic sutures can be placed around the duct and catheter, these often prove awkward and time consuming to use. Most surgeons have employed surgical clips to secure the catheter. Once the catheter is in place, a laparoscopic clip applier is introduced through the upper midline cannula. A single clip is then loosely applied around the duct and catheter. This is necessary not only to secure the catheter within the duct but also to prevent extravasation of contrast.

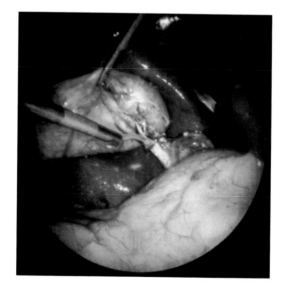

When this method is used, the wide flange of the Taut cholangiogram catheter may help prevent inadvertent dislodgment of the catheter. A major disadvantage of this technique is that one of the lateral cannulas must be used to introduce the catheter into the abdominal cavity. A second cannula and instrument are also required to guide the catheter into the duct. Therefore only one grasping forceps is available to provide exposure of the cystic and common bile duct. Occasionally this may prove inadequate, especially in patients with extensive inflammatory adhesions near the neck of the gallbladder or in very obese individuals. Although the upper midline sheath may be used to temporarily insert a retraction instrument, it must be removed later since this cannula is used to insert the clip applier or sutures to secure the catheter within the duct. If proper exposure cannot be maintained with one grasping forceps, it may be necessary to insert a fifth cannula. This portal may then be used to introduce the cholangiogram catheter or for placement of the second retraction instrument. An additional 5 mm abdominal puncture causes little if any additional postoperative discomfort or cosmetic disfigurement and should be used if it will facilitate the exposure.

Another option is to puncture the anterior abdominal wall with a standard IV needle and sheath, remove the needle, and insert the catheter through the remaining sheath.

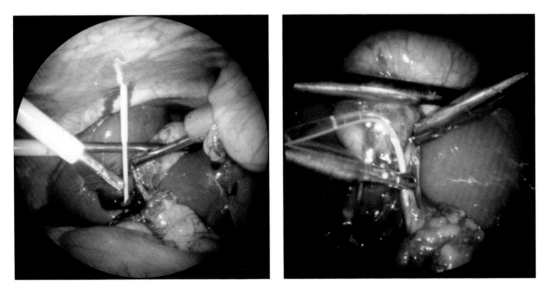

This direct puncture technique does not require repositioning or removal of instruments and thereby saves time. It also allows both lateral cannulas to be used to introduce grasping forceps on the gallbladder and maintain exposure. To prevent excessive air leak it is important that the diameter of the catheter and the IV sheath are similar. Therefore catheters with a wide flange cannot be used.

Although each of the techniques described has its advantages and disadvantages, the final decision will ultimately depend on instrument availability, experience, and personal preference.

INTRAOPERATIVE MANAGEMENT OF CHOLEDOCHOLITHIASIS

As mentioned previously, all patients are screened for choledocholithiasis preoperatively. If common duct stones are suspected, ERCP is performed. When stones are identified within the common bile duct, endoscopic retrieval is usually successful. If this is not feasible, the patient may require an open laparotomy and common bile duct exploration. This should, however, be an uncommon occurrence. More controversial is the management of common bile duct stones discovered during operative cholangiography. Currently, several different therapeutic options are available. The laparoscopic procedure may be converted to a laparotomy and common bile duct exploration. Alternatively, the laparoscopic cholecystectomy may be completed and the patient followed up using ERCP. If choledocholithiasis is confirmed, a sphincterotomy and stone extraction are performed. A third and more liberal approach is to complete the laparoscopic cholecystectomy and perform ERCP on selected patients only.

Aborting the laparoscopic procedure to perform an open common bile duct exploration on the basis of an abnormal cholangiogram appears to be the most conservative therapeutic approach. The vast majority of these patients, however, can undergo postoperative ERCP and successful removal of common bile duct stones. Although this is an invasive procedure with a major complication rate of approximately 1% to 2%, it is usually tolerated far better than an open laparotomy and common bile duct exploration.[2] Patients with very large stones or other pathologic conditions that would make such an approach unsuccessful should have been detected during the preoperative evaluation. Therefore the likelihood of encountering a patient unable to undergo successful endoscopic stone retrieval and requiring an interval laparotomy and duct exploration should be extremely uncommon. However, our patients are always informed of this possibility.

At the University of Maryland Medical Center we recommend completing the laparoscopic procedure and selectively obtaining a postoperative ERCP. The vast majority of our patients with abnormal operative cholangiograms were found to have normal-sized ducts with only a small defect(s) visible on the x-ray film. Previous experience has shown that small stones should clear the common bile duct without major sequelae.[6] This would appear to be especially true if the patient has not had prior symptoms of choledocholithiasis. In addition, the incidence of false positive laparoscopic cholangiograms may be slightly higher than encountered with the open procedure. During laparoscopic surgery the abdomen is distended under pressure with CO_2. Opening the cystic duct and introducing a catheter may allow gas bubbles to enter the biliary tract. Although this is not a common event, it should be considered when interpreting the cholangiogram. Therefore it is our recommendation that when the operative cholangiogram demonstrates only a small defect within a normal-sized common bile duct, the laparoscopic procedure should be completed. The patient is then told that another endoscopic procedure may be necessary in the future. If larger stones are found within a dilated common bile duct (suggesting obstruction), we advise the patient to undergo ERCP during the same hospitalization.

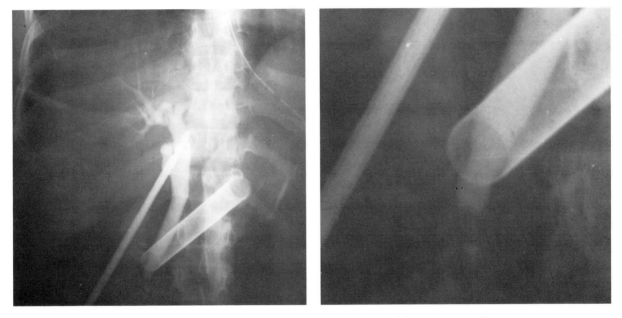

Dilated common bile duct with two stones visible near ampulla.

In our series of over 175 patients undergoing laparoscopic cholangiograms only 12 patients were found to have one or more defects within the common bile duct suggesting the possibility of choledocholithiasis. Two of these patients underwent ERCP and sphincterotomy during the same hospitalization. The remaining 10 patients were told the findings and possible therapeutic options. With a normal-sized duct, small stones (<2 to 3 mm diameter), and no prior history of stone passage, the subsequent risk of developing an acute obstruction of the common bile duct was considered minimal. These patients were followed up closely for any subsequent biliary complaints. Only two individuals developed symptoms suggestive of possible persistent common bile duct stones. Both of these patients underwent successful sphincterotomy and stone extraction. The majority of our patients with abnormal cholangiograms thus avoided an additional expensive and invasive procedure.

Most laparoscopic surgeons in the United States advise their patients to undergo routine ERCP if a positive cholangiogram is obtained. Very few recommend aborting the laparoscopic procedure and performing an open common bile duct exploration. No information is available as to how many surgeons recommend selective postoperative ERCP under such circumstances. Unfortunately experience is insufficient at this time to determine which of these three approaches is the safest and most cost effective.

When laparoscopic cholecystectomy was first introduced in 1987, therapeutic options were limited to those described above. The treatment of common bile duct stones during laparoscopic surgery has been the focus of intense clinical investigation. Laparoscopic choledochoscopy and even common bile duct exploration have recently been described in selected patients.[7] The most established method involves the introduction of a flexible choledochoscope into the common bile duct. Several models have controllable, deflectable tips that facilitate cannulation of the duct and allow for the manipulation of the scope within the biliary tree.

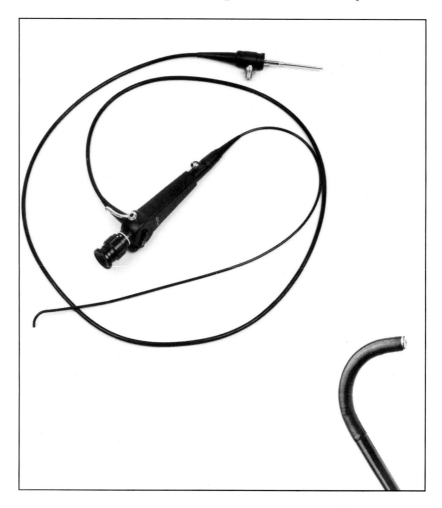

At the present time the safest approach to the common bile duct appears to be through the cystic duct. This technique avoids extensive dissection of the common bile duct and minimizes the risk of major biliary or vascular injury. A fiberoptic choledochoscope is usually inserted through the most lateral 5 mm laparoscopic cannula (anterior axillary site) and directed into the cystic duct opening and then into the common bile duct to visualize any stones within the ducts.

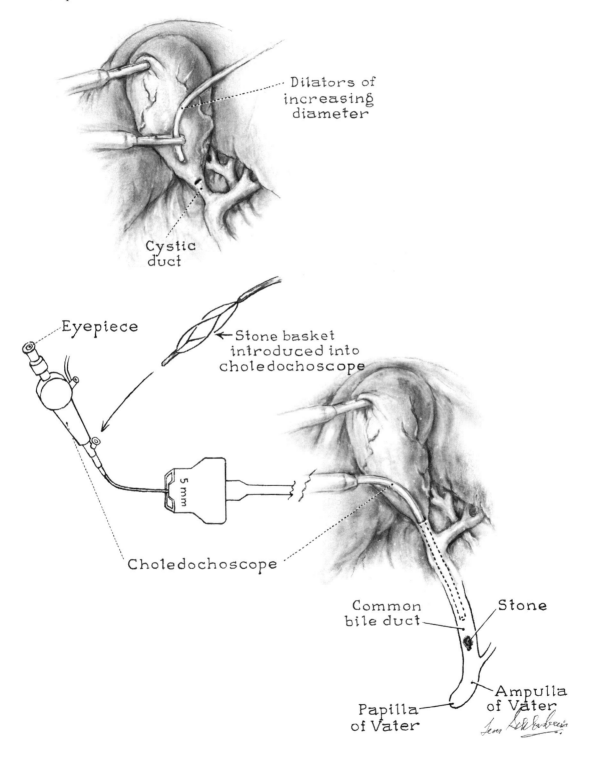

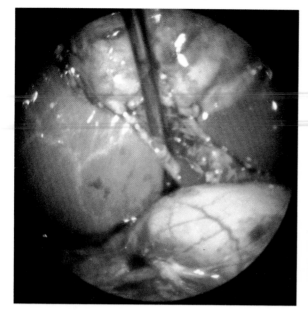

Insertion of flexible choledochoscope into
opening made in cystic duct.

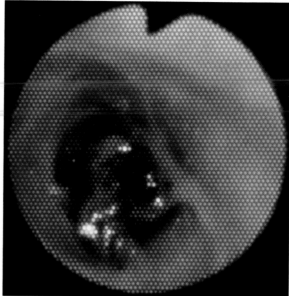

Choledochoscopic image of small stone in
distal common bile duct.

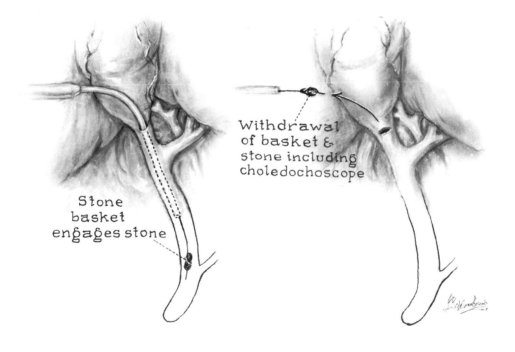

Stone
basket
engages stone

Withdrawal
of basket &
stone including
choledochoscope

A working channel through the choledochoscope allows for continuous saline irrigation to facilitate visualization. Occasionally it is helpful to pass a guidewire through the channel of the scope and guide it into the cystic and common bile ducts. The choledochoscope is then passed over the wire and into the common bile duct. This same lumen may also be used to introduce instruments such as an endoscopic stone basket, which may allow the surgeon to remove common bile duct calculi.

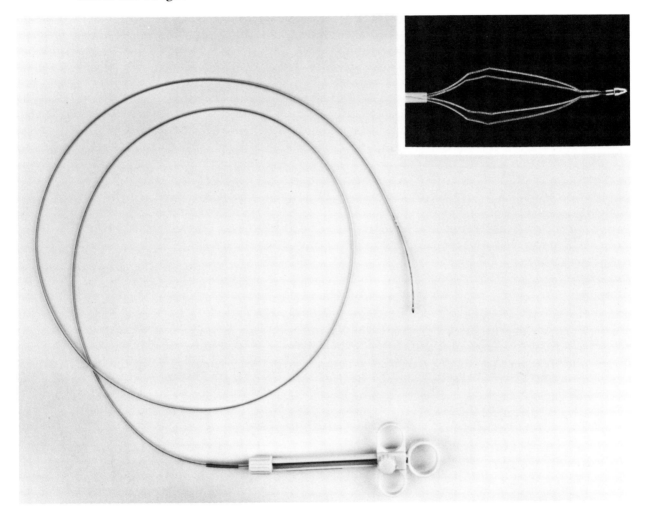

The small size of the working channel does not allow for the removal of most of these stones; therefore the choledochoscope must be removed as each stone is secured. If the stone is too large to be removed through the cystic duct lumen, lithotripsy of the stone may be performed using a mechanical, electrical, or laser energy source. Crushing forceps may be inserted through the working channel of the choledochoscope; however, these may prove difficult to use with larger stones. An electrohydraulic lithotriptor (Calcutript; Karl Storz Endoscopy, Culver City, Calif.) can deliver an energy source through a small guidewire, which can easily fragment larger stones. This wire is passed through the working channel of the choledochoscope and under direct vision guided to the stone.

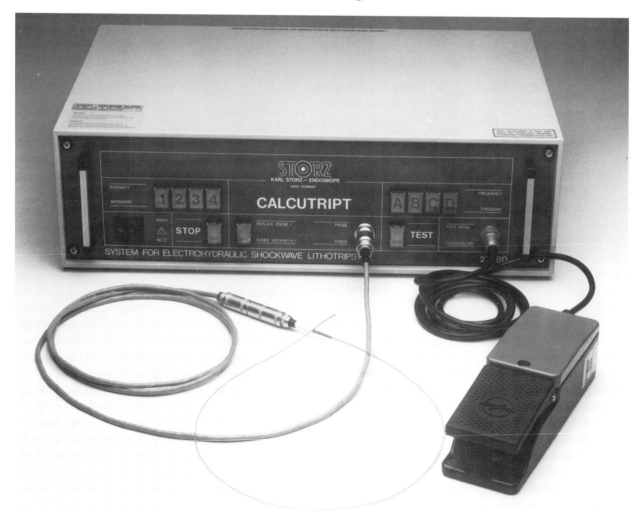

The pulsed-dye laser (Candela Laser Corporation, Wayland, Mass.) may also be used to fracture larger common bile duct stones.

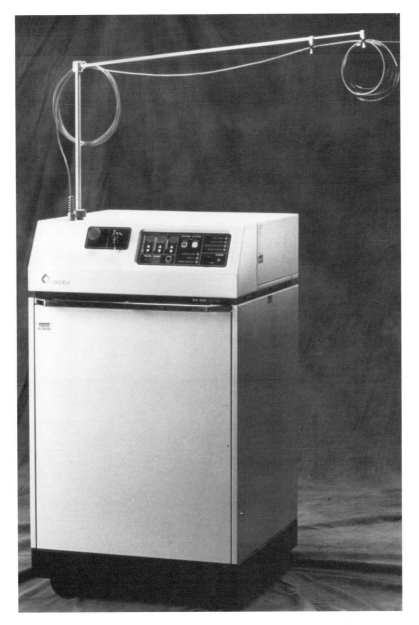

Light energy is delivered through a small quartz fiber, which is also guided through the working channel of the choledochoscope. With the endoscope the quartz fiber is placed in direct contact with the stone and the stone fractured. The pulse duration is so short that minimal heat is generated, thereby posing little risk of ductal injury. The fragmented pieces are then removed with the stone basket or irrigated through the ampulla and into the duodenum.

One current limitation of existing choledochoscopes is the size of the instrument. Endoscopes that have controllable tips and working channels range from 2.5 to 5.0 mm in diameter. Occasionally this size of endoscope may be too large to introduce through the cystic duct. Smaller choledochoscopes are available but are not equipped with a working channel or flexible controls, thus limiting their usefulness. Special cystic duct dilators have recently been developed to aid in the passage of larger choledochoscopes through smaller caliber cystic ducts.

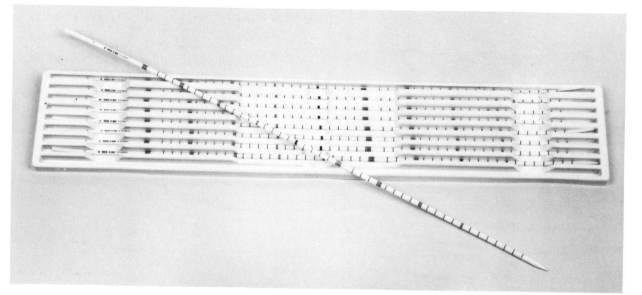

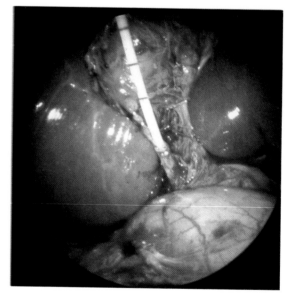

These dilators are passed through either the midline or lateral cannula and directed into the ductal opening. Gradually increasing diameter dilators are inserted until the cystic duct opening will accommodate the choledochoscope.

The major disadvantage of exploring the biliary tract with a choledochoscope introduced through the cystic duct is that it is not always possible to access the common hepatic and intrahepatic ducts. The sharp angle between the cystic and common hepatic duct often prevents the surgeon from directing the scope into the more proximal ducts. The use of excessive force in attempting to guide the choledochoscope in this direction may result in ductal injury. If the stone is not accessible with the choledochoscope or proves impossible to retrieve, the surgeon may elect to simply place a guidewire into the cystic duct, across the common bile duct, and into the duodenum. Postoperatively this will facilitate cannulation of the ampulla and bile ducts with the duodenoscope. This should increase the likelihood of a successful endoscopic sphincterotomy and stone extraction.

Direct common bile duct exploration under laparoscopic guidance has been reported.[7] Current limitations of this technique include a lack of instrumentation specifically developed to intubate and explore the bile duct, the clinical and technical experience necessary to safely dissect the common bile duct, and the ability to close the choledochotomy with sutures under laparoscopic guidance. Many of these problems are currently being addressed, and it is clear that many significant advances in laparoscopic bile duct surgery will be made in the near future.

REFERENCES

1. Zucker KA, Bailey RW, Gadacz TR, Imbembo AL. Laparoscopic guided cholecystectomy. Am J Surg 161:36-44, 1991.
2. Cotton PB, Williams CB. Duodenoscopic sphincterotomy. In Cotton PB, Williams CB, eds. Practical Gastrointestinal Endoscopy. Oxford: Blackwell, 1984, pp 86-97.
3. Salzstein EC, Evani SV, Mann RW. Routine operative cholangiography. Arch Surg 107:289-291, 1973.
4. Levine SB, Lerner HJ, Leifer ED, Lindheim SR. Intraoperative cholangiography. A review of indications and analysis of age-sex group. Ann Surg 198:692-697, 1983.
5. Mills JL, Beck DE, Harford FJ. Routine operative cholangiography. Surg Gynecol Obstet 161: 343-346, 1985.
6. Bergdahl A, Holmund S. Retained bile duct stones. Acta Chir Scand 142:122-131, 1976.
7. Petlin J. Laparoscopic management of choledocholithiasis. Surg Laparosc Endosc (in press).

CHAPTER 11

Laparoscopic Appendectomy

Eddie Joe Reddick, M.D.
William B. Saye, M.D.

Appendectomy for acute appendicitis is one of the most frequently performed operations by general surgeons. Appendectomy during the routine treatment of right lower quadrant pain and endometriosis is also becoming commonplace. The laparoscope appears to be an excellent instrument for managing both of these problems.

Kurt Semm from Kiel, Germany, reported the first case of an appendix removed solely with laparoscopic methods in 1983.[1] The appendix was not acutely inflamed, and in fact Semm did not recommend this procedure in the setting of acute inflammation. It was not until 1987 that the first report of laparoscopic surgery for acute appendicitis was published.[2] Several large clinical series of laparoscopic appendectomy have since been published, and many surgeons are now performing this procedure in the acute setting.[3-5] Gotz, Pier, and Bacher[3] have recently published a series of 400 patients undergoing laparoscopic appendectomy. In only 12 patients was the laparoscopic procedure converted to an open laparotomy because of operative complications (i.e., bleeding) or dense adhesion formation that precluded a safe dissection. Acute appendicitis was confirmed by histopathologic findings in 72% of patients and chronic inflammation in 14%; a normal appendix was removed in less than 12%. In two patients, postoperative abscess formation (both occurring in patients initially operated on for perforated appendicitis) required interval laparotomy. There were only 14 patients with wound infections, and these were limited to areas of cellulitis surrounding the umbilical puncture site. These infections were treated with antibiotics alone and did not require opening the incision. Although this and other publications discuss the cost-benefit considerations of laparoscopic vs. open appendectomy, actual data regarding reductions in hospital stay and health care expense are not available as yet. These reports do, however, document the safety of this procedure as well as the apparent reduction in postoperative wound complications.

TECHNIQUE

As an end organ the appendix lends itself to easy removal by the laparoscope. The blood supply of the appendix must be controlled and divided as well as its attachment to the cecum. The latter must be controlled in such a fashion as to prevent any leakage of fecal material. Both of these tasks are easily performed with current laparoscopic instrumentation.

After establishing pneumoperitoneum, a 10 mm trocar is inserted through the umbilicus. If there has been previous surgery or there are signs of acute peritonitis, the abdomen may be more safely entered using the Hasson technique (see Chapter 5). The Hasson technique also permits the removal of a swollen, inflamed appendix because of the slightly larger fascial opening associated with this procedure.

A 10 mm forward-viewing laparoscope is placed through the umbilical sheath with a video camera mounted for visualization. A second puncture (5 mm) is placed 1 to 2 cm superior to the symphysis pubis in the midline.

The placement of the third trocar and sheath (5 mm) may vary. This cannula may be placed either low in the right lower quadrant or in the midline 2 cm below the umbilicus. If all three cannulas lie along the midline, the surgeon will have all of the instruments in the same plane as his camera. However, if the trocars are placed too close together, the instruments and laparoscope can hit one another during the operative procedure. If the third trocar is inserted in the right lower quadrant, instrument interference will pose less of a problem. Although either the right lower quadrant or infraumbilical site will provide adequate exposure in most patients, we prefer to place the third trocar through the right lower quadrant.

Occasionally a fourth puncture (5 mm) may be required, especially with a retrocecal appendix. This trocar may be placed in the right upper quadrant and used to introduce a bowel grasping forceps to elevate the cecum superiorly. Dividing the inferior and lateral peritoneal bands will mobilize a retrocecal appendix sufficiently to complete the laparoscopic appendectomy.

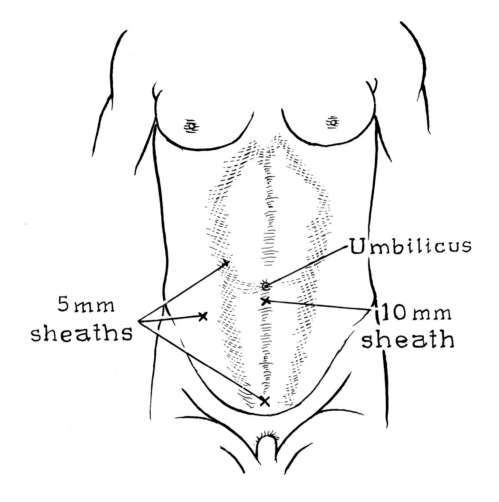

5 mm
sheaths

Umbilicus

10 mm
sheath

After all of the laparoscopic sheaths are in place, the appendix is identified and grasped with the right lower quadrant forceps. This places tension on the mesoappendix, which facilitates dissection of the vessels.

If the tip of the appendix is too swollen or inflamed to safely grasp with the forceps, a pretied chromic EndoLoop (Ethicon, Inc., Sommerville, N.J.) may be placed around the tip of the appendix for traction.

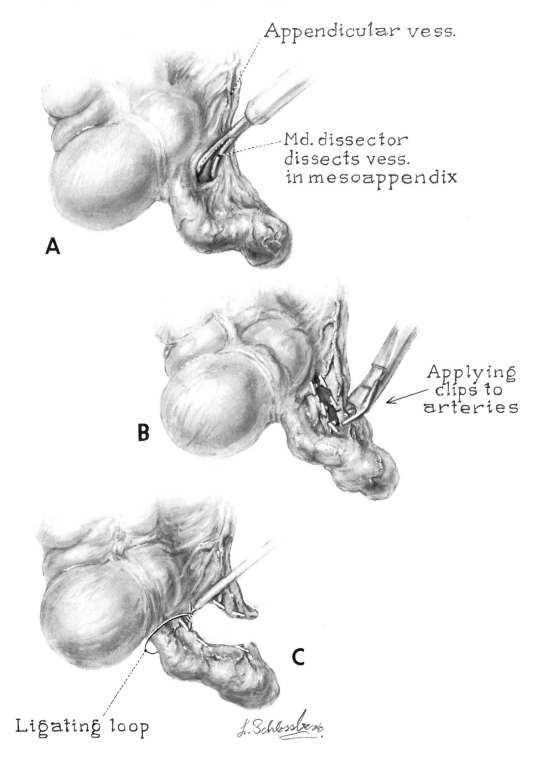

Appendicular vess.

Md. dissector
dissects vess.
in mesoappendix

A

Applying
clips to
arteries

B

C

Ligating loop

L. Schlossberg

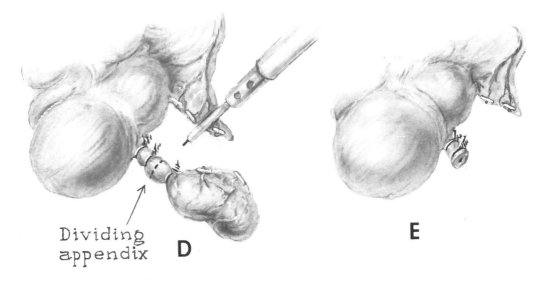

Dividing appendix **D**

E

Atraumatic forceps are introduced through the suprapubic port, and blunt dissection is used to open a plane between the vessels of the mesoappendix. Alternatively, a laser fiber may be inserted through the suprapubic port and used to create small openings in the mesoappendix. The lateral pelvic wall should be used to absorb any forward scatter of laser energy.

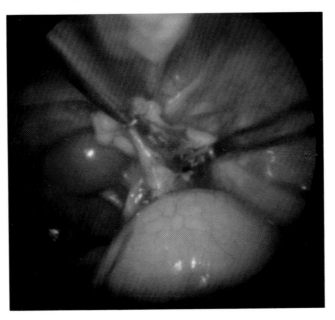

Operative photograph of forceps dissecting vessels of mesoappendix.

If adequate tension cannot be placed on the mesoappendix via the right lower quadrant port, the right upper quadrant port may be inserted to apply cephalad traction on the cecum.

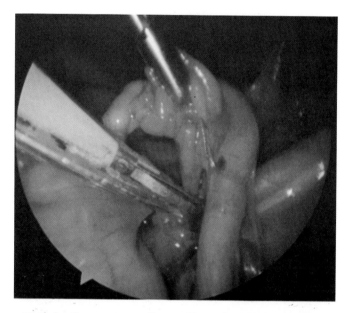

Vessels of mesoappendix are ligated with 9 mm clips.

The 10 mm scope is removed from the umbilical port, and a 5 mm forward-viewing diagnostic scope with attached camera is inserted through the suprapubic port. A clip applier is inserted through the umbilical port, and titanium clips are applied to the vessels of the mesoappendix using the previously formed openings in the mesentery. The vessels of the meso-appendix are ligated with 9 mm titanium surgical clips. This may take only a single clip or may require multiple clips, depending on the anatomy of the appendiceal blood supply.

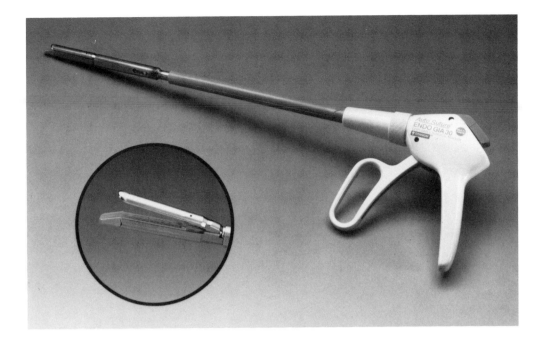

A multiloaded instrument will prevent delays due to reloading the single-fire instruments. A recently developed laparoscopic stapling device (Endo GIA; United States Surgical Corporation, Norwalk, Conn.) may also be used to divide the mesoappendiceal vessels. This instrument is 30 mm long and fires a triple row of hemostatic staples. A cutting blade is incorporated within the instrument to divide the tissue between the rows of staples.

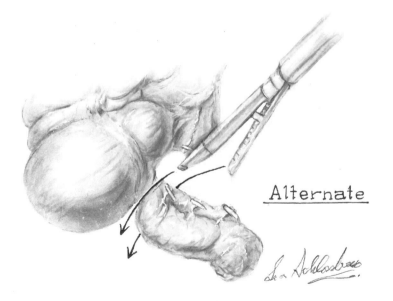

Tension is placed on end of appendix and laparoscopic stapler placed across mesoappendix and/or base of appendix.

The 5 mm laparoscope is removed, and the 10 mm laparoscope is reinserted through the umbilical sheath. The laser fiber is reinserted through the suprapubic port and is used to transect the mesoappendix from the appendix. The hemostatic properties of the laser will control most of the bleeding from the appendiceal surface, whereas the clips provide hemostasis of the vessels themselves. With the appendix completely freed from the mesoappendix, three chromic EndoLoops are placed near the appendiceal base.

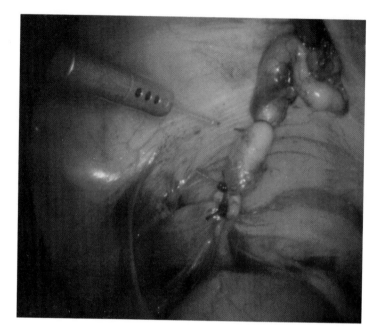

These pretied sutures are introduced through the suprapubic port (see pp. 230 and 231). Two sutures are placed near the cecum and the third approximately 1 cm distally. The laser fiber is inserted through the suprapubic sheath and the appendix divided between the two proximal and the more distally placed sutures. Spillage from the appendix is controlled by the distal EndoLoop. The high temperatures produced by the laser energy beam will destroy the appendiceal mucosa as the transection is performed. This should reduce the chance of later mucocele formation. Alternatively, the Endo GIA may be used to divide the base of the appendix (see p. 233). Recent data on open appendectomies have failed to show that invagination of the appendiceal stump has any advantage over simple ligation and division,[6] and thus it is probably not necessary during laparoscopic surgery. However, Semm[1] has described a laparoscopic suturing technique that incorporates the appendiceal stump into the wall of the cecum.

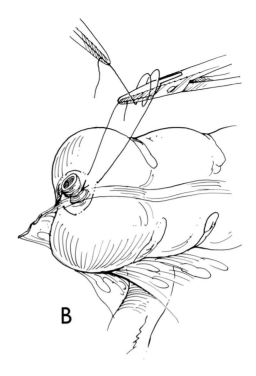

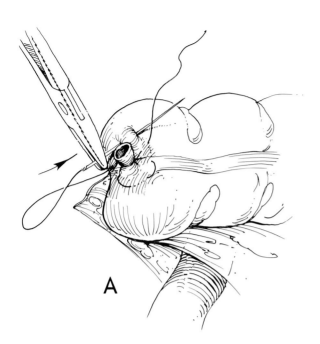

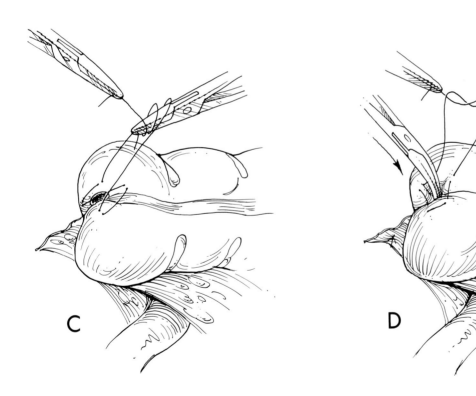

Modified from Semm K. Operative Manual for Endoscopic Abdominal Surgery (Friedrick ER, translator and editor). Chicago: Year Book, 1986.

The transected appendix is secured by the right lower quadrant grasping forceps. The 10 mm laparoscope is removed from the umbilical sheath, and the 5 mm scope is inserted through the suprapubic port. A 10 mm forceps is placed through the umbilical port and the base of the appendix grasped. The appendix is removed from the abdominal cavity through the umbilical cannula. If the appendix is too large to pull through this sheath, the umbilical cannula and the appendix may be removed together. An alternative method is to replace the 10 mm diagnostic scope with a 10 mm operating laparoscope. This scope has a smaller optical lens system but incorporates a 5 mm working channel within the same tube. The appendix can be grasped by a forceps through the operating scope and extracted as the scope is pulled out of the umbilical trocar. With either of these techniques the contaminated tissue is prevented from coming into contact with the abdominal wall, decreasing the risk of wound infection. Occasionally patients will have a very swollen and inflamed appendix that will not pull through the 10 mm umbilical cannula. In this situation the 10 mm umbilical cannula may be removed and the fascial opening dilated to accommodate a larger 20 mm appendiceal trocar and sheath (Karl Storz Endoscopy, Culver City, Calif.). This instrument was designed to allow removal of these enlarged appendices without contaminating the abdominal wound.

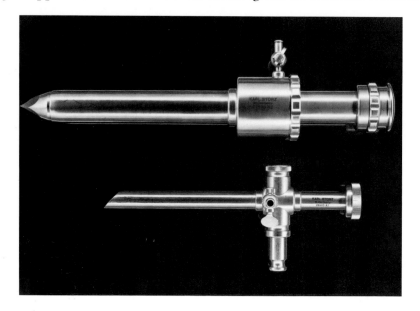

The umbilical fascial opening is closed with a figure-of-eight absorbable suture and all of the skin incisions closed with subcuticular stitches. Plastic dressings are placed over the wounds.

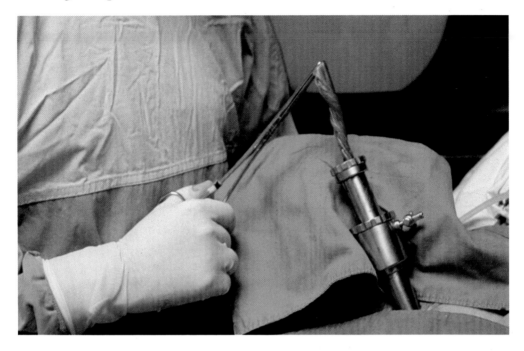

POSTOPERATIVE CARE

Patients may resume a regular diet when fully recovered from anesthesia. A 1.5 mg scopolamine patch placed behind the patient's ear in the recovery room will decrease postoperative nausea. Pain after laparoscopic appendectomy is usually minimal and in most patients can be managed by oral analgesics alone. Patients may shower immediately after surgery since their wounds are covered with plastic dressings. As there are no significant muscular or fascial defects, patients may return to their normal activities without restrictions within 48 hours.

DISCUSSION

Although most open appendectomies for acute appendicitis are performed through 2 to 4 cm incisions, frequently the opening will have to be enlarged for adequate exploration and removal of the appendix. Enlargement of the incision and forceful retraction lead to greater tissue trauma and anoxia, thereby increasing the risk of wound infections. Larger incisions also cause more pain and therefore require longer hospital stays as well as delay the patient's return to normal activities.

Many patients, especially females, present with atypical right lower quadrant pain dictating an operation to rule out appendicitis. In as many as 20% or more of these cases the problem will be a gynecologic disorder or some other condition totally unrelated to the appendix. It is sometimes difficult, if not impossible, to adequately examine both the right and left adnexa with the typical 2 to 4 cm incision used for the traditional open appendectomy.

Laparoscopic surgery is performed through three small abdominal incisions. Generally these do not have to be extended for the appendectomy, although on occasion a fourth puncture may be necessary. Patients experience less pain, length of hospitalization is often decreased, and routine activities are resumed earlier. To minimize the cosmetic disfigurement, the umbilical scar is generally well hidden within the skin folds of the umbilicus, and the suprapubic incision is placed just at or below the hairline. The other incisions are only 5 mm in size and create minimal scarring. Cosmetically the small residual scars are more acceptable than that resulting from a standard McBurney incision.

The laparoscope also provides excellent visualization of the pelvic organs, the large and small intestine, and most of the other intra-abdominal organs. In those situations in which appendicitis is not the culprit, the disease process may often be managed with laparoscopic surgery. In patients with chronic lower abdominal pain associated with endometriosis, the appendix may be involved by the endometrial process. Occasionally it may prove necessary to remove the appendix to decrease the diagnostic dilemma if lower abdominal pain recurs. The appendix may then be removed at the same time the endometrial implants are being ablated laparoscopically.

CONCLUSION

Laparoscopic laser appendectomy can be performed safely in most patients with acute appendicitis, thereby decreasing the chance of wound infection and facilitating the rapid return to full activities. The laparoscope may also be used to examine the appendix in those patients in whom the diagnosis of acute appendicitis is less clear. If a diseased appendix is then found, it should not be necessary for the surgeon to withdraw the laparoscope and perform an additional abdominal incision. Laparoscopic appendectomy may also be performed in conjunction with treatment for endometriosis and other gynecologic disorders.

Although the current data are limited, laparoscopic appendectomy appears to be a safe and effective alternative to open appendectomy. The role of laparoscopic surgery for the patient with routine appendicitis is still unclear. Additional clinical trials will be necessary for a full evaluation in this setting.

REFERENCES

1. Semm K. Endoscopic appendectomy. Endoscopy 15:59-64, 1983.
2. Schrieber J. Early experience with laparoscopic appendectomy in women. Surg Endosc 1:211-216, 1987.
3. Gotz F, Pier A, Bacher C. Modified laparoscopic appendectomy in surgery. Surg Endosc 4:6-9, 1990.
4. Gangal HT, Gangal MH. Laparoscopic appendectomy. Endoscopy 19:127-129, 1987.
5. Mouret P, Marsaud H. Appendicectomies per laparoscopic technique and evaluation. Surg Endosc (in press).
6. Engstrom L, Fenyo G. Appendicectomy: An assessment of stump invagination. A prospective trial. Br J Surg 72:971-972, 1985.

CHAPTER 12

Laparoscopic Pelvic Lymphadenectomy

Thierry G. Vancaillie, M.D.
William W. Schuessler, M.D.

Pelvic lymphadenectomy was once integral to the management of patients with malignancy of the lower urogenital tract when attempts were made to remove all of the affected tissue.[1,2] The myth that radical surgery was curative persisted for several decades, leading to extremely crippling and morbid procedures. Surgeons and radiotherapists alike have claimed to have found the best approach for treatment of cancer of the lower genito-urinary tract for both men and women. However, apart from differences in distribution of recurrent disease, no clear advantage of either radical surgery or radiation therapy has been documented. What we have learned is that survival depends on the extent and aggressiveness (grade) of the tumor at the time of diagnosis. Emphasis has, therefore, been correctly placed on the early detection of malignancy. This has been achieved mainly through public education and screening programs such as cervical Papanicolaou smears and transrectal ultrasonography of the prostate.

Patients with cancers of the bladder and prostate have markedly different survival rates if regional lymph node metastasis has occurred at the time of diagnosis.[3] For bladder cancer, a single positive lymph node may well dictate that a surgeon should resort to palliative therapy (chemotherapy or radiotherapy) rather than a curative therapy (radical cystoprostatectomy). For prostate cancer, potentially curative local procedures (external beam radiotherapy) or excellent palliative (orchiectomy) therapies are available for patients with positive lymph nodes. If there is no evidence of lymph node involvement, a curative surgical procedure (radical prostatectomy) may be indicated. Therefore a positive lymph node found on pelvic lymphadenectomy may change the course of treatment for the patient with bladder or prostate cancer.

Lymphadenectomy by laparotomy, however, is associated with significant morbidity and even mortality. In patients with prostate cancer, lymphadenectomy alone has an early postoperative complication rate varying from 12% to 24% (Table 12-1). When combined with radical prostatectomy, the complication rate is, as would be expected, slightly higher (17% to 33%). Is this an acceptable price to pay for a noncurative procedure? The answer is not a clear "yes" or "no." Pelvic lymphadenectomy provides important information for devising an effective therapeutic program tailored to the individual patient. On the other hand, does a strictly staging operation warrant an average hospital stay of 6.8 days and substantial risks (i.e., blood transfusions, thromboembolic accidents, wound infections, lymphocele, etc.)[9]? In view of these disadvantages many investigators have sought alternative methods for the detection of lymphatic spread of malignant cells.

Imaging methods such as CT, MRI, and contrast lymphography have proved to be of limited usefulness. A "negative" imaging study has no clinical significance because microscopic invasion of lymph nodes cannot be visualized by any method currently available. The increasing focus on early diagnosis of malignant lesions through screening programs has made microscopic lymphatic disease a more important issue. Invasive imaging procedures encompass the various techniques of guided needle aspiration for cytologic examination.[10] The information obtained is more valuable than that from imaging studies because the likelihood of a false positive

Table 12-1. Early Postoperative Complication Rates of Surgical Interventions in Patients With Prostatic Cancer

Author	Lymphadenectomy Only		Lymphadenectomy and Prostatectomy	
	No. of Patients	%	No. of Patients	%
McLaughlin et al.[4]	7/30	23	10/30	33
Nicholson and Richie[5]	—		8/47	17
Ray et al.[6]*	12/50	24	—	
McCullough, McLaughlin, and Gittes[7]	6/30	20	9/30	30
Lieskovsky, Skinner, and Weisenburger[8]	2/17	12	13/65	20

*Transperitoneal approach.

result is drastically reduced by the availability of a tissue sample. Still, there is the specter of an unknown incidence of false negative results. This false negative index is estimated to be as high as 15%. Although the morbidity associated with guided needle aspiration is extremely low, this advantage is offset by the relative worthlessness of a negative result.

A third line of clinical research is directed toward developing a surgical procedure with fewer complications than those reported for traditional laparotomy and lymphadenectomy. Such a surgical procedure, called pelvioscopy,[11,12] was first developed in Denmark in the 1970s. This procedure consisted of inserting a mediastinoscope through a small incision medial to the iliac crest and dissecting into the retroperitoneal space. Hald and Rasmussen[11] reported on an initial small series of 12 patients with prostate or bladder cancer. The chief (and real) advantage was the short duration (average 20 minutes) of the surgery. However, only one pelvic sidewall was explored. The main disadvantage is that the procedure is based on sampling palpable lymph nodes. Therefore no nodal tissue was obtained in 4 out of 12 patients. A modification of this technique is performed in France by Salvat and Dargent[13] in women with cervical malignancy. They make one single incision in the midline suprapubically and gain access to both pelvic sidewalls. The midline incision, however, limits the accessibility of the proximal part of the iliac vessels. The advantages are, again, short operating time and the possibility of using only a local anesthetic. However, the same disadvantage is obvious: this is a sampling technique, not a complete resection. Fuerst[14] developed the idea of marking the lymph nodes by interstitial injection of a dye, isosulfan blue, which then highlights the nodes through lymphatic absorption. The dye differentiates nodes from fatty tissue, thereby enabling directed biopsy. After an initial report of an animal experiment in 1985, no further data have been published.

The next procedure developed was one in which the small incisions used for pelvioscopy were retained, but the procedure was extended for excision of complete chains of lymph nodes rather than random sampling. Querleu[15] in France was the first to perform laparoscopic pelvic lymphadenectomy in a systematic fashion as a staging procedure for women with cervical malignancy. This procedure is truly a hybrid inasmuch as some advantages of minimally invasive surgery, such as reduced postoperative morbidity, apply, whereas the same objective is attained as in classic surgery.

There is no major difference in technique for males and females. However, gynecologic oncologists in the United States have expressed little interest since abdominal hysterectomy is the standard treatment for cervical malignancy in its early stages. The radical approach combining abdominal hysterectomy with lymphadenectomy still prevails. In Europe there is greater experience with vaginal surgery for cervical malignancy. This explains why our European colleagues are more receptive to the idea of performing laparoscopic pelvic lymphadenectomy prior to vaginal hysterectomy or radiation (depending on histologic findings). The benefit of this approach is lower postoperative morbidity.

TECHNIQUE

Depending on training patterns, specialties are likely to be biased as to whether they consider laparoscopy to be a major or minor procedure. Interns in obstetrics and gynecology have been exposed to laparoscopic procedures for sterilization and diagnosis and are aware of the minimal surgical risk it entails. Urologists, however, do not tend to view it as a "minor" procedure. It is unlikely that laparoscopy will become a minor procedure performed by first-year urology residents. Rather, it will likely be considered a more difficult intervention to be reserved for the chief resident.

Because of endosurgery's complexity and advanced instrumentation, the technical demands placed on the surgeon have drastically increased. A great many variables require constant attention: light intensity, CO_2 absorption, water pressure, laser safety, and many more. To cope with this situation, a team approach is ideal. The team includes a circulating nurse, operating room technician, surgeon, assistant, anesthesiologist, radiologist, as well as pathologist. Let us not forget that the purpose of the intervention is to provide the pathologist with a valuable specimen! Cooperation is the key to proper management of the patient with cancer of the lower urogenital tract. Some aspects of this team approach need to be emphasized.

Anesthesia

Anesthesia is the subject of Chapter 4, but certain aspects should be stressed here. Less muscle relaxation is needed for laparoscopy than for open surgery. The level of anesthesia required is not as great. Other aspects are specific to laparoscopic procedures, foremost of which is the use of CO_2 gas. Tens of liters of CO_2 will be used during the procedure. One of the side effects of large volumes of gas is that the patient cools off rapidly! A monitoring system needs to be instituted. Both pulmonary and vascular CO_2 partial pressures must be monitored constantly. A low tidal volume is necessary so that respiratory movements do not interfere with the surgery. Insufflation leads to an increase of expiratory partial CO_2 pressure. These two factors, therefore, impose the necessity of hyperventilation.

Numerous changes in the patient's position for optimal access and the increased intra-abdominal pressure resulting from insufflation interfere with venous return, diastolic filling pressures, etc. Close cardiac surveillance, with more liberal use of arterial and central venous lines, allows the anesthesiologist to deal better with hemodynamic variations.

Instrumentation

No instruments, no surgery; it is that simple. Some surgeons may envision performing open surgery with one set of instruments for the duration of their career. This is unlikely to happen with laparoscopy, for obvious reasons. The instruments are more elongated and the moving parts smaller; in short, they are less sturdy because of technical restrictions. Damage can be minimized if one person, as member of the team, takes care of the instruments and replaces malfunctioning equipment before it breaks down. We have found it extremely beneficial to assign one member of the surgical team to be responsible for maintenance of the equipment and to assist as a surgical technician during the procedure.

Circulating Nurse

Before surgery can begin, many switches have to be turned on and many dials set correctly. It will not take long for the operating room personnel to realize how important it is to have all hardware well organized to avoid jumping over and under hoses, electrical lines, foot pedals, and other operating room hazards. This is not to imply that the arrangement of the operating room setup is inflexible, but it is important to position the hardware so that all regulators can be reached easily. The setup in our operating suite is shown on p. 246.

The circulating nurse needs to know exactly how to connect the various cables and hoses before any procedure is started. "In service" becomes a critical part of successful endosurgery. It is also wise for the surgeon, assistant, and, in fact, every single person in the room to understand the functioning of each piece of equipment.

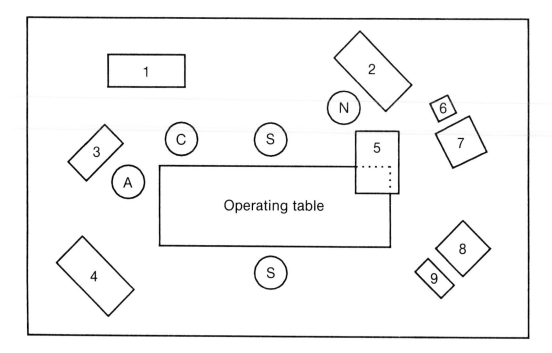

1 - Operating table with instruments for emergency laparotomy
2 - Operating table with laparotomy instruments
3 - Anesthesia cart
4 - Anesthesia machine
5 - Mayo stand with most frequently used laparoscopy instruments
6 - Equipment to preheat endoscopes
7 - Hardware cart with TV monitor
8 - Hardware cart with TV monitor
9 - Laser

A - Anesthesiologist   N - Surgical technician
C - Camera holder/assistant   S - Surgeons

Patient Positioning

Proper positioning and, even more important, the constant need to change the patient's position are of utmost importance in endosurgery. Whatever endosurgical procedure is being performed, physical and technical restrictions are imposed on the number and movement of ancillary instruments. One can compensate for these technical restrictions by changing the position of the operating table. This includes the Trendelenburg, reverse Trendelenburg, and lateral tilt positions. The objective of any change in position is to bring the operative field in front of the surgeon, limiting extreme lateral movements. The ideal position for a patient undergoing endosurgical pelvic lymphadenectomy is a dorsal recumbent position with elevation of the pelvis. The pelvic forward tilt can be obtained by placing a roll of towels underneath the buttocks of the patient prior to disinfection. The arms of the patient should be aligned alongside the trunk. This allows maximum mobility for the surgeon and assistants. The anesthesiologist needs to adjust to the use of long intravenous lines that disappear under the drapes for the rest of the intervention. The ideal position for lymphadenectomy of the right obturator fossa is a 10-degree Trendelenburg position with a 30-degree left lateral tilt. The surgeon standing to the left of the patient then has the most direct approach to the right obturator fossa. Restraining straps must, of course, be placed at the level of the patient's shoulders and upper thigh.

Incisions

Insufflation is carried out using a Veress needle introduced through an incision inside the umbilicus, not beneath it (p. 248). If previous surgery has left a midline scar, which is often the case in the elderly patient, insufflation is performed at a site away from the scar, along the mammillary line, either left (preferably) or right, depending on the location of the scar. Insufflation is continued until the intra-abdominal pressure reaches approximately 15 mm Hg. Higher pressure will compress the large veins and interfere with the hemodynamic homeostasis. The amount of gas required to reach the 15 mm Hg mark is variable, ranging from 2.5 to 7.0 L. A lack of resistance to insufflation is the best indicator that the Veress needle is well positioned. The main trocar ("first-puncture" trocar and trocar for the telescope) is inserted through the umbilicus at the same site used to introduce the Veress needle. In some unusual circumstances (umbilical hernia, plastic surgery, scar, etc.) the trocar is inserted away from the umbilicus. However, it is wise to remain close to the umbilicus; otherwise one of the two pelvic sidewalls will be difficult to visualize properly.

Introduction of the Veress needle and first-puncture trocar are truly blind procedures and, as such, are subject to complications such as bowel perforation and vascular injury (see Chapter 16). Routine placement of a gastric tube will reduce the risk of inadvertent intragastric insufflation. Also, an empty stomach reduces the volume of the abdominal contents and therefore improves visualization.

Visualization is also improved by use of a mechanical bowel preparation (e.g., Go-LYTELY, magnesium sulfate, or Reglan) and replacement of N_2O by air for anesthesia. N_2O accumulates in the bowel lumen, reducing the intra-abdominal "operating volume." Abstaining from dairy products for 2 days prior to surgery also reduces intraluminal gas. All these seemingly insignificant details greatly improve access and visualization of the operating field and are therefore of critical importance.

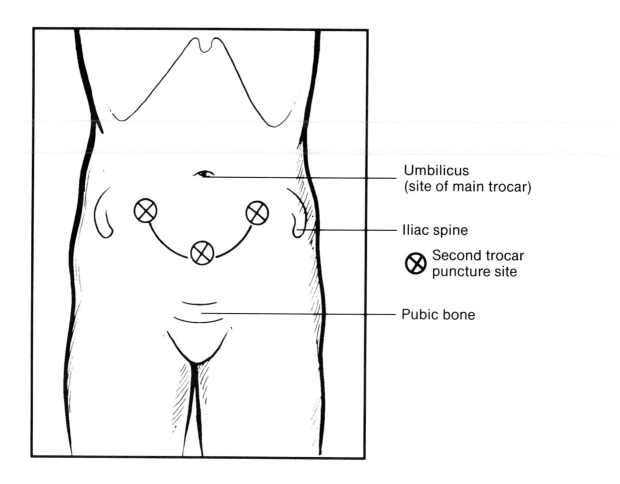

The second-puncture or accessory trocars are introduced along a semicircular line halfway between the umbilicus and pubis or iliac spine.

Injury to the epigastric vessels during this maneuver can be avoided by direct visualization of these vessels through the laparoscope. Currently we use three ancillary trocars: one suprapubic and two lateral. The suprapubic and contralateral trocars are used by the surgeon to operate on either the right or the left pelvic sidewall. The ipsilateral trocar is used by the assistant.

Landmarks

The transperitoneal endoscopic access is certain to be disconcerting to the urologist at first. The perspective is completely different than via the retroperitoneal route. Careful inspection of pelvic and abdominal cavities is of paramount importance prior to proceeding with the surgery. The landmarks immediately visible are the umbilical ligaments, the internal inguinal rings, the epigastric vessels, and the vas deferens (or round ligament).

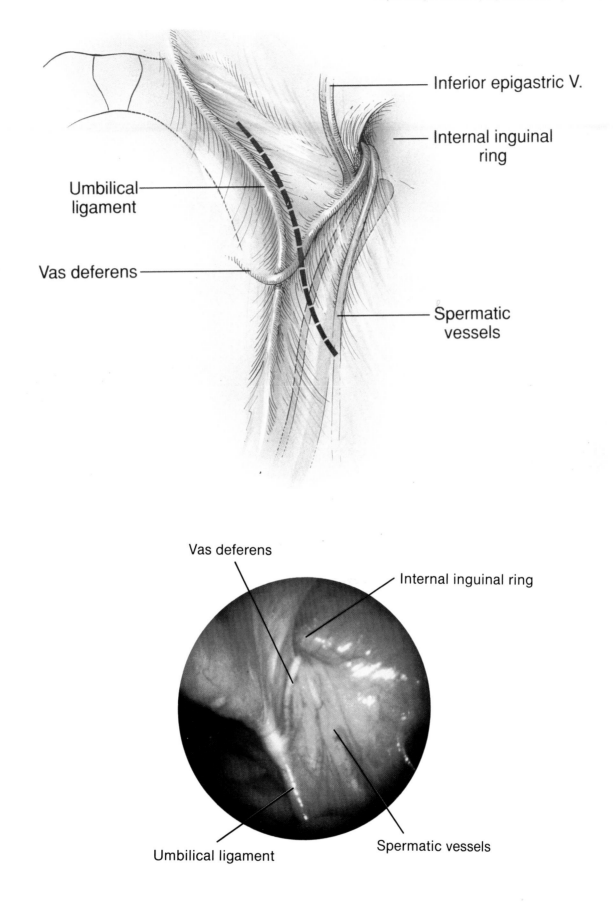

Inferior epigastric V.

Internal inguinal ring

Umbilical ligament

Vas deferens

Spermatic vessels

Vas deferens

Internal inguinal ring

Umbilical ligament

Spermatic vessels

The external iliac vessels themselves are not well delineated, especially in the obese patient. When we were apprentices we tried to gain access to the obturator fossa along the medial aspect of the external iliac vein. This approach proved useless for all landmarks were lost. The umbilical ligament (obliterated umbilical artery) offers not only a welcome and constantly present landmark, but also a good site for applying forceps. This orientation also provides the surgeon with the welcome knowledge that immediately lateral to the umbilical ligament is a space without any vital structure: the paravesical space through which he will be able to reach the next landmark—the pubic bone—a landmark that can be seen and felt. The pubic bone is an important landmark because it will allow location of both the external iliac vein and the obturator nerve. Visual landmarks prevail over tactile landmarks in endosurgery. Indeed, tactile information, upon which many surgeons have based their skills, is significantly reduced!

"Limited" Lymphadenectomy (Obturator Chain)

The surgeon standing on the left side of the patient starts operating on the right pelvic sidewall. His left hand manipulates a grasping forceps introduced through the suprapubic port; his right hand operates a cutting instrument through the left lateral trocar. The assistant standing on the right side of the patient maneuvers a grasping forceps used for retraction to improve exposure. The initial incision of the peritoneum is made immediately lateral to the umbilical ligament, starting at the level of the internal inguinal ring, which obviously lies in a plane above the pubic bone (see p. 249). The incision is carried downward and cephalad, crossing the vas deferens; the direction of the cut is then changed to a less steep, downward one, deviating laterally and cephalad in the direction of the iliac bifurcation. This change of direction is mandated by the course of the ureter, which is parallel but usually below the hypogastric vessels. In some, but not all, patients the ureter can be visualized through the peritoneum. This initial incision can be made with a CO_2 or fiber laser or with scissors.

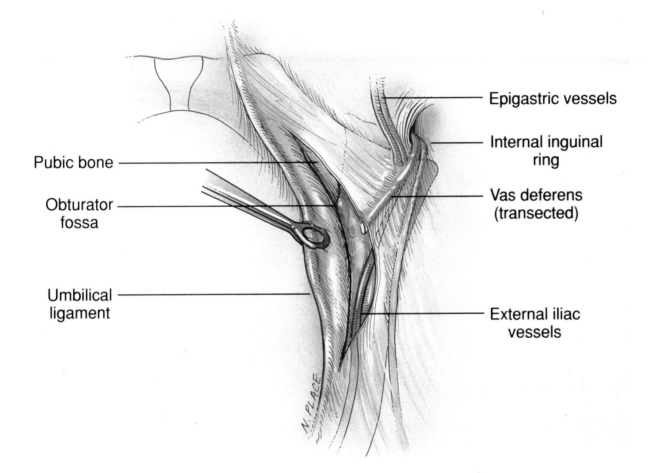

Epigastric vessels

Internal inguinal ring

Pubic bone

Vas deferens (transected)

Obturator fossa

Umbilical ligament

External iliac vessels

The next step is to coagulate and cut the vas deferens (or round ligament). This allows maximum retraction of the medial peritoneal edge toward the midline and thus offers better access to the obturator fossa. The peritoneum is bluntly dissected off the sidewall to expose the obturator fossa and iliac vessels. Then the pubic bone is located.

A forceps placed along the umbilical ligament gently probes the paravesical space and quickly identifies the bone. Meticulous dissection of the bone will help in identifying the other anatomic structures. Once the pubic bone is identified, the dissecting forceps is directed downward and slightly laterally to unroof the obturator fossa. No vital structures are at risk as long as the dissecting instrument is kept away from the sidewall.

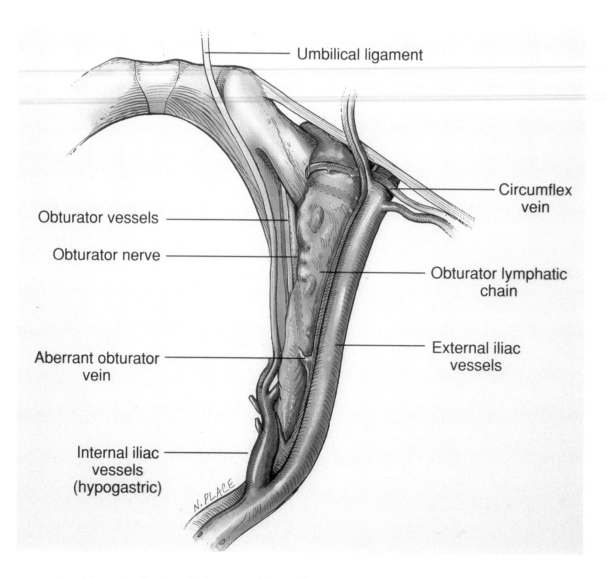

- Umbilical ligament
- Circumflex vein
- Obturator vessels
- Obturator nerve
- Obturator lymphatic chain
- External iliac vessels
- Aberrant obturator vein
- Internal iliac vessels (hypogastric)

N. PLACE

At this point it should be possible to distinguish the vital structures of the sidewall: the external iliac vein and artery and the obturator nerve. The lymphatic chain lies in between. The assistant should at this point retract the external iliac vessels to allow the surgeon better access to the lymphatic tissue. The nodal tissue is grasped approximately 3 cm proximal to the pubic bone. At this level there is less risk of injuring the circumflex vein or an aberrant obturator vein.

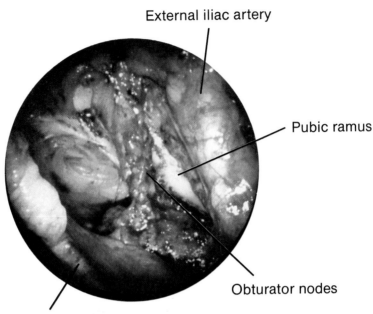

External iliac artery

Pubic ramus

Obturator nodes

Umbilical ligament

Dissection is continued alongside the medial aspect of the external iliac vein until the obturator nerve is visualized. The nodal tissue is then detached from the iliac vein and the pubic bone. During this maneuver the circumflex vein can be visualized in most cases. About half the time it is possible to spare the vein; otherwise it is transected after coagulation or clip application. The lymphatic chain can be further dissected off the sidewall or first transected at the level of the pubic bone after positive identification of the obturator nerve.

During cephalad dissection of the nodal tissue an aberrant obturator vein may be encountered at approximately 3 to 4 cm distal from the iliac bifurcation. Because of the optical magnification provided by the endoscope, it is usually not difficult to identify this aberrant vessel. Next comes the cephalad transection of the lymphatic chain at the junction of external iliac vein and obturator nerve. At this moment the surgeon is under the greatest tension because the area is difficult to reach and is close to the internal iliac vein. One of the technical difficulties during endosurgical lymphadenectomy is the inability to maintain a strong grasp of the nodal tissue during blunt dissection at the proximal end. It is helpful to loosen the lymphatic chain all around as extensively as possible before blunt transection of the proximal end is attempted. This represents the end of "limited" pelvic lymphadenectomy. The nodal tissue is left in the obturator fossa until after completion of the opposite side. The procedure for the left side is similar to that for the right, except that the surgeon now stands on the right side of the patient and the assistant on the left. We have found it beneficial to operate with two surgeons, each functioning alternatively as principal surgeon and then assistant so that they are not forced to change sides during surgery. Changing positions alters the optical perspective. Another difference between left and right is that there are almost always adhesions between the sigmoid colon and left pelvic sidewall, probably because of subclinical peridiverticulitis. It is necessary in most cases to dissect those adhesions free prior to opening the peritoneum. Alternatively, the peritoneum can be incised above the pelvic brim and folded downward and medially. In so doing, the sigmoid is also separated from the sidewall.

When the dissection is completed on both sides, the tissue is removed through a 10 mm port, which is either the first-puncture trocar or one of the ancillary trocars. If tissue is removed through the first-puncture trocar, a 5 mm zero-degree endoscope is inserted through an ancillary trocar for visualization. The nodal tissue is grasped with either a large spoon forceps or with a regular grasping forceps introduced through a reducing sleeve. In some cases the lymphatic tissue can be removed only in bits and pieces, a frustrating experience but nonetheless necessary until more adequate instrumentation is available.

"Extended" Lymphadenectomy (Obturator and Iliac Chain)

"Extended" lymphadenectomy involves the resection of all nodal and fatty tissue from the iliac bifurcation to the pubis between the ureter and genito-femoral nerve. This includes meticulous dissection of the external iliac artery, external iliac vein, hypogastric artery, and ureter in addition to the dissection previously described as "limited" lymphadenectomy. At our thirty-first procedure we added this extended dissection on the right side as part of a prospective study to evaluate the diagnostic value and morbidity of extended lymphadenectomy. Once the obturator nodal tissue has been removed, the anatomy of the pelvic sidewall can be clearly distinguished. The iliac and hypogastric vessels as well as the ureter can be identified more easily than when the peritoneum was intact. The bottom of the surgical field has already been defined by dissection of the obturator nerve. For further resection, the lateral limits of the field must be defined based on the ureter and the genitofemoral nerve. These two latter structures form a V, which delineates the dissection. The angle of the V is located at the common iliac artery, and the distal border is formed by the pubic bone.

The umbilical ligament, the fourth branch of the hypogastric artery, is again a welcome landmark. Gentle traction on the ligament will mobilize the artery and thereby facilitate differentiation from the ureter. Indeed, arterial pulsations are less easily visualized than palpated. Moreover, atherosclerosis, present to some degree in every elderly patient, further reduces the possibility for visual identification of arterial pulsations. Once the ureter and hypogastric artery have been identified, the peritoneal incision is extended cephalad 1 to 2 cm beyond the common iliac artery. The peritoneum is dissected off the external iliac vessels. The assistant holds and retracts this peritoneal flap. The fatty tissue lateral to the iliac vessels is bluntly divided until the genitofemoral nerve is identified. This dissection is carried out along the entire length of the external iliac artery. At the distal end care must be taken to avoid injuring the epigastric and circumflex vessels. Cloquet's ganglion can be identified in some patients when the lymphatic chain is grasped and traction exerted in a cephalad direction. It is doubtful that removal of Cloquet's ganglion adds significantly to the prognostic value of pelvic lymphadenectomy. It undoubtedly adds a definite surgical risk because of the proximity of the epigastric and circumflex vessels. The ganglion itself is also well vascularized. We resect the ganglion only when we are able to completely dissect it off the surrounding vascular structures. Most often it is left in place. Once the lateral and distal dissections are completed, attention is directed to the iliac artery. The adventitia is incised with scissors over the entire exposed length and the fatty tissue retracted medially. Then the artery is gently held to the side to allow blunt dissection of the groove between artery and vein. Further dissection involves the adventitia of the hypogastric artery down to the insertion of the umbilical ligament. The medial lateral border, delineated by the ureter, is dissected bluntly. We do not routinely denude the ureter. This represents the end point of "extended" lymphadenectomy on one side.

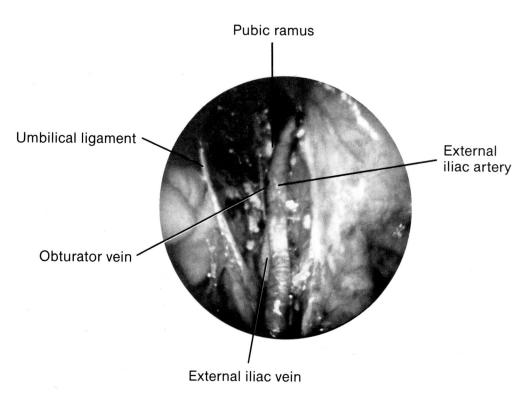

The samples are removed in the manner previously described. The peritoneal incisions are not closed. Indeed, we assume that when the abdomen is deflated, the edges of the incisions approximate. Incomplete occlusion of the peritoneal incision during healing may help avoid the formation of lymphocele.

After the peritoneal cavity is deflated, the 10 mm incisions are closed with a single stitch through the fascia. The advantage of subcutaneous absorbable suture material is that it need not be removed. The smaller incisions are simply approximated at the skin. The patient is then extubated and transferred to the recovery room. Although the intervention appears minimal since there is no large wound dressing, it should be emphasized that the patient has indeed undergone major surgery. In addition, many patients with lower genitourinary tract malignancy are elderly, necessitating strict monitoring of vital signs. Further postoperative care comprises administration of antibiotics (cephalosporins) and restriction of physical activities for 7 days. The patient is allowed to return home after 23 hours' observation, but a longer stay may be advisable, depending on the patient's general status. A follow-up visit is scheduled in 4 to 5 days to discuss further treatment.

Anatomopathologic Sampling and Evaluation

Ideally, the dissection of each sidewall results in two distinct pieces of tissue. However, it is sometimes difficult to avoid disruption of the samples, especially during extended lymphadenectomy. It is therefore advisable to remove the obturator node sample prior to extending the dissection to avoid confusion. Proper labeling of the specimen is, of course, mandatory. It has also been our experience that close collaboration with the pathologist is of utmost importance. One pathologist handles all our samples personally and communicates directly with the surgeon. Examination of the samples is as follows. The specimens are immediately transferred to the laboratory. The pathologist dissects any identifiable lymph nodes and labels them appropriately. The remaining fat is embedded en bloc. Every lymph node is cut at several levels and the middle levels examined first. All tissue is processed, without exception, allowing for accurate staging.

STUDY DESIGN AND OBJECTIVES

It should be noted that all patients in this series were recruited after routine transrectal ultrasonography of the prostate. Palpable lesions were the exception rather than the rule. The first 12 patients were selected because they had no surgical and anesthetic risks. Thereafter, lymphadenectomy was offered to all patients, regardless of their history and physical condition. After the first 30 procedures two more changes were introduced: extended lymphadenectomy on the right side and the methodology for anatomopathologic sampling and evaluation, as described previously. We intend to follow the current protocol for at least 50 cases.

The objectives of this study are to answer the questions: (1) Does laparoscopic lymphadenectomy provide sufficient material for histologic examination? (2) Is morbidity as low as for other laparoscopic procedures?

RESULTS

The first question can be answered affirmatively. Nodal tissue was obtained in all cases. The variability in the total number of nodes sampled in patients was large, but this is of limited importance. In particular, there seemed to be no difference in the number of nodes removed on the left and right sides. A discrepancy between sides could be interpreted as the result of technical difficulties and therefore cast doubt on the value of the procedure. It can be seen from the data in Table 12-2 that there were significantly more lymph nodes identified in the last six cases. The surgical technique did not change per se, aside from the inclusion of the right iliac lymphatic chain. The important change was the establishment of a strict protocol for histologic evaluation of the sample.

Intraoperative morbidity is extremely low thus far. Blood loss did not exceed 100 ml in any case. Laparotomy for repair of inadvertent damage was not required. One procedure was interrupted because hypercarbia occurred that could not be corrected by hyperventilation (patient No. 33). We still do not know whether this isolated case represented an instrument malfunction or a true complication.

Early postoperative morbidity included one case of acute urinary retention with prostatitis and one case of low-grade fever of unknown origin. One patient, not included in the series reported here, developed peritonitis secondary to an occult perforation of the small bowel. Five previous abdominal surgeries had caused dense adhesions. It is assumed that the small bowel was injured during lysis of these adhesions. This injury went unnoticed and subsequently led to peritonitis.

Only one late complication occurred: a hernia through a 10 mm suprapubic incision that resolved spontaneously. No lymphocele or chronic lymphedema of the lower extremities has occurred thus far (longest follow-up is 12 months).

Table 12-2. Results of Laparoscopic Pelvic Lymphadenectomy in 36 Patients

Patient No.	Age (yr)	Gleason Grade[16]	Volume (cm²)	PAP (mg/ml)	PSA (mg/ml)	OR Time (min)	Hospital Stay (days)	Right Obturator	Right Iliac Nodes	Left Obturator
1	75	6	0.45	0.4	6.1	160	1	2	—	4
2	76	3	NA	0.7	1.1	153	7	9	—	12
3	72	9	8.28	31.0	90.0	195	4	4	—	6
4	74	7	1.45	0.9	12.0	100	2	12	—	7
5	89	5	0.11	0.5	5.5	190	1	10	—	9
6	57	5	3.60	3.0	15.1	205	9	6	—	3
7	63	7	1.58	0.3	1.4	120	1	13	—	9
8	75	7	4.00	1.5	24.0	145	1	5	—	7
9	68	6	0.16	0.1	6.8	145	1	5	—	6
10	61	6	NA	1.0	8.2	145	1	7	—	7
11	72	4	0.22	1.1	1.9	125	1	11	—	7
12	68	5	1.92	1.9	11.0	90	1	7	—	8
13	64	7	1.80	10.8	75.4	225	1	8	—	7
14	75	6	0.18	0.4	3.3	230	1	7	—	5
15	71	7	1.15	2.2	30.0	220	1	4	—	5
16	76	5	0.17	0.6	2.1	175	1	5	—	2
17	67	6	2.81	0.9	23.0	115	1	9	—	6
18	75	6	0.80	0.6	12.0	190	1	4	—	2
19	72	7	2.35	2.8	36.0	240	1	3	—	3
20	75	4	1.34	0.3	12.8	100	2	3	—	3
21	78	3	0.53	0.3	1.9	120	1	3	—	1
22	79	7	0.39	0.3	12.0	95	7	3	—	3
23	64	6	1.80	0.4	12.0	90	1	5	—	5
24	71	5	5.13	NA	41.8	200	1	5(+)	4(−)	3(−)
25	82	6	1.55	0.7	16.0	135	1	5	—	4
26	69	7	0.45	0.5	10.0	115	1	5	—	4
27	84	6	1.15	2.2	16.6	140	3	6	—	5
28	75	NA	0.18	0.9	7.5	80	2	2	—	3
29	63	6	1.27	0.3	2.9	140	2	10	—	7
30	76	6	0.32	0.5	10.0	110	2	4	—	3
31	70	6	7.56	5.1	124.0	165	2	16(−)	14(+)	5(+)
32	64	7	3.72	1.2	22.0	235	2	11	18	9
33	74	9	NA	0.8	25.0	150	1	11	—	10
34	70	5	0.38	0.6	1.5	255	2	6	8	3
35	68	5	0.72	2.6	33.0	120	4	5	9	11
36	76	7	1.47	0.7	11.0	165	2	22	7	9

PSA = prostate-specific antigen; PAP = prostatic acid phosphatase.

No thromboembolic accidents have occurred, which is attributable we believe to the fact that patients are not restricted from physical mobilization in the immediate postoperative period. Postoperative pain is minimal and easily managed with oral medication as early as 4 hours postoperatively. Although ambulation is restricted, especially in elderly patients, active mobilization in bed is encouraged. Thrombosis prevention devices are now used routinely in patients 60 years or older. Since this rule has been added to our protocol only recently, we cannot evaluate its effectiveness at this time.

It is somewhat premature at this stage to try to evaluate extended lymphadenectomy in terms of its prognostic value. However, we know that extending the lymphadenectomy has prolonged the length of the surgical procedure an average of 30 minutes and patients tend to stay in the hospital for a longer time. It appears that morbidity is greater with extended laparoscopic lymphadenectomy. Whether this will be balanced by a more reliable prognosis remains to be determined.

CONCLUSION

Laparoscopic lymphadenectomy provides tissue samples comparable to those obtained at open surgery. Our series is relatively small, but there is no doubt that the incidence of complications, whether intra- or postoperative, may be described as infrequent compared to that after open surgery. Laparoscopic lymphadenectomy is therefore an extremely valuable prognostic intervention to precede definitive treatment of malignancies of the lower urogenital tract.

REFERENCES

1. Wertheim E. The extent of the abdominal operation for carcinoma. Am J Obstet Gynecol 66:169-177, 1912.
2. Meigs JV. Carcinoma of the cervix—The Wertheim operation. Surg Gynecol Obstet 78:192-199, 1944.
3. Gervasi LA, Mata J, Easley JD, Wilbanks JH, Seale-Hawkins C, Carlton CE, Scardino PT. Prognostic significance of lymph nodal metastases in prostate cancer. J Urol 142:332-336, 1989.
4. McLaughlin AP, Saltzstein SL, McCullough DL, Gittes RF. Prostatic carcinoma: Incidence and location of unsuspected lymphatic metastases. J Urol 115:89-94, 1976.
5. Nicholson TC, Richie JP. Pelvic lymphadenectomy for stage B_1 adenocarcinoma of the prostate: Justified or not? J Urol 117:199-201, 1977.
6. Ray GR, Pistenma DA, Castellino RA, Kempson RL, Meares E, Bagshan MA. Operative staging of apparently localized adenocarcinoma of the prostate: Results in fifty unselected patients. I. Experimental design and preliminary results. Cancer 38:73-83, 1976.
7. McCullough DL, McLaughlin AP, Gittes RF. Morbidity of pelvic lymphadenectomy and radical prostatectomy for prostatic cancer. J Urol 117:206-207, 1977.

8. Lieskovsky G, Skinner DG, Weisenburger T. Pelvic lymphadenectomy in the management of carcinoma of the prostate. J Urol 124:635-638, 1980.

9. Grossman IC, Carpiniello V, Greenberg SH, Malloy TR, Wein AJ. Staging pelvic lymphadenectomy for carcinoma of the prostate. J Urol 124:632-634, 1980.

10. Correa RJ Jr, Kidd CR, Burnett L, Brannen GE, Gibbons RP, Cummings KB. Percutaneous pelvic lymph node aspiration in carcinoma of the prostate. J Urol 126:190-191, 1981.

11. Hald T, Rasmussen F. Extraperitoneal pelvioscopy: A new aid in staging of lower urinary tract tumors. A preliminary report. J Urol 124:245-248, 1979.

12. Iversen P, Bak M, Juul N, Laursen F, van der Maase M, Nielsen L, Rasmussen F, Torp-Pedersen S, Holm HH. Ultrasonically guided ^{125}iodine seed implantation with external radiation in management of localized prostatic carcinoma. Urology 34:181-186, 1989.

13. Salvat J, Dargent C. Panoramic retroperitoneal pelviscopy. Presented at the symposium on Laparoscopic Surgery: The American Experience. Baltimore: Aug. 11-13, 1988.

14. Fuerst DE. Laparoscopic examination of pelvic lymph nodes. Urology 26:482-483, 1985.

15. Querleu D. Laparoscopic pelvic lymphadenectomy. Presented at the Thirteenth International Workshop on Reconstructive Pelvic Surgery in Gynecology, Leuven, Belgium: Aug. 31-Sept. 2, 1989.

16. Gleason DF. Histologic grading and clinical staging of prostatic carcinoma. In Tannenbaum M, ed. Urologic Pathology: The Prostate, 1st ed. Philadelphia: Lea & Febiger, 1977, p 171.

CHAPTER 13

Laparoscopic Truncal and Selective Vagotomy

Jean Mouiel, M.D.
Namir Katkhouda, M.D.

Experience gained from laparoscopic appendectomy, adhesiolysis, and cholecystectomy has made possible the use of this technology for the treatment of acute and chronic duodenal ulcer disease. Laparoscopic vagotomy procedures are now being offered to patients at the Hôpital St. Roch in Nice, France, and more recently in North America.[1,2] Although to date our largest experience with laparoscopic ulcer surgery has involved posterior truncal vagotomy with anterior seromyotomy, both truncal and selective procedures will be described in this chapter. In addition, our experience with emergency laparoscopic management of perforated duodenal ulcer is presented.

TRUNCAL VS. SELECTIVE VAGOTOMY

Although we prefer to use selective vagotomy for patients undergoing elective duodenal ulcer surgery, we also advise that surgeons become skilled in the technique of abdominal truncal (complete) vagotomy with dilatation of the pylorus. In our experience this operation has proved easier to perform than selective vagotomy and will probably be the laparoscopic acid-reducing procedure initially performed by most surgeons. The immediate and long-term results of truncal vagotomy in patients with intractable or complicated ulcer disease are known to be quite satisfactory despite the relatively small incidence of postgastrectomy complications. Although many gastroenterologists and surgeons now consider highly selective vagotomy to be the procedure of choice for patients with intractable ulcer disease, truncal vagotomy continues to play an important role.[3]

PATIENT SELECTION

The preoperative evaluation of patients with duodenal ulcer disease scheduled to undergo laparoscopic surgery is comparable to that for traditional surgery. The absolute and relative contraindications for laparoscopic vagotomy are nearly identical to those described for cholecystectomy (see Chapter 8). Candidates for elective surgical therapy are, in general, individuals in whom the ulcer diatheses has proved resistant to medical therapy.

In our first series of seven patients the average length of intensive medical therapy prior to laparoscopic surgery was 3.7 years.[1] At the present time individuals are considered candidates for elective laparoscopic surgery if they continue to complain of recurrent ulcer symptoms despite full compliance with medical management for at least 2 years. In addition, these patients should be followed with regular and well-documented endoscopic or radiologic examinations and have no intercurrent complications at presentation. Surgery may also on occasion be recommended for patients who cannot correctly comply with therapeutic advice or cannot be followed regularly because of geographic or socioeconomic reasons.

The preoperative workup includes screening for surgical risk factors (i.e., cardiovascular or pulmonary disease) as well as a thorough evaluation of the ulcer disease. The latter usually requires endoscopic, laboratory, and acid secretory studies. If clinically indicated, a serum gastrin level should be obtained to exclude the possible presence of a gastrinoma. Endoscopy should be performed to visualize the area of disease directly and to determine if scarring or stenosis of the pylorus or duodenum has occurred. In addition, endoscopy excludes other disorders of the upper gastrointestinal tract (gastric carcinoma, esophageal reflux, etc.) in which symptoms may mimic those of peptic ulcer disease. Acid secretory tests include measurement of unstimulated or basal acid output (BAO) and peak acid output (PAO) following administration of pentagastrin (6 μg/kg). Most patients refractory to medical treatment will show marked hyperacidity. Secretory studies are also useful to demonstrate postoperative reduction of acid output and provide a means to assess the effectiveness of the vagotomy.

TECHNIQUE
Complete Truncal Vagotomy

As in traditional open surgery, general anesthesia and endotracheal intubation are advised. We do not routinely insert bladder catheters for upper abdominal laparoscopic procedures; however, nasogastric aspiration is necessary to ensure that the stomach is empty. We generally insert both a nasogastric tube and a fiberoptic gastroscope. The latter not only distends the esophagus but may also be used to transilluminate and identify important anatomic landmarks such as the gastroesophageal junction. Occasionally it may prove difficult to insert both of these devices because of the relatively small diameter of the upper esophagus. In this event a smaller caliber pediatric endoscope may be used.

The patient is placed in the supine position with legs spread apart to facilitate the two-team approach. This is similar to the technique described by Dubois et al.[4] for laparoscopic cholecystectomy.

The operating surgeon stands between the legs of the patient; an assistant is stationed at the patient's left side. A second assistant is positioned on the patient's right. The operating room is set up so that the light source, insufflator, and video monitors are in direct view of the entire surgical team, anesthesiologists, and operating room staff. An electrocautery unit and YAG laser systems are also available. The patient is prepared and draped as for open laparotomy. Surgical instruments required to perform the traditional procedure are kept within the operating room in case laparoscopic surgery is deemed impossible or hazardous and thus an open procedure is required.

Pneumoperitoneum is established using CO_2; the intraperitoneal pressure is maintained at or below 14 mm Hg. The insufflation needle is usually introduced through the umbilicus. After the abdomen has been fully distended, a total of five punctures are made.

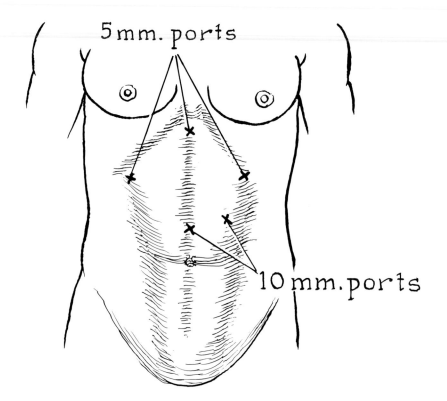

The first trocar (10 mm) is inserted approximately 5 cm above the umbilicus and is used to introduce the forward-viewing laparoscope and video camera. Then, under direct vision, the remaining trocars are inserted through the abdominal wall. A 5 mm trocar and cannula are inserted just below and to the right of the xiphoid and are used for introducing blunt-nosed retractors or aspiration-lavage probes. Five-millimeter trocars are also placed along the right and left mammillary lines and allow for the insertion of grasping forceps or needle holders. The fifth puncture is a 10 mm trocar placed to the left of the laparoscope and through the rectus muscle. This is the operating cannula through which a hook coagulator, scissors, collagen applicator, and hemostatic clip appliers are later introduced.

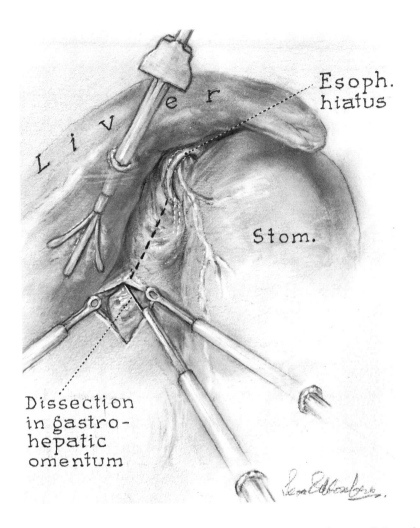

The operative procedure is similar in many ways to the traditional open operation. The abdominal cavity is first explored with the video laparoscope to determine if the laparoscopic approach is feasible. A full survey of the hiatal region is performed by retracting the left lobe of the liver with a palpation probe or fanlike retractor.

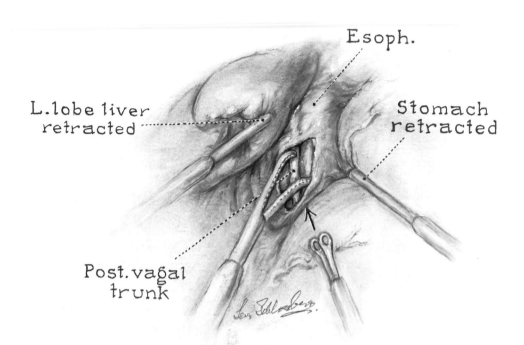

The lesser sac is entered through an opening in the pars flaccida and nervosa, which allows the surgeon to dissect cephalad along the lesser curvature to the hiatal region. The left gastric vein is usually encountered during this dissection and is divided between clips or sutures as necessary. The essential landmark of the region is the right crus of the diaphragm, which can be retracted along with the proximal stomach to the patient's left while the coagulator/dissector hook is used to open the pre-esophageal peritoneum. This allows visualization of the mesoesophagus where the posterior vagus nerve can be found.

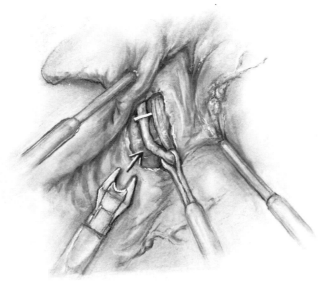

The esophagus is retracted to the left with a blunt probe, and the inferior margin of the hiatus is dissected with the hook probe until the nerve is identified.

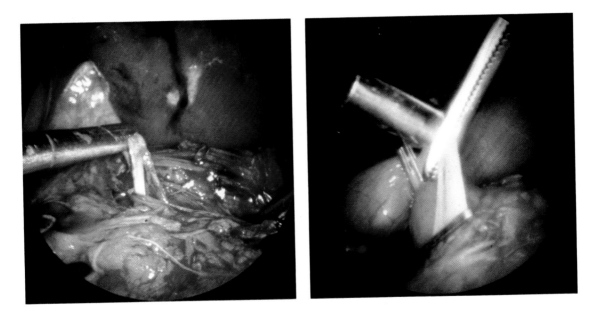

Gentle traction is exerted on the nerve while it is dissected free from the surrounding tissues.

The nerve is then transected between two surgical clips and a small fragment retrieved for histologic examination.

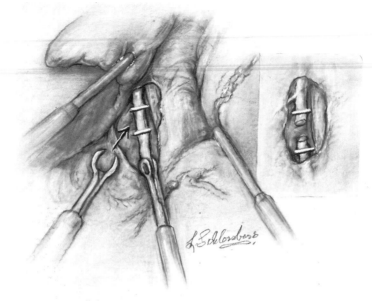

The next step is to divide the anterior vagus nerve. The pre-esophageal peritoneum is incised with the hook-coagulator until the left crus of the diaphragm is reached. The anterior vagus nerve can be easily identified and snared with the hook dissector. The nerve is then divided between two surgical clips.

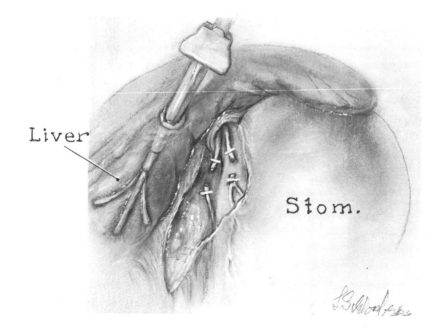

Vagotomy is complete once Grassi's criminal branch is identified and divided as well as any other aberrant branches along the left margin of the esophagus. The entire circumference of the esophagus may be examined by retracting first the left and then the right margins of the esophagus to either side, thus exposing the posterior aspect.

We also routinely perform pneumatic dilatation of the pylorus to avoid potential problems with gastric emptying after a truncal vagotomy. This partially ruptures the oblique and circular muscles of the pylorus and results in a widely patent channel.[5] The laparoscope and video camera are left within the abdomen while a flexible gastroscope is positioned within the pylorus.

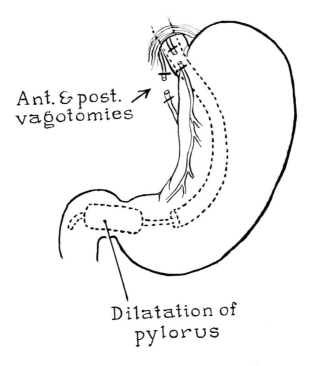

A 16 mm pyloric balloon is inserted through the working channel of the endoscope and inflated to 45 psi. Proper positioning of the balloon is confirmed laparoscopically, and a careful examination is performed to ensure that a dilatation-induced perforation has not occurred.

Hemostasis must be confirmed; if necessary, additional titanium clips are applied. A closed suction drainage catheter can be inserted through the right lateral cannula and positioned near the hiatus if indicated (see p. 171). The pneumoperitoneum is completely deflated, the trocars are removed, and the puncture holes are closed. We generally infiltrate the puncture sites with a long-acting local anesthetic agent to minimize postoperative pain.

Posterior Truncal Vagotomy and Anterior Seromyotomy (Taylor's Procedure)

Selective or parietal cell vagotomy is associated with ulcer recurrence rates as high as 20%.[3,6] Inadequate denervation of the parietal cell mass is believed to be the most common cause of failed selective vagotomy. Extensive dissection and division of vagal nerve fibers near the antrum and pyloric channel, on the other hand, may lead to gastric stasis. Problems in predicting the extent of vagal denervation led Taylor, Gunn, and MacLeod[7] to the procedure known as posterior truncal vagotomy with anterior seromyotomy. The effectiveness of anterior seromyotomy was based on the anatomic observation that the anterior vagus nerve courses obliquely through the seromuscular layers of the stomach before innervating the fundic parietal cell mass. Dividing the seromuscular layer of the stomach along the lesser curvature would thus assure complete fundic denervation. According to Taylor's original description, the myotomy was begun approximately 6 cm proximal to the pylorus and 1.5 cm from the lesser curve. He believed this technique diminished both the risk of injury to the nerve of Latarjet and ischemic necrosis of the stomach. The myotomy was extended proximally as far as the gastroesophageal junction. Taylor preferred dividing the longitudinal and circular muscle fibers and leaving the deeper, thin layer of oblique muscle intact. Later, Kahwaji and Grange[8] proposed extending the length of the myotomy proximally to include the gastric cardia. This modification was designed to ensure complete denervation of the gastroesophageal junction and gastric cardia. Subsequent investigations have shown that anterior seromyotomy does not alter gastric motility or emptying.[9] Vasovagal nerve arcs appear to conduct impulses from the anterior to the posterior antrum.[10] Therefore a gastric emptying procedure such as pyloroplasty or balloon dilatation is not necessary. Taylor et al.[11] reported a 6% incidence of recurrent duodenal ulcer in 77 patients followed up 4½ years after the procedure.

In performing Taylor's procedure with the laparoscope the lesser curvature is exposed and opened in the same manner as described for truncal vagotomy. The posterior vagus nerve is dissected free from the posterior aspect of the esophagus and divided between surgical clips. The anterior lesser curve seromyotomy is then performed beginning at the cardia and extended to within 6 cm of the pylorus.

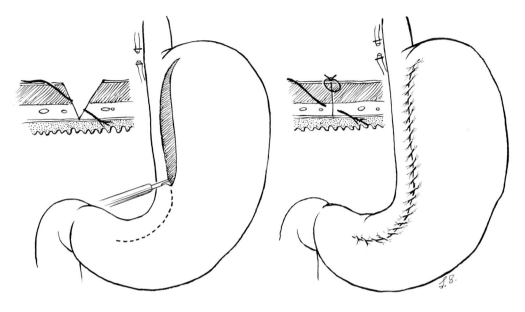

This point is recognized by the branching of the nerve of Latarjet (the "crow's foot"). The seromyotomy is maintained at a distance of 1.5 cm from the lesser curve. Care is taken not to penetrate the gastric mucosa. The magnification afforded by the video laparoscopic imaging system appears to minimize this risk. A standard monopolar cautery hook instrument is used to perform the seromyotomy (see Chapter 2). A running 3-0 or 2-0 monofilament suture (i.e., overlap suture) is then used to approximate the seromuscular defect to minimize the risk of perioperative bleeding and tissue adhesions. A fibrin sealant (Tissucol; Immuno Corporation, Vienna, Austria) is applied over the suture line to further ensure hemostasis.

Posterior Truncal Vagotomy and Anterior Selective Vagotomy

Recently Bailey, Flowers, and Graham[2] reported the technique of laparoscopic posterior truncal vagotomy and anterior selective vagotomy. This procedure is based on the operation originally described in 1978 by Hill and Barker.[12] These earlier investigators reported a 73% reduction in basal acid output and a 65% reduction in stimulated acid secretion in the first 20 patients to undergo this procedure. They also found that the mean gastric emptying time in these patients was nearly identical to that in a group of unoperated controls.

Bailey and co-workers performed their procedure using a five-puncture technique similar to that described previously. The only differences are that the primary 10 mm trocar and cannula are inserted closer to the umbilicus, and the second accessory 10 mm puncture is placed through the right midabdomen rather than the left.

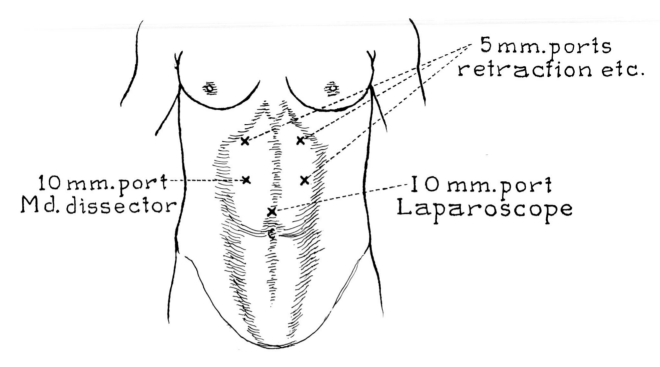

The left lobe of the liver is mobilized by dividing the left triangular ligament. A fanlike retractor is then used to hold the liver laterally. A 48 Fr dilator is used to distend the esophagus and place the stomach on tension. This also results in the greater curvature of the stomach being pushed laterally (to the patient's left) and posterior. The lesser curvature is pulled medially and anteriorly, thus facilitating exposure of the anterior vagal nerve fibers. The esophagus is retracted to the left with a blunt probe and the lesser omentum opened. The posterior vagus nerve is dissected from the posterior mesoesophagus and divided between titanium clips (Endo-Clip; United States Surgical Corporation, Norwalk, Conn.). When pathologic examination has confirmed that the specimen is of neural origin, attention is directed to the anterior vagus nerve. The nerve is identified near the anterior aspect of the esophagus and placed on tension with a blunt probe inserted through the subxiphoid cannula. The serosa is carefully opened with Semm hook scissors along the lesser curvature of the stomach. Individual branches of the anterior vagus nerve are then easily displayed as they enter the stomach.

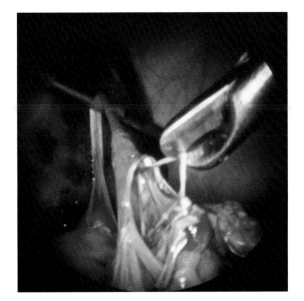

Titanium clips are applied to each branch and then divided using Semm hook scissors.

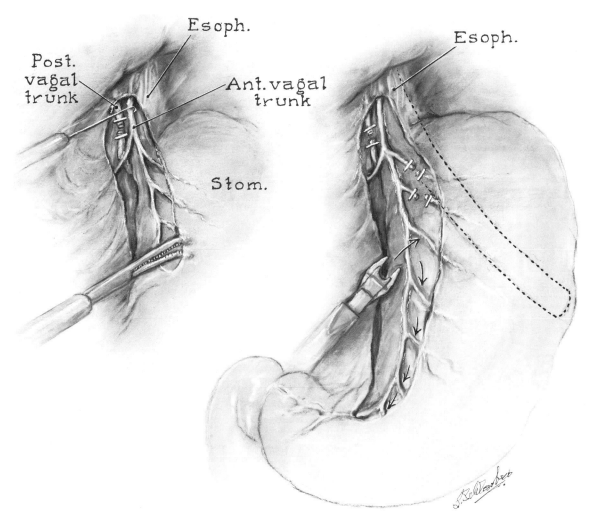

The magnification and clarity of the laparoscopic image often enables the nerve to be dissected separate from the adjacent blood vessels. The branches of the nerve of Latarjet innervating the gastric antrum are easily identified and preserved. With the anterior vagus nerve on tension and retracted to the patient's right, the entire gastroesophageal area is carefully dissected to divide any vagal branches innervating the cardia.

MANAGEMENT OF PERFORATED DUODENAL ULCER

In the emergency setting, laparoscopic surgical intervention may also be indicated for patients seen within 12 hours of duodenal ulcer perforation. In addition to closing the perforation, either a truncal or selective vagotomy may be performed, depending on the operative findings and the experience of the surgeon. If the patient is seen more than 12 hours after perforation, management should be restricted to simple closure of the duodenal perforation.

Acute duodenal perforations are usually anterior and are easily identified through the laparoscope. Often gastric fluid can be seen escaping from the opening. The entire abdominal cavity is examined to determine the degree and extension of peritonitis. Abdominal fluid is obtained for bacterial cultures and sensitivity (i.e., antibiotic) testing. After the peritoneal cavity has been irrigated copiously, the perforation may be closed in either of two ways. Simple closure can be achieved by using a laparoscopic needle holder with a 20 mm straight needle attached to a 15 cm long threaded suture material. Two or three sutures are placed with knots tied intracorporeally (i.e., instrument tie) or extracorporeally, approximating the omentum over the site of perforation with each suture. A collagen/fibrinogen mixture may then be sprayed over the operative site. The perforation can also be closed by using a combined endoscopic and laparoscopic approach as shown on p. 277.

A grasping instrument is inserted via the operating channel of the flexible gastroscope and out through the duodenal opening. The grasping forceps are used to pull a segment of omentum over the duodenal opening. The omentum is then secured to the duodenum by laparoscopic sutures as described earlier. A drain placed through the trocar in the right hypochondrium is maintained under 30 mm H_2O negative pressure (i.e., closed suction drainage). The pneumoperitoneum is desufflated and the abdominal punctures closed as previously described.

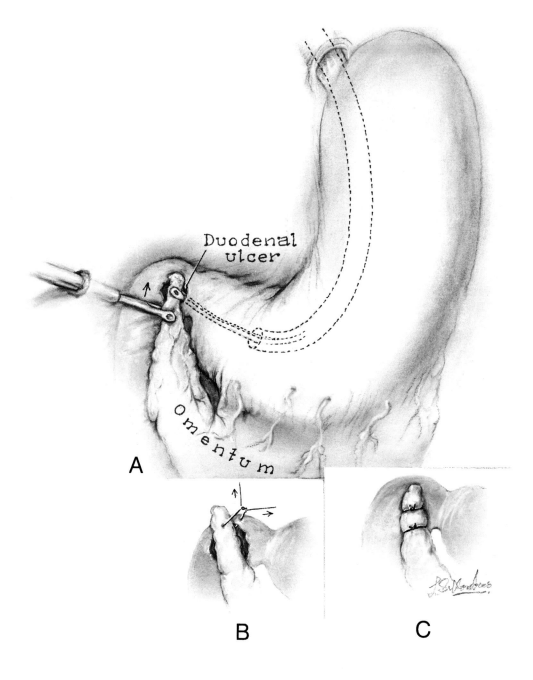

Duodenal ulcer

Omentum

A

B

C

POSTOPERATIVE CARE

The nasogastric tube is left in place for a minimum of 24 hours following vagotomy alone and 48 hours after closure of an acute duodenal perforation. The patient is discharged 48 to 72 hours after vagotomy and 5 days after simple closure for perforation. Although antibiotics are not used routinely for vagotomy, they are given prophylactically if the patient is suspected of having a perforation. Similar to the experience with laparoscopic cholecystectomy, postoperative pain is minimal and may be nonexistent with injection of local anesthesia into the puncture holes. When required, nonsteroid analgesics can be prescribed.

Repeat endoscopy is performed 4 to 6 weeks after surgery to confirm healing of the ulcer. Postoperative secretory studies are also performed to document reduction in acid output.

RESULTS

As of November 1990, we have performed 30 operations for duodenal ulcer at the Hôpital St. Roch. Twenty-two of these procedures were performed in patients with chronic duodenal ulcer disease intractable to medical treatment and eight for acute perforations. Results are comparable to those we obtained in patients undergoing elective open vagotomy procedures. All endoscopic evidence of duodenal ulcer disease was found to have disappeared 1 month after the laparoscopic procedure. Postoperative acid secretion (BAO and PAO) was reduced by 80%. No mortality or serious morbidity was seen in these first 30 patients. One patient, however, must be considered as an operative failure. This patient required surgical correction of gastroesophageal reflux 2 months after vagotomy. The outcome was eventually satisfactory.

CONCLUSION

We began laparoscopic surgical treatment of duodenal ulcer disease 2 years ago concomitant with laparoscopic cholecystectomy. This new approach to ulcer disease appears promising since it allows the laparoscopic surgeon to perform either complete truncal vagotomy, posterior truncal vagotomy and anterior seromyotomy, or posterior truncal vagotomy and anterior selective vagotomy. Although most patients are managed appropriately with short-term administration of H_2 blockers, proton pump inhibitors, or other medical regimens, a significant number of patients will require continuous therapy or will fail initial therapy. In these individuals a laparoscopic procedure that may offer an 85% chance or greater of controlling their ulcer disease without lifelong medication may be appealing, especially if it affords a minimal disruption of their life-style.

Nevertheless, these new laparoscopic techniques need to be evaluated further for long-term effectiveness. We have begun a multicenter controlled trial not only to evaluate the results of laparoscopic surgery but also to compare them with standard medical therapy. Both long-term results and cost-effectiveness are being addressed. Only then will it be possible to truly inform the patient of new therapeutic alternatives using noninvasive procedures.

REFERENCES

1. Katkhouda N, Mouiel J. Treatment of chronic duodenal ulcer with posterior truncal vagotomy and anterior seromyotomy without laparotomy using video coelioscopy. Am J Surg (in press).
2. Bailey RW, Flowers JL, Graham SM. Combined laparoscopic cholecystectomy and selective vagotomy. Surg Laparosc Endosc (in press).
3. Elfberg BA, Nilsson F, Selking O. Parietal cell vagotomy and truncal vagotomy in elective duodenal ulcer surgery: Results after six to twelve years. Upsala J Med Sci 94:129-136, 1989.
4. Dubois F, Icard P, Berthelot G, Levard H. Coelioscopic cholecystectomy. Preliminary report of 36 cases. Ann Surg 211:60-62, 1990.
5. Taylor TV. Experience with the lunder quist ownman dilator in the upper gastrointestinal tract. Br J Surg 70:445, 1983.
6. Macintyre IMC, Millar A, Smith AN, Small WP. Highly selective vagotomy 5-15 years on. Br J Surg 77:65-69, 1990.
7. Taylor TV, Gunn AA, Macleod DAD. Anterior lesser curve seromyotomy and posterior truncal vagotomy in the treatment of chronic duodenal ulcer. Lancet 2:846-848, 1982.
8. Kahwaji F, Grange D. Ulcère duodénal chronique. Traitement par séromyotomie fundique antérieure avec vagotomie tronculaire postérieure. Press Med 16:28-30, 1987.
9. Taylor TV, Holt S, Heading RC. Gastric emptying after anterior lesser curve seromyotomy and posterior truncal vagotomy. Br J Surg 72:620-622, 1985.
10. Daniel EE, Sarna SK. Distribution of excitatory vagal fibres in canine gastric wall to control motility. Gastroenterology 71:608-611, 1976.
11. Taylor TV, Lythgoe JP, McFarland JB, Gilmore IT, Thomas PE, Ferguson GH. Anterior lesser curve seromyotomy and posterior truncal vagotomy versus truncal vagotomy and pyloroplasty in the treatment of chronic duodenal ulcer disease. Br J Surg 77:1007-1009, 1990.
12. Hill GL, Barker CJ. Anterior highly selective vagotomy with posterior truncal vagotomy: A simple technique for denervating the parietal cell mass. Br J Surg 65:702-705, 1978.

CHAPTER 14

Laparoscopic Inguinal Hernia Repair

Giovanni M. Salerno, M.D.
Robert J. Fitzgibbons, Jr., M.D.
Charles J. Filipi, M.D.

Approximately 500,000 patients have inguinal hernia repairs each year.[1] Modern-day inguinal hernia repair has been dominated by the extraperitoneal groin approach as initially proposed by Bassini in 1884. He revolutionized the treatment of inguinal hernia by introducing the concept of reconstruction of the floor of the inguinal canal. Modifications of his original hernia repair were proposed by Bull and Cooley, Ferguson, Halsted, and more recently McEvedy and McVay to avoid testicular complications and to further reduce the postoperative recurrence rate.[2]

Despite these modifications, inguinal herniorrhaphy has not reached perfection. The abundance of literature dealing with various sutures and suturing techniques, prosthetic materials, and new herniorrhaphy modifications underscore this. In a recent collected series from around the world in which the Bassini repair and a variety of its modifications were used to repair inguinal hernias, the postoperative recurrence rates varied from 0% to 7% for indirect, 1% to 10% for direct, and 5% to 35% for recurrent hernias.[3] In addition to recurrence, painful postoperative neuromas, spermatic cord injury, and postoperative epididymitis or orchitis are occasionally seen with the classic extraperitoneal herniorrhaphy using the groin approach. Finally, the conventional operation is painful and is associated with a significant loss of hours on the job, especially when the patient's occupation involves heavy lifting.

Transabdominal repair of an inguinal hernia is not a new concept. Most surgeons will readily perform such a procedure in a patient with an inguinal hernia at the conclusion of another operation requiring a laparotomy if the patient's condition is stable. The morbidity associated with conventional laparotomy makes transabdominal inguinal hernia repair as a primary procedure impractical. However, the recent introduction of therapeutic laparoscopy in general surgery has generated renewed interest in this approach.

HISTORICAL PERSPECTIVE

The American surgeon Henry Marcy realized that failure to close the internal ring or low ligation of an indirect inguinal hernia sac predisposed the patient to recurrence. Even with the most accurate reconstruction, suturing one or more musculoaponeurotic layers to the inguinal ligament was doomed to failure if the reconstruction did not include closure of the internal ring or high hernial sac ligation.[4,5] Marcy[6,7] was the first to describe a procedure that achieved high hernia sac ligation and inguinal ring closure through a transabdominal approach. In 1932 the transabdominal approach was modified by LaRoque, who referred to it as the intra-abdominal method. He made an inguinal skin incision higher than usual, opened the peritoneum, and dissected the hernia sac from within the abdominal cavity. This was followed by closure of the inguinal hernia defect from within the peritoneal cavity.[8] LaRoque believed intra-abdominal repair had several advantages such as accurate diagnosis of indirect, direct, or femoral hernias; rapid dissection of the sac without spermatic cord trauma; and safe resection of gangrenous bowel or omentum. Unfortunately, although he performed 1700 of these procedures, accurate follow-up data are lacking.

The usefulness of incidental indirect inguinal hernia repair from within the abdominal cavity at the time of a laparotomy performed for unrelated diseases was recognized by Andrews, another American surgeon, in 1924.[9] Andrews closed the inguinal hernia defect by placing sutures in the peritoneum and fascia from within the peritoneal cavity. He thought this was a far more effectual method for repair of an indirect inguinal hernia than other methods at that time.

THE GER PROCEDURE

In 1982 Ger[10] described the management of a variety of abdominal wall hernias through a transabdominal approach in a series of 13 patients who underwent laparotomy primarily for other intra-abdominal conditions (8 indirect, 2 direct, 2 umbilical, and 1 femoral). The Ger procedure for repair of a groin hernia is similar to the one described by Marcy[6] and later modified by LaRoque.[8] However, it differs in that the hernia sac is neither dissected, ligated, nor reduced but instead stainless steel Michel clips

(3 × 15 mm) are used to close the peritoneal opening of the sac. Only one recurrence was noted in this series of 13 patients operated on using this technique, the longest follow-up being 44 months.[10] Interestingly, the last patient in Ger's report had the inguinal hernia defect repaired with the clips placed under laparoscopic guidance. The staples were applied with a special stapling device inserted through a second laparoscopic cannula. The patient was followed up for 3 years without evidence of recurrence.

More recently, Ger et al.[11] published a study in dogs with congenital indirect inguinal hernias. The purpose of this investigation was to test his newly conceived laparoscopic approach to inguinal hernia. Of the 15 beagle dogs in the study population, the first three animals underwent standard laparotomy and stapling of the peritoneal opening under direct vision and the remaining dogs had closure of the same opening under laparoscopic guidance after insufflation of nitrous oxide to establish pneumoperitoneum. Care was taken to leave small gaps between staples to avoid the formation of a hydrocele. Once again a custom-designed stapler was used for this procedure.

All 12 dogs undergoing laparoscopic repair of a congenital indirect inguinal hernia were cured. Examination of en bloc inguinal specimens showed that if the staples were properly applied, they "sunk" below the peritoneum and disappeared. Superficial application of staples resulted in staple migration with loss of effective closure. Examination of the processus vaginalis with probes showed that in five dogs the sac was obliterated and in eight dogs its size was considerably reduced. Ger et al. proposed the following advantages of laparoscopic repair of a groin hernia: (1) small puncture wounds; (2) minimal dissection; (3) less chance of injury to the spermatic cord; (4) decreased incidence of ischemic orchitis; (5) decreased incidence of bladder injury; (6) no ilioinguinal postoperative neuralgia; (7) outpatient procedure; (8) ability to achieve a very high closure of the peritoneal sac; (9) minimal postoperative discomfort; (10) faster recovery time; (11) simultaneous intra-abdominal diagnostic laparoscopy; and (12) ability to diagnose and treat bilateral groin hernias without extensive dissection.

PROSTHETIC REPAIR OF GROIN HERNIAS

In an attempt to further reduce the recurrence rate after inguinal hernia repair, the concept of "tension-free" hernia repair was introduced. Lichtenstein et al.[12] postulated that the prime etiologic factor in hernia repair recurrence is suturing together, under tension, structures that are not normally in apposition. This tension violates a basic surgical principle of wound healing. They introduced the tension-free prosthetic hernioplasty that uses prosthetic mesh in groin hernia repair as a substitute for the classic inguinal floor reconstruction.

Prosthetic surgical techniques were originally used only for repair of recurrent or unusually large hernias. However, there is now a trend to employ these techniques in patients undergoing repair of direct and indirect groin hernias for the first time. Lichtenstein et al.[12] reported no recurrence (follow-up of 1 to 5 years) and no prosthetic infection in 1000 consecutive cases. Stoppa and Warlaumont[13] investigated the preperitoneal prosthetic repair of groin hernias in first-time operations and showed lower rates of postoperative wound infection and decreased number of days away from work when compared with the standard technique. The authors reported a recurrence rate of 1.4% in 572 prosthetic hernia repairs. Nyhus et al.[14] have also evaluated the preperitoneal prosthetic repair of first-time operated direct inguinal hernias, recurrent combined groin hernias, and recurrent femoral hernias (a total of 203 procedures). They reported similar encouraging results with a recurrence rate of 1.7%.

COMBINED LAPAROSCOPIC APPROACH AND PROSTHETIC REPAIR

It is logical to postulate the advantages of a combined laparoscopic approach and tension-free prosthetic technique. Under laparoscopic vision a synthetic mesh prosthesis could be fixed to the peritoneal surface with metal clips to accomplish closure of the internal inguinal ring and to strengthen the weak inguinal floor. This laparoscopic placement could conceivably be the same for direct, indirect, or even femoral hernias. The repair would incorporate the advantages of the intra-abdominal approach without the morbidity associated with conventional laparotomy.

Recently Popp[15] reported the repair of a coincidental direct inguinal hernia discovered at the time of a laparoscopic myomectomy with the use of a 4 × 5 cm oval dehydrated dura mater patch. A laparoscopic suturing technique with extracorporeally tied knots was used to fix the patch in place. Based on this experience, Popp thought laparoscopic repair of abdominal wall hernias was technically feasible but was concerned about the possibility of intra-abdominal adhesions resulting in bowel obstruction and other complications.

Three additional methods dealing with laparoscopic repair of indirect groin hernias deserve consideration. In the technique developed by Leonard Schultz of Minneapolis, Minnesota, the peritoneal sac is incised at the internal inguinal ring opening. The sac is then pulled back by traction and blunt dissection and is cut at the ring opening. After laparoscopic examination of the inguinal canal for hemostasis, a polypropylene patch is inserted into the canal and the peritoneal opening is closed with staples. To date, 30 patients have been operated on using this technique. The longest follow-up has been 8 months, and one recurrence has been diagnosed (personal communication, 1990). The technique proposed by Harry Reich of Kingstone, Pennsylvania, is based on the insertion of a polypropylene mesh "plug" into the inguinal sac followed by simple closure of the peritoneal opening with sutures (personal communication, 1990). A combination of these methods has been adopted by Corbitt[16] in West Palm Beach, Florida. The hernia is reduced and the sac is pulled into the peritoneal cavity. The hernia sac is then opened near the apex, allowing the cord structures to be identified. A 2 × 5 inch piece of polypropylene is rolled into a plug and inserted through the internal ring and the inguinal canal. A 2-inch square mesh is placed over the internal ring and the peritoneum closed over it with a laparoscopic stapling instrument (Endo GIA; United States Surgical Corporation, Norwalk, Conn.). Corbitt has performed 30 of these procedures with no recurrences, although the length of follow-up has been limited thus far. These procedures, however, must be investigated further before they can be proposed as valid alternatives to present methods of inguinal hernia repair.

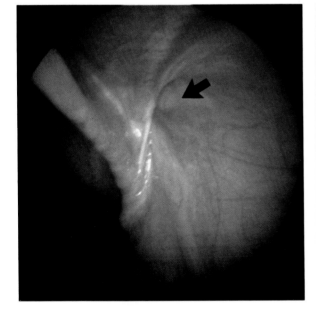

Laparoscopic appearance of right indirect hernia in a 40-year-old man.

Marlex mesh in place over right inguinal hernia defect prior to peritoneal closure.

STUDY DESIGN AND OBJECTIVES

Laparoscopic inguinal hernia repair is currently under investigation at the Creighton University Laboratory of Experimental Laparoscopic Surgery. The current protocol has been designed to investigate the laparoscopic placement of a nonabsorbable prosthesis using an intra-abdominal approach with a simple onlay technique. The procedure does not include ligation of the hernia sac or surgical apposition of peritoneal or musculo-aponeurotic structures; it is theorized that the prosthesis will effectively accomplish both goals. In effect, the laparoscopic approach of Ger will be combined with the tension-free principles proposed by Lichtenstein et al. The potential advantages are as follows: (1) only a few additional minutes are required to apply the patch and secure it in place; (2) less postoperative discomfort will result since no groin tissue is dissected; (3) absence of surgically apposed tissue that must heal will permit immediate return to work without restriction; (4) long-term postoperative complications specifically related to the groin incision will be eliminated; (5) because the cord structures are not disturbed, no testicular complications will occur; and (6) bilateral groin hernias can be treated during the same operation because of the lack of tension. It is anticipated that the repair would be applicable to all types of groin hernias: femoral, direct, and indirect. Potential disadvantages are (1) adhesions with bowel obstruction; (2) difficult-to-treat infections because of the intra-abdominal location of the prosthesis; and (3) erosion of the prosthetic material into organs or blood vessels.

The investigation addresses the following questions:
- Can an inguinal hernia be successfully repaired using a transabdominally placed prosthetic material without ligation of a peritoneal sac or tissue apposition?
- Can a technique be developed to quickly, accurately, and reproducibly place the prosthetic material laparoscopically?
- Can a metal clip applier or stapling device be developed to facilitate fixation of the prosthesis?
- Is polypropylene mesh (Prolene) or expanded polytetrafluoroethylene (PTFE) weave (Gore-Tex soft tissue patch) a better prosthetic material and what will be the rate of adhesion formation to each?
- Will oxidized regenerated cellulose (Interceed) decrease the rate of adhesions to the prosthesis?

TECHNIQUE

The male pig is an excellent model because large bilateral congenital indirect inguinal hernias are frequently found at laparotomy.

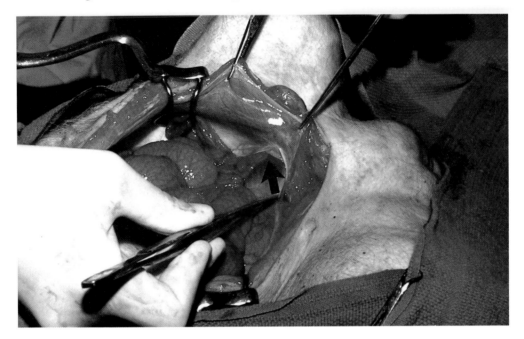

The study is being conducted in three phases. In the first phase, pigs with inguinal hernias undergo laparotomy, and a 6 × 5.5 cm patch of polypropylene mesh is sutured to the peritoneal surface of the groin. The inguinal defect is overlapped generously with the prosthesis, which is carried over the femoral vessels. The opposite side (or the smaller of the two hernias if the hernia is bilateral) is similarly covered with polypropylene mesh, but in addition, an absorbable adhesion barrier made of oxidized regenerated cellulose is sutured to the abdominal side of the prosthesis.

Assuming the results of the first phase suggest that the project should be continued, the second and third phases will determine the feasibility of laparoscopic placement of a polypropylene or expanded PTFE weave prosthesis with or without the oxidized regenerated cellulose adhesion barrier. A stapling device designed to secure the prosthesis to the peritoneal surface that can be introduced through a laparoscopic cannula is currently under development. Preliminary results from our laboratory have been encouraging.

The initial intention was to use preperitoneal placement of a prosthetic material because of our concern about the sequela related to adhesions of abdominal organs to an intra-abdominally placed prosthesis. The technique, which was developed by one of the authors (C.J.F.), included an initial hydrodissection of the preperitoneal space around the internal inguinal defect. A cannula releasing a high-pressure saline solution was inserted into the preperitoneal space transcutaneously. Insertion of the cannula and preperitoneal hydrodissection were carried out under direct vision through a laparoscope placed intra-abdominally via a 10 mm cannula inserted immediately above the umbilicus. The laparoscopic view of the abdominal wall below shows the hernia defect.

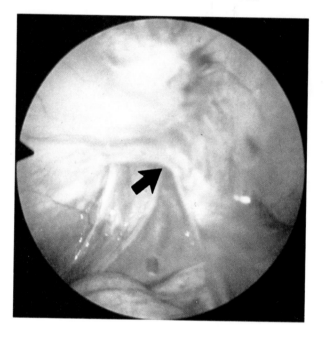

The saline solution was then removed from the preperitoneal space and replaced with CO_2 using a Veress needle. A 10 mm cannula was introduced into the preperitoneal space to permit the introduction of a laparoscope with attached camera. The view of the dissected preperitoneal space with the laparoscope in the preperitoneal space shows the inguinal hernia defect as well as the inferior epigastric vessels (*E.V.*).

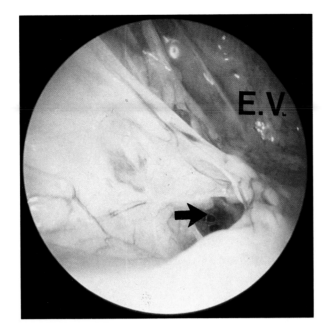

Two additional 5 mm cannulas were also placed in the preperitoneal space to allow the introduction of grasping instruments. A 6 × 11 cm piece of polypropylene mesh was rolled onto itself and then inserted through the 10 mm cannula into the preperitoneal space. The mesh was unrolled and applied to the hernia defect and allowed to overlap the cord structures and the abdominal wall. It was secured in place using a titanium clip applier. At the end of the procedure all instruments were withdrawn, the pneumo-preperitoneum was released, and the animals were awakened.

Technical problems made laparoscopic preperitoneal herniorrhaphy difficult. First, the hydrodissection of the preperitoneal space often led to peritoneal perforation, which limited the size and the duration of the working pneumopreperitoneum. Second, the mesh prosthesis was difficult to handle because of the small working space and confusing spacial orientation. And third, the procedure was time consuming. These difficulties prompted us to abandon laparoscopic preperitoneal hernia repair and to concentrate on an intra-abdominal approach. The current technique for laparoscopic placement of the intra-abdominal prosthesis is as follows:

Preliminary pneumoperitoneum is produced with CO_2 using a Veress needle. A 10 mm laparoscopic cannula is inserted transabdominally just above the umbilicus. A laparoscope and attached video camera are then inserted. A 6 × 5.5 cm piece of polypropylene mesh is rolled onto itself and inserted into the abdomen through a 10 mm cannula placed above the groin on the side to be repaired. A second 5 mm cannula is placed in a symmetric position above the contralateral groin. Grasping instruments are inserted through both cannulas. Under direct laparoscopic vision the mesh is unrolled and applied against the abdominal wall, covering the peritoneal opening of the inguinal defect. A grasper is used to hold both the peritoneum and an edge of the prosthesis together while titanium clips are applied with a laparoscopic clip applier to fix the prosthesis to the peritoneum. The instruments are withdrawn, and the pneumoperitoneum is released.

RESULTS

The animals were sacrificed and an autopsy performed at the fourth postoperative week. Examination of the abdominal cavity of the pig has shown the polypropylene prosthesis entirely attached to the underlying peritoneum and the inguinal hernia defect closed. Surprisingly, few adhesions to the prosthesis have been noted to date. In this case an 11 × 6 cm prosthesis was used. However, we subsequently found the 6 × 5.5 cm prosthesis to be adequate.

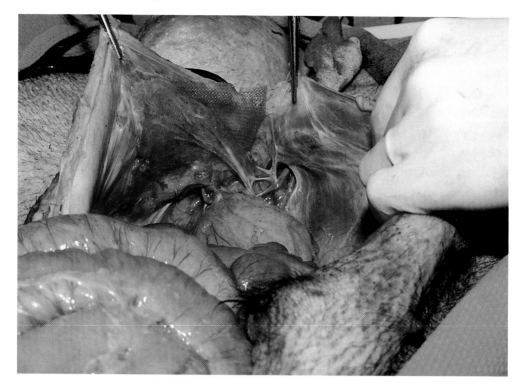

Pathologic examination of transversus muscle and peritoneum from the area of prosthetic implantation revealed a matured granulation response characterized by overgrowth of the polypropylene mesh by peritoneum with reestablishment of mesothelium on the new parietal peritoneal surface. This finding, however, differs from data reported in the literature by others.[17] The mesothelium showed focal chronic inflammation and thickening. Empty circular spaces indicate polypropylene fibers surrounded by flattened lining cells and a narrow rim of chronic inflammation characterized by histiocytes and foreign body giant cells. The remainder of the peritoneum was not inflamed. Polypropylene material remaining after sectioning appears as bright objects in spaces at upper left and lower right.

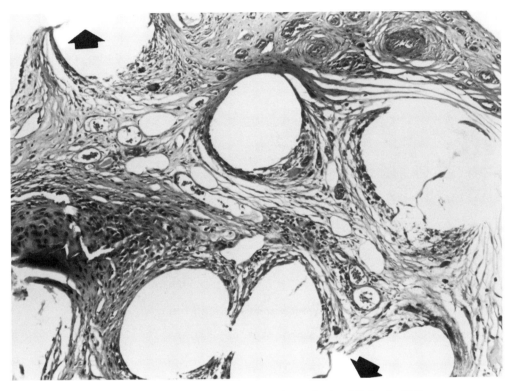

Hematoxylin and eosin stain under polarized light (×100)

Mesothelial proliferation can be seen at parietal peritoneal surfaces.

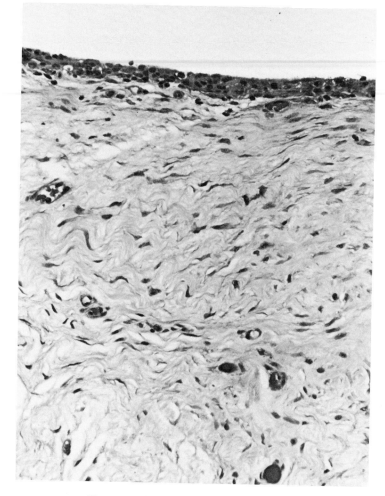

Hematoxylin and eosin stain (×430)

CONCLUSION

Laparoscopic repair of an inguinal hernia is an intriguing concept. The principal benefits would be decreased postoperative pain and earlier return to employment. In addition, the local groin complications occasionally encountered after conventional extraperitoneal inguinal hernia repair, such as neuromas and spermatic cord or testicular problems, might be avoided. Clearly, however, the approach is investigational. In addition to the complications normally associated with laparoscopy, other potential problems included adhesions of intra-abdominal organs to the hernia repair site and infection, especially if prosthetic material is used. Reports of laparoscopic inguinal hernia repair performed in humans are largely anecdotal. Meaningful data dealing with recurrence rates or morbidity will not be available until a standardized technique is developed and subjected to controlled clinical trials. Further laboratory evaluation is warranted. At the present time patients undergoing laparoscopic inguinal hernia repair should be informed that the procedure is still in the developmental stage.

George A. McClellan, M.D., Department of Pathology, Creighton University School of Medicine, assisted in examining the histologic specimens.

REFERENCES

1. Selected data on hospitals and use of services. In Polister P, Cunico E, eds. Socio-Economic Factbook for Surgery, 1989. Chicago: American College of Surgeons, pp 25-42.
2. Reed RC. Historical survey of the treatment of hernias. In Nyhus LM, Condon RE, eds. Hernia. Philadelphia: JB Lippincott, 1989, pp 1-17.
3. Condon RE, Nyhus LM. Complications of groin hernias. In Nyhus LM, Condon RE, eds. Hernia. Philadelphia: JB Lippincott, 1989, pp 253-269.
4. Marcy HO. A new use of carbolized catgut ligatures. Boston Med Surg J 85:315-316, 1871.
5. Griffith CA. The Marcy repair of indirect inguinal hernias: 1870 to present. In Nyhus LM, Condon RE, eds. Hernia. Philadelphia: JB Lippincott, 1989, pp 106-118.
6. Marcy HO. The cure of hernia. JAMA 8:589-592, 1887.
7. Marcy HO. Hernia. New York: Appleton, 1892.
8. LaRoque GP. The intra-abdominal method of removing inguinal and femoral hernia. Arch Surg 24:189-203, 1932.
9. Andrews E. A method of herniotomy utilizing only white fascia. Ann Surg 80:225-238, 1924.
10. Ger R. The management of certain abdominal hernias by intra-abdominal closure of the neck. Ann R Coll Surg Engl 64:342-344, 1982.
11. Ger R, Monroe K, Duvivier R, Mishrick A. Management of indirect inguinal hernias by laparoscopic closure of the neck of the sac. Am J Surg 159:371-373, 1990.
12. Lichtenstein IL, Shulman AG, Amid PK, Montllor MM. The tension-free hernioplasty. Am J Surg 157:188-193, 1989.
13. Stoppa RE, Warlaumont CR. The preperitoneal approach and prosthetic repair of groin hernia. In Nyhus LM, Condon RE, eds. Hernia. Philadelphia: JB Lippincott, 1989, pp 199-225.
14. Nyhus LM, Pollak R, Bombeck TC, Donahue PE. The preperitoneal approach and prosthetic buttress repair for recurrent hernia. Ann Surg 208:733-737, 1988.
15. Popp LW. Endoscopic patch repair of inguinal hernia in a female patient. Surg Endosc 4:10-12, 1990.
16. Corbitt JD. Laparoscopic herniorraphy. Surg Laparosc Endosc (in press).
17. Law NW, Ellis H. Adhesion formation and peritoneal healing on prosthetic materials. Clin Materials 3:95-101, 1988.

Laparoscopic Guided Intestinal Surgery

Avram M. Cooperman, M.D.
Karl A. Zucker, M.D.

Until June 1988 laparoscopic guided gastrointestinal surgery was but a vision to some surgeons, an inane idea to others, and a non-thought for most. The explosive growth of laparoscopic cholecystectomy has been unprecedented, and now, the extension of surgical laparoscopy beyond the biliary tract is a reality. As described in previous chapters, procedures such as laparoscopic appendectomy, truncal and selective vagotomy, inguinal hernia repair, and pelvic lymphadenectomy have become established clinical procedures. Preliminary applications of laparoscopy to small bowel and colon surgery have recently emerged. Although infrequently requiring operative intervention, the small bowel's mobility and long mesentery make it particularly amenable to laparoscopic intervention. In addition, the high incidence of colon disease provides an ample base for surgeons to develop new and innovative laparoscopic procedures for the large bowel.

Currently, the most limiting aspect of laparoscopic intestinal surgery is the lack of appropriate instruments. Manufacturers of laparoscopic equipment have shown little interest in developing instruments that are radically different from existing devices or from those currently used in open procedures. Unfortunately existing surgical techniques of bowel resection and hand-sewn anastomoses are not easily performed through the laparoscope. Now, however, the competitive forces involved in what promises to be a large and lucrative market have prompted corporations to develop new and innovative instruments. The recent introduction of laparoscopic stapling devices, noncrushing bowel clamps, as well as larger laparoscopic cannulas has made laparoscopic intestinal surgery a reality. Although still limited in application, some of the laparoscopic intestinal procedures currently in use as well as the instruments presently available and under development will be described in this chapter.

LAPAROSCOPIC SMALL BOWEL SURGERY

The small bowel appears to be ideally suited for laparoscopic surgery. Its smaller diameter (as compared to the colon) and long mesentery allow for easy mobilization and access via the laparoscope. Unfortunately (at least for the enthusiastic laparoscopic surgeon) there are relatively few indications for operative intervention in the small bowel. Our experience with laparoscopic small bowel surgery thus far has been limited to various procedures involving enteral alimentation. This includes laparoscopic jejunostomy tube placement and Roux-en-Y cutaneous jejunostomy. Although the preferred method of providing enteral alimentation for those individuals unable to swallow remains percutaneous endoscopic gastrostomy (PEG) tube placement, a small number of patients are not candidates for this procedure. The presence of significant gastroesophageal reflux or gastric outlet obstruction (either functional or mechanical) may preclude this approach. In addition, patients who have previously undergone extensive upper abdominal surgery, including partial gastrectomy, may not be ideal candidates for PEG placement. In these latter individuals a laparoscopic approach to enteral nutrition may be preferable to open gastrostomy or jejunostomy tube placement. Generally, patients requiring enteral access for long-term alimentation are poor operative risks for traditional surgery. These individuals often have extensive head and neck tumors, esophageal malignancies, or major neurologic dysfunction (acute or chronic). Therefore a minimally invasive operation such as laparoscopic jejunostomy tube placement may be associated with fewer complications than surgical procedures requiring an open laparotomy.

Jejunostomy Tube Placement

As with all patients undergoing laparoscopic surgery, the patient and/or the family must be informed of the possibility that an open laparotomy may be required. Thus these procedures are always performed in a sterile operating room environment with appropriate anesthesia coverage (a general anesthetic is recommended). If patients have not had a midline abdominal incision previously, the initial access for insertion of the insufflation needle is the supraumbilical site. A small incision is made in the upper folds of the navel, and the insufflation needle is inserted directly into the peritoneal cavity. Proper placement of the needle should be confirmed as described in Chapter 8. The abdomen is distended with 3 to 4 L of CO_2, and the needle is replaced with a 10 mm laparoscopic trocar and cannula. The patient is then placed in a 20- to 30-degree reverse Trendelenburg position.

If the patient has had an abdominal procedure near the umbilicus before, the open laparoscopic technique may be used (see Chapter 5), or an alternative site for insufflation needle insertion may be chosen. The right midclavicular site will usually provide adequate access for jejunostomy tube placement. Initially the abdominal cavity is surveyed with the video laparoscope to determine the feasibility of jejunostomy tube placement. Extensive adhesions in the upper abdomen may preclude identification of the jejunum and proper placement of the feeding tube. Accessory 5 mm laparoscopic trocars and cannulas are then inserted in the left midabdomen and in the upper midline, approximately 5 cm from the xiphoid.

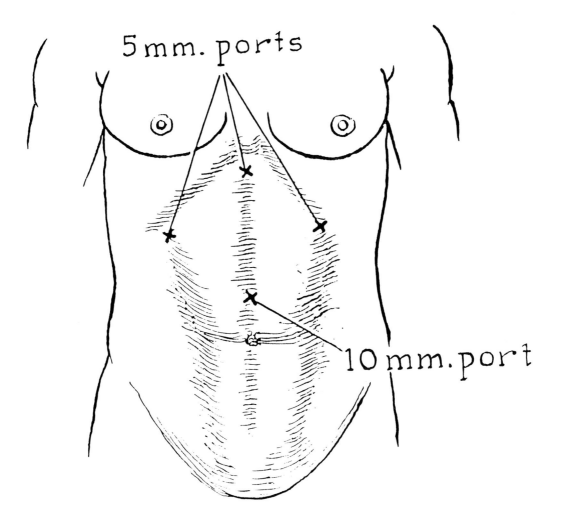

The proximal jejunum is identified near the ligament of Treitz and followed for 60 to 100 cm. The small bowel should be manipulated with a combination of blunt probes and specially designed bowel grasping forceps (Dorsey intestinal clamp; American Surgical Instruments, Pompano, Fla.).

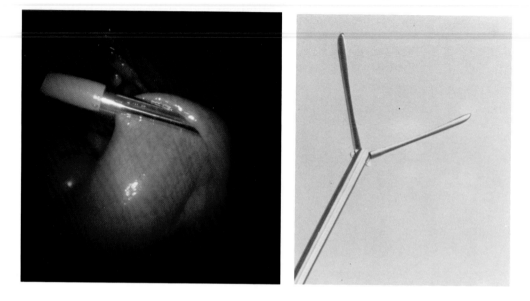

If the proximal jejunum can be successfully identified and mobilized to the anterior abdominal wall, the 10 mm umbilical cannula is removed and replaced with a specially designed 20 mm cannula. The skin incision should be continued within the folds of the navel. The umbilical fascial opening may be enlarged under direct vision by simply extending the incision or by using the obturator of the larger cannula to dilate the fascial defect. Care must be taken not to overenlarge the fascial opening since this may result in a persistent gas leak and difficulty in maintaining adequate pneumoperitoneum. If necessary, one or more fascial purse-string sutures may be used to seal a gas leak around the umbilical opening.

Previous experience with laparoscopic cholecystectomy and appendectomy has shown that the umbilical fascial opening may be enlarged as much as 3 to 4 cm with no significant additional postoperative morbidity or cosmetic disfigurement. It is important, however, to avoid incising the adjacent rectus abdominis muscle to avoid any such complaints.

A 20 mm metal cannula is currently available that was originally designed for removal of very swollen and inflamed appendices (Karl Storz Endoscopy, Culver City, Calif.). A movable diaphragm within the sheath prevents loss of CO_2. The long length of the cannula (200 mm), however, can limit the length of intestine that can be eviscerated. Shorter disposable fiberglass cannulas available in 20, 30, and 40 mm diameters are currently being developed.

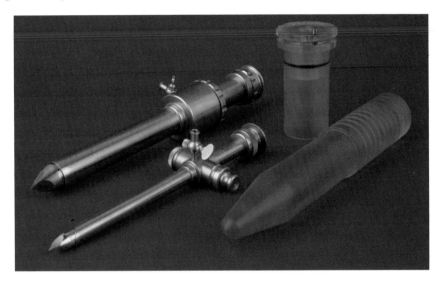

**A 20 mm diameter laparoscopic cannula (left),
a standard 10 mm instrument (center), and a prototype 30 mm
disposable cannula and obturator (right).**

These later devices are designed with an inner sleeve that will accept a standard sized (11 or 12 mm) cannula, which permits the use of a wide range of different sized instruments. The flapper valve of the smaller cannula prevents loss of pneumoperitoneum.

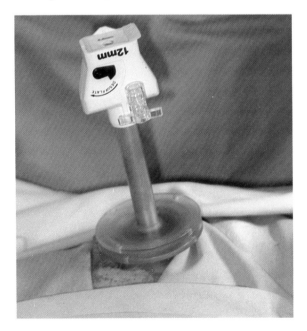

After the 20 mm laparoscopic cannula is inserted, a 5 mm laparoscope and video camera are introduced through the upper abdominal cannula. The jejunum is grasped with a noncrushing bowel clamp and pulled gently through the sheath and out of the abdomen.

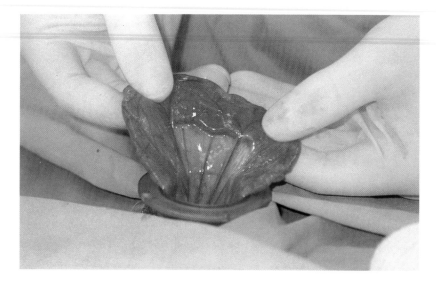

An appropriate reducing sleeve or converter may be necessary because most grasping instruments are 5 mm in diameter. The jejunostomy tube can be placed through the left midabdominal cannula and brought out alongside the segment of small bowel. To facilitate evisceration of the jejunum, CO_2 is released from the peritoneal cavity to reduce the distance between the mesentery and the abdominal wall. The tube is placed within the lumen using either the Stamm or Witzel technique. We prefer the Witzel approach to minimize the likelihood of leakage around the catheter or inadvertent removal. Two or more seromuscular sutures may be placed near the jejunostomy tube insertion site to allow for later attachment to the anterior abdominal wall. The jejunum is dropped back inside the peritoneal cavity and pneumoperitoneum reestablished. The jejunum is brought to the anterior abdominal wall by pulling on the jejunostomy tube. A laparoscopic suture holder is inserted through the upper midline sheath and used to secure the bowel to the peritoneum with the previously applied sutures.

The left midabdominal cannula is removed, leaving the jejunostomy tube in place. The tube may then be sewn to the skin. The abdominal cavity is reexamined and the remaining cannulas removed. The umbilical fascial defect is closed with two or three interrupted sutures. The 5 mm upper abdominal fascial openings do not require closure. The skin incisions may be approximated with sutures or skin staplers.

Roux-en-Y Cutaneous Jejunostomy

An alternative method of providing long-term enteral alimentation is the creation of a cutaneous Roux-en-Y jejunostomy. With this procedure intermittent jejunostomy feedings may be given by simply intubating the stoma. This operation may be indicated in those patients in whom enteral alimentation is expected to be prolonged to avoid complications such as removal of the catheter, leakage around the catheter, and infection.

The four-puncture technique described earlier is used; however, a 10 mm left midabdominal trocar and sheath are used rather than the 5 mm size. Pneumoperitoneum is established, and a 10 mm laparoscope and camera are inserted through the supraumbilical cannula. The proximal jejunum is again identified, and a site approximately 60 to 100 cm from the ligament of Treitz is mobilized to the anterior abdominal wall. The umbilical fascial defect is enlarged to accommodate a 30 mm laparoscopic sheath. The segment of jejunum is then brought out through this cannula as the CO_2 is released.

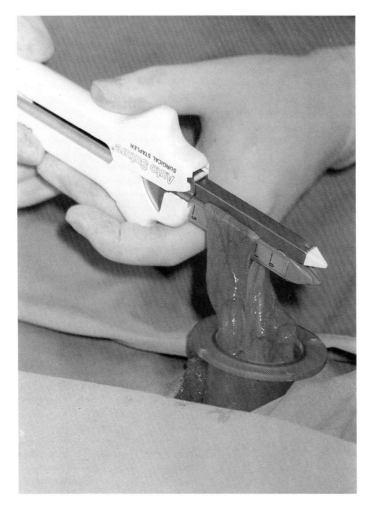

The jejunum is divided with an intestinal stapling device, and an extracorporeal jejunojejunostomy is performed to reestablish gastrointestinal continuity. This leaves an isoperistolic jejunal limb approximately 30 cm in length.

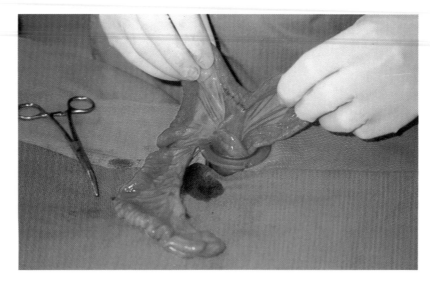

The jejunal mesentery is removed from the distal end to facilitate jejunostomy formation. Sutures are positioned to allow the jejunal limb to be secured to the peritoneum and to close the space along the lateral abdominal wall. The small bowel is placed back into the abdomen and the peritoneum distended with CO_2. A reducing sleeve is inserted into the umbilical cannula and the jejunal limb held in place with a clamp inserted through the left midabdominal sheath. The left abdominal sheath is then removed, allowing the jejunal limb to be pulled out of the abdomen.

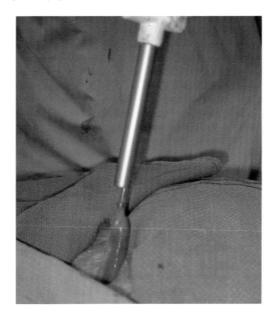

The skin and fascia may have to be slightly enlarged to accommodate the jejunal segment. The small bowel is fixed to the fascia so that approximately 1 cm protrudes above the skin. A continuous or running mucocutaneous absorbable suture completes the jejunostomy. The internal sutures are completed and the cannulas removed.

Intracorporeal Intestinal Anastomosis

The previous laparoscopic techniques depend on mobilization of bowel segments outside of the peritoneal cavity for placement of catheters or intestinal anastomosis (extracorporeal surgery). Obviously this limits possible future applications of laparoscopic surgery if extracorporeal manipulation may not be feasible. An alternative method currently being developed employs internal laparoscopic stapling devices (Endo GIA; United States Surgical Corporation, Norwalk, Conn.).

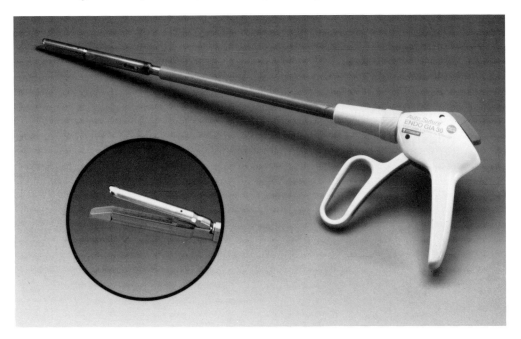

This instrument is similar to intestinal stapling devices used in open surgery. The laparoscopic version has been designed to fit through a 12 mm cannula and will be available in 30 and 60 mm lengths.

This instrument makes intracorporeal bowel surgery possible. Small or large bowel can now be divided within the abdomen without spillage of intestinal contents. The Endo GIA may be used to divide mesentery in the same fashion as that used to control the mesoappendix during appendectomy (see Chapter 11). The stapling device may also be used to perform a side-to-side intestinal anastomosis; however, the small enterotomies made for instrument insertion must be closed by hand.

Use of an endoscopic stapling device in laparoscopic intestinal surgery has thus far been limited to a number of experimental protocols. As of November 1990, extensive clinical trials involving the use of this instrument were under way; the results should be available soon.

LAPAROSCOPIC COLON SURGERY

Laparoscopic colon surgery has potential (1) for diagnostic purposes, (2) for localization and mobilization of segments of bowel and performing extracorporeal anastomoses, and (3) for resecting and anastomosing intra-abdominal segments of colon totally within the abdomen. The first two applications are presently possible; the third is in the developmental stage.

When large sessile polypoid lesions with foci of invasive cancer are detected with the colonoscope, segmental resections of the colon are often necessary to ensure that the deep margins are free of tumor and regional nodes are not involved. The long abdominal incision utilized to explore the abdomen in some instances can be significantly reduced with the aid of the laparoscope. During the initial colonoscopy the lesion to be removed is infiltrated with methylene blue to facilitate later identification by the laparoscopist. The abdomen is distended with CO_2 and a 10 mm trocar and sheath inserted just above or below the umbilicus. A complete intra-abdominal examination with the video laparoscope is performed with a careful assessment for the presence of local or regional metastasis. If the lesion is in a mobile or redundant segment of colon, a short abdominal incision is made directly over the lesion and the segment of bowel delivered out of the abdomen. Alternatively, a 30 or 40 mm trocar and sheath may be used to extract the colon. This device has the option of maintaining pneumoperitoneum while securing the segment of bowel. Ideally the larger cannula is inserted through the umbilical fascial opening; however, it may be placed directly over the segment of colon if required. The blood supply and lateral margins are secured with hemostats, surgical clips, or staplers. Either a hand-sewn or stapled anastomosis is performed outside the body. The bowel is then replaced within the abdominal cavity and the small incision closed.

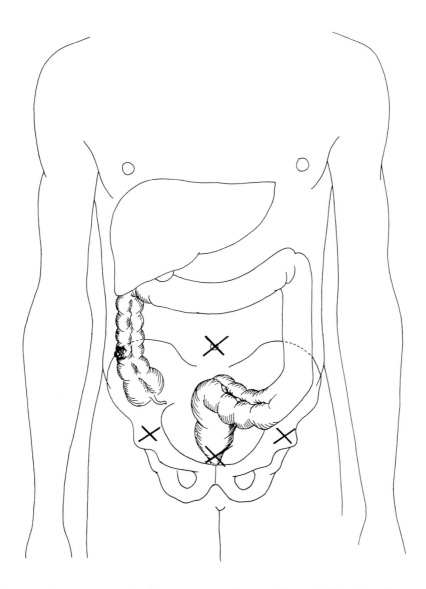

The diseased segment of colon may not be easily mobilized to the anterior abdominal wall. Often extensive dissection is needed to free the colon from surrounding tissues. This involves mobilizing the bowel through three accessory ports introduced at convenient locations. Five-millimeter trocars are inserted in the right and left lower abdominal quadrants, and the third accessory cannula is placed just above the symphysis pubis.

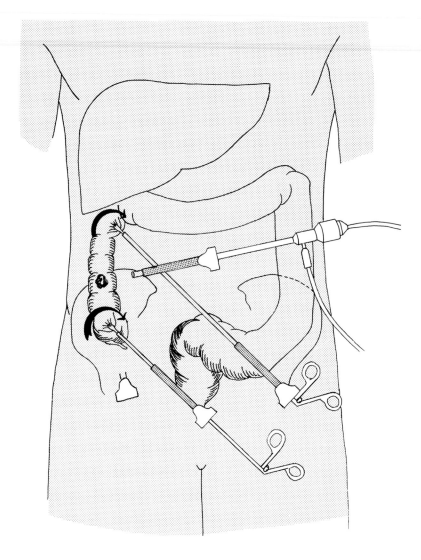

For polypoid lesions of the right colon, the cecum and ascending colon are grasped proximally and distally and rotated toward the midline. The spatulated cautery or laser is introduced through the right lower abdominal cannula and is used to incise the avascular plane lateral to the ascending colon. This dissection has proved easier for the right colon than for the descending and/or sigmoid colon.

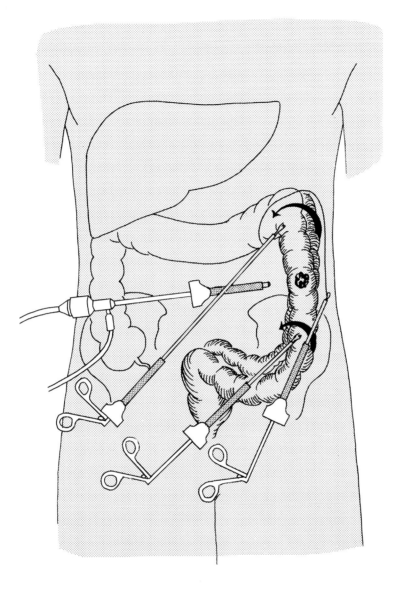

To mobilize segments of the left colon, bowel grasping forceps are inserted through the lower midline and right lower abdominal cannulas. Dissection is then accomplished using the left lower abdominal cannula. Placing the patient in a lateral tilt with the table in the Trendelenburg position will allow the small bowel to be positioned out of the way.

The mobilized segment can then be delivered onto the abdominal wall and the blood supply controlled by clamps or sutures or with clips.

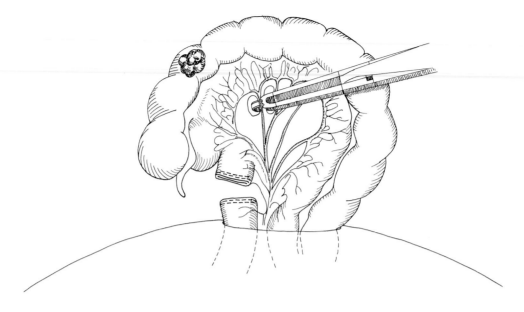

Again this may be accomplished using a small mini-laparotomy or via a large laparoscopic cannula. The bowel is then transected and reapproximated with staplers or by hand.

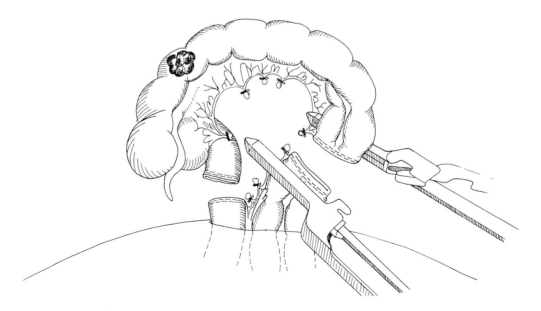

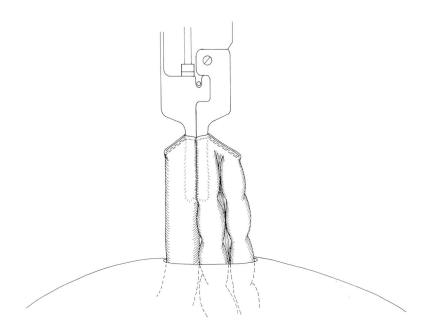

Even very long segments of colon have been safely removed with this laparoscopic-assisted technique. Recently a complete right hemicolectomy was performed on two patients with the specimens removed from the abdomen through a 5 cm abdominal incision (M. Jacobs, personal communication, 1990).

Lahey and colleagues from Rochester, New York, have described a technique of laparoscopic resection of the sigmoid colon and rectum using a standard EEA stapler (P. Lahey, personal communication, 1990). The left colon is mobilized in a manner similar to that described above. The left lower abdominal puncture is then dilated to accept a 12 mm cannula. This allows the insertion of a laparoscopic stapling device (Endo-GIA), which is then used to divide the bowel proximal and distal to the segment to be resected. The blood supply is controlled by firing the stapler across the mesocolon. The 12 mm cannula is removed and the puncture site dilated further to remove the specimen and to eviscerate the proximal end of the divided bowel. The anvil of the EEA stapling instrument is inserted into the lumen and a purse-string suture applied. The colon is returned to the abdominal cavity and the fascial defect closed with a purse-string suture. The EEA instrument is then inserted through the rectum and joined to the anvil. The staplers are fired and the instrument removed. The anastomosis is checked by inspecting the rings of tissue within the stapling device and by infusing methylene blue through the rectum. A multicenter trial has begun to evaluate the efficacy of this laparoscopic procedure.

Similar to small bowel surgery, intracorporeal resection and anastomosis may soon be possible using devices such as the Endo GIA. However, improvements in laparoscopic sutures or stapling devices will be necessary to safely approximate the small colostomies necessary to introduce this instrument as well as to adequately control the large vessels within the mesentery.

CONCLUSION

Laparoscopic gastrointestinal surgery is still in its infancy. Current applications for biliary tract disease represent only a small portion of the potential for this new surgical discipline. Widespread application of this technique to other abdominal visceral surgical procedures is imminent. The colon and small bowel lend themselves readily to laparoscopic surgery because lesions are frequently small, the bowel is mobile and has ample mesentery, and the blood supply is via a long pedicle that facilitates exposure and dissection.

The development of instruments such as laparoscopic staplers, atraumatic graspers, and bowel clamps has broadened the indications for surgical laparoscopy to the treatment of various disorders of the large and small bowel. Alternative methods of promoting intestinal bonding such as fibrin glue and laser welding may further expand the role of laparoscopic intestinal surgery.

CHAPTER 16

Complications of Laparoscopic General Surgery

Robert W. Bailey, M.D.

Published reports dealing with laparoscopic gynecologic surgery support the contention that such procedures are not associated with a significantly greater incidence of complications than similar operations performed via laparotomy. However, they indicate that a large proportion of the complications that do occur are related to physician training.[1,2] Most complications have occurred in cases where the laparoscopic surgeon has performed fewer than 250 procedures.[1-3]

Potential complications of laparoscopic-directed surgery must include, at the very least, the same complications encountered during the performance of a similar procedure via laparotomy. There is, however, a distinct and identifiable incidence of complications related specifically to laparoscopy. Large clinical series reporting on the morbidity and mortality associated with general surgical procedures performed under laparoscopic guidance have not yet been completed. Available data from the gynecologic literature, therefore, forms most of our current knowledge of complications associated with laparoscopic surgery.

The mortality rates for laparoscopic gynecologic procedures (diagnostic and therapeutic) are extremely low, ranging from 0% to 0.5%, with most surveys reporting much less than 0.1%.[1-5] A recent compilation of over 145,000 laparoscopic gynecologic procedures (both diagnostic and therapeutic) demonstrated a mortality rate of 0.01%.[3] In these reports there is a surprisingly low incidence of deaths related to cardiovascular and pulmonary complications. This may be at least partially explained by the fact that the vast majority of gynecologic laparoscopic procedures are performed on younger women. Statistics for older persons who undergo laparoscopic gastrointestinal procedures (i.e., cholecystectomy) may differ significantly.

Therefore it may be unwise to compare overall operative mortality in future published series from general surgeons to that documented in the gynecologic literature.

The incidence of laparoscopic-related morbidity is estimated to be less than 4%.[1,2,4-8] The more common complications encountered during laparoscopic pelvic procedures are summarized in Table 16-1.

Most series in which laparoscopic complications are reported, however, are retrospective and therefore may underestimate the true incidence. A recent prospective study indicates a 2.3% and 5.1% incidence of major and minor complications, respectively, occurring during diagnostic and therapeutic laparoscopic procedures over a 7-year period.[6] A mortality of 0.5% was also reported in this study. The authors point out that their prospective complication rate was five to seven times higher than the incidence reported in previous retrospective series on laparoscopic surgery.

Infection rates for general surgical procedures performed using video-directed laparoscopy should not be greater than those encountered during open laparotomy. Overall, the incidence of intra-abdominal and wound infections is less than 1.4 in every 1000 laparoscopic gynecologic procedures performed.[2] Early reports on laparoscopic appendectomy and cholecystectomy suggest that the incidence of wound infections may in fact be slightly lower than for the same procedure performed via laparotomy.[9,10] Presumably this correlates with the smaller operative incisions and the removal of infected tissues via the laparoscopic cannula, thus avoiding contact with the abdominal wall (i.e., laparoscopic appendectomy; see Chapter 11).

Table 16-1. Incidence of Complications of Laparoscopy*

Complication	Rate (%)
Pneumoperitoneum related	0.7
Hemorrhage	0.6
Perforating injuries	0.3
Infection	0.1
Intestinal burns	0.05
Cardiac arrest	0.03

*Modified from Phillips JM. Complications in laparoscopy. Int J Gynaecol Obstet 15:157-162, 1977.

Any laparoscopic procedure will be associated with an identifiable incidence of complications that are related specifically to laparoscopy, regardless of the operation being performed. Some of the more common complications encountered during laparoscopic surgery will be discussed briefly followed by a description of operative complications associated specifically with laparoscopic cholecystectomy. Extensive reviews of laparoscopic-related morbidity and mortality are available in the gynecologic literature.[1,2,8,11]

COMPLICATIONS RELATING TO INSUFFLATION AND TROCAR INSERTION

The most obvious difference between traditional surgery and laparoscopic surgery is the need to establish pneumoperitoneum. Several factors should be considered when choosing the appropriate gas for insufflation. The cardiovascular and respiratory side effects, the degree of peritoneal irritation (resulting in postoperative discomfort), and whether the gas will support combustion must all be considered when choosing an appropriate insufflation agent. Carbon dioxide, room air, oxygen, and nitrous oxide have all been used for establishing pneumoperitoneum. CO_2 is the preferred agent for most laparoscopic procedures because it is readily available, inexpensive, rapidly absorbed, and will suppress combustion. This latter property is extremely important in procedures that use electrocautery or lasers. The high diffusion coefficient of CO_2 may also lessen the severity of any gas emboli introduced into the vascular system. Its rapid clearance from the bloodstream results in an extremely fast rate of excretion from the body. On the other hand, the rapid diffusion properties of CO_2 allow it to be readily absorbed across the peritoneum, which may result in a rise in PCO_2 and a fall in pH. CO_2 retention, however, does not usually represent a significant management problem because it can be easily corrected with controlled ventilation. One disadvantage of CO_2 is that it may make the patient more prone to cardiac dysrhythmias than other agents.[8,12] One study reported a 17% incidence of dysrhythmias (mostly ventricular) when CO_2 was used as the insufflation agent as compared to 5% with nitrous oxide.[13] Fortunately these rhythm disturbances are usually transient and rarely affect the patient's clinical status.

Nitrous oxide is also used for laparoscopic insufflation, generally for diagnostic procedures performed under local anesthesia. Its anesthetic properties allow for adequate distention of the abdomen without causing the awake patient undue discomfort. Most laparoscopic surgeons, however, are hesitant to use nitrous oxide because it will support combustion. Since many laparoscopic procedures utilize electrocautery or laser energies, the use of any flammable gas is contraindicated. Room air and oxygen have also been used on occasion for diagnostic laparoscopic procedures but should be avoided because of the higher risk of fatal gas emboli and their ability to support combustion.

CO_2 must be introduced into the peritoneal cavity according to very strict guidelines to avoid complications. Details of the proper technique for insufflation are presented in Chapters 5 and 8. Complications may occur when using either the percutaneous or open technique (i.e., Hasson technique) of insufflation. The most common difficulty when attempting percutaneous insufflation is improper placement of the needle. Several maneuvers are recommended to confirm proper positioning of the needle prior to starting gas flow (see Chapter 8). The majority of surgeons currently use specially designed insufflation needles with blunt stylets. This blunt tip retracts over the sharp needle after entering the peritoneal cavity, thereby minimizing the risk of laceration or perforation of underlying structures (see Chapter 2). Perforation of the stomach, small bowel, colon, bladder, or major vascular structures, however, may still occur. Insertion of the insufflation needle into one of these organs can be easily detected by saline irrigation and aspiration through the needle with a syringe. Routine use of nasogastric and urinary catheters will lessen the risk of injury to the stomach and bladder and will facilitate laparoscopic visualization of the upper and lower abdomen.

If the insufflation needle has perforated the bladder or gastrointestinal tract, it should be immediately removed and discarded. A new needle may then be inserted at another location, or the surgeon may choose to perform an open laparoscopy (see Chapter 5). Following successful insufflation, the injury may be examined with the laparoscope and a decision made as to the appropriate management. Because of the small size of the insufflation needle the majority of such injuries do not require operative intervention. Occasionally minor insufflation needle injuries may be repaired using laparoscopic suturing or stapling techniques. This type of intervention, however, requires considerable skill and practice.

The site of injury should be reexamined at the end of the laparoscopic procedure to ensure that further visceral contamination or bleeding is not occurring. If there is any question regarding the nature of the injury, a laparotomy should be performed and the perforation examined directly.

The insufflation needle may also be inadvertently positioned within the omentum, mesentery, or retroperitoneum. The pressure reading through the needle should increase rapidly (well above 15 mm Hg) since the CO_2 is being pumped into a relatively closed space. After the laparoscope has been inserted, gas may occasionally be seen within the mesentery, omentum, or retroperitoneum. This will resolve without serious sequelae and should not be a major concern.

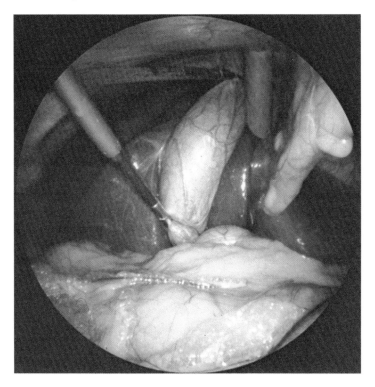

Gas trapped within leaves of omentum following peritoneal insufflation.

Visualization of the porta hepatis may be compromised, however, if a large amount of CO_2 has been pumped into the omentum or mesentery. A careful examination should be made to ensure that the needle did not also perforate a major blood vessel or other visceral structures.

An unusual complication of insufflation needle placement is massive distention of the preperitoneal space. If the tip of the needle is placed between the fascia and peritoneum, this space may expand enough to contain 3 to 4 L of gas.

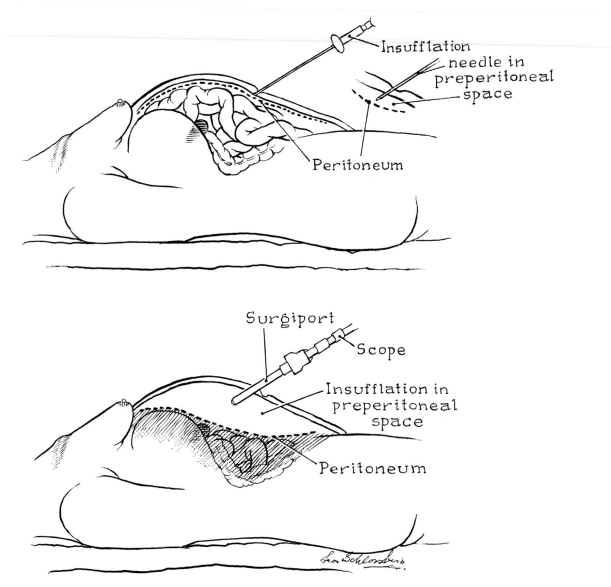

If this space expands symmetrically, the abdomen will appear distended as after correct peritoneal insufflation. It will also respond with convincing tympany as the surgeon percusses the abdomen. This complication is identified when the cannula and laparoscope are inserted into this space. The peritoneum can easily be observed intact above the viscera. This layer should be carefully opened with laparoscopic scissors and the tip of the cannula guided beneath it. CO_2 is then insufflated into the true peritoneal cavity. An intravenous needle and catheter may be placed percutaneously into the distended preperitoneal space to assist in collapsing it.

On occasion gas may dissect along fascial planes into the thoracic or pelvic regions, resulting in pneumomediastinum or subcutaneous and scrotal emphysema. This situation is more likely to occur in the presence of high intra-abdominal pressures (>16 mm Hg) resulting from either external compression on the abdomen (i.e., an assistant leaning on the abdomen) or excessive gas flow into the abdomen. The latter may occur with a faulty insufflation device or as a result of additional gas being instilled to cool the tip of a laser fiber. Scrotal emphysema, pneumomediastinum, and sub-cutaneous emphysema will resolve spontaneously and, in our experience, have not resulted in significant morbidity. We do recommend that patients with pneumomediastinum receive broad-spectrum antibiotics until the gas is reabsorbed, generally within 24 to 48 hours.

Gas emboli entering the vascular system has been reported to occur in approximately 1 in every 65,000 cases.[8] These emboli may result from either direct placement of the insufflation needle into a blood vessel or CO_2 entering venous channels that were severed or otherwise exposed during the operative dissection.[14] Such emboli, especially those occurring when the insufflation needle has been placed directly within a major vascular structure, may be fatal unless detected rapidly. Initial treatment consists of immediate cessation of insufflation and the release of all gas from the abdominal cavity. Additional therapeutic maneuvers may also be required based on the patient's clinical status (see Chapter 4).

Increased intra-abdominal pressure after insufflation may cause respiratory compromise, especially in patients with diminished pulmonary reserves. This problem may be compounded by excessive pneumoperitoneum (>15 mm Hg). The use of controlled or assisted ventilation with general anesthesia will minimize this risk; however, the anesthesiologist should monitor continuously for any changes in ventilatory pressures.

Patients undergoing laparoscopic surgery with thoracic epidural or local anesthesia are more susceptible to pulmonary compromise resulting from the abdominal distention (see Chapter 4). During these procedures the abdominal pressure should be maintained at 10 mm Hg or less. Patients should be constantly monitored for subtle signs of respiratory difficulty and CO_2 retention.

In addition to massive emboli, cardiovascular collapse during laparoscopy may also result from a profound vasovagal response or impairment of venous return to the heart.[12,15,16] Appropriate treatment involves immediate cessation of insufflation, withdrawal of all gas from the abdomen, and taking the patient out of the steep reverse Trendelenburg position (if performing cholecystectomy or vagotomy). Standard measures to maintain cardiovascular stability are then applied. Fortunately such major disturbances in the patient's hemodynamic status are rare. Minor alterations, on the other hand, are not uncommon during laparoscopic procedures. Changes in blood pressure, heart rate, cardiac output, and venous return to the heart have all been reported.[12,16-19] A more detailed discussion of the identification and treatment of gas embolism and other causes of cardiovascular complications is found in Chapter 4.

Insufflation of CO_2 into the peritoneal cavity is also associated with postoperative shoulder pain. This referred pain is believed to be the result of direct irritation of the diaphragm by CO_2 or the rapid stretching associated with insufflation. This pain is usually described as an arthralgic-like discomfort in one or both shoulders. It may occur in as many as one third of patients but is usually severe in less than 5%. The symptoms generally respond well to oral analgesics and/or anti-inflammatory medication and often resolve spontaneously within 24 to 48 hours after surgery. The frequency and severity of the shoulder pain can be decreased by removing all of the CO_2 from the abdomen at the conclusion of the laparoscopic procedure. Slow insufflation of the peritoneal cavity (1.0 to 1.5 L/min) when initially establishing the pneumoperitoneum may also reduce this complaint. After the abdomen is fully distended, the insufflator can then be switched to high flow (>6.0 L/min) to maintain the pneumoperitoneum. This is especially helpful when performing laparoscopic surgery under regional and local anesthesia. In our experience, acute shoulder pain during the operative procedure is the greatest limitation of performing laparoscopic cholecystectomy in the awake patient.

Insertion of laparoscopic trocars and cannulas is another source of operative complications. Injuries to the gastrointestinal tract,[20-22] major abdominal blood vessels,[23-26] and urinary tract[27-30] have all been described. The overall frequency of major complications related to trocar insertion alone ranges from approximately 1 in every 500 to 1 in every 2000 cases.[1-8,11] Injuries usually occur during "blind" insertion of the first trocar. The likelihood of such injuries is increased if there are underlying adhesions from prior abdominal surgery. Segments of mesentery and bowel may be fixed to the anterior abdominal wall and therefore more easily injured during trocar insertion. If the patient has had prior surgery near the site of trocar placement, the surgeon may elect to perform open laparoscopy (see Chapter 5). With this technique the peritoneal cavity is entered under direct vision, which should prevent injury. This open laparoscopic technique, however, may prove difficult in the face of extensive adhesions, and bowel injuries may still occur when entering the peritoneal cavity.[31,32] An alternative approach is to insert the insufflation needle at a site distant from the prior surgical incision. If laparoscopic cholecystectomy is performed in a patient with an existing midline incision, the needle can be placed in the right upper quadrant through either the anterior axillary or midclavicular site. Following insufflation, the needle is removed and replaced with a 5 mm trocar and cannula. A 5 mm laparoscope is then placed through the cannula and the abdominal cavity examined. With this approach the optimal sites for additional trocar placement can be assessed.

A thorough search for intra-abdominal injuries should be made immediately following trocar insertion and introduction of the laparoscope. If an injury is found, appropriate surgical management should be instituted. Following successful placement of the umbilical trocar and sheath, subsequent accessory trocars are inserted under laparoscopic guidance. This allows the surgeon to direct the accessory trocar tip away from underlying tissues. One of the more common causes of trocar injury is the so-called uncontrolled entry. This may occur when the surgeon applies increasing force to the trocar while attempting to enter the abdominal cavity. When the sharp tip finally penetrates the fascia, there is a sudden loss of resistance, and the instrument may forcefully enter the peritoneal cavity. The tip of the trocar may then lacerate or perforate underlying structures. This type of injury may be more common with reusable metal laparoscopic trocars. Repeated use of this type of instrument will result in a blunt trocar tip that increases the amount of force required to penetrate the fascia. Disposable laparoscopic trocars and cannulas offer several distinct advantages over reusable metal trocars. These devices are intended for single use only and threfore do not have the opportunity to become dull from repeated use. The disposable trocars are also equipped with plastic safety shields that advance over the end of the sharp tip once it has penetrated the peritoneum. This shield minimizes the risk of visceral injury even if the trocar is inserted too vigorously into the abdomen.

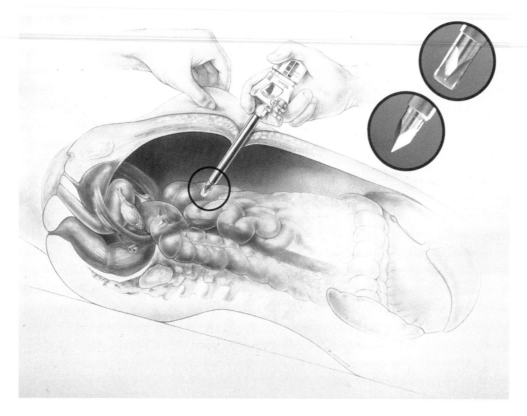

These disposable trocars, however, will not prevent an intestinal or mesenteric injury if they are inserted into a site where bowel has adhered to the abdominal wall. The trocar tip must traverse an empty space for the safety shield to fully advance over the sharp end.

Unlike insufflation needle injuries, perforation of a major blood vessel, bladder, or gastrointestinal tract with a 5 mm, 10 mm, or larger trocar should be managed by immediate laparotomy and repair. The trocar and cannula should be left in place while opening the abdomen to minimize further contamination or bleeding. In addition, it may prove difficult to later identify with certainty the site of injury once the trocar has been removed. The risk of a trocar injury to the gastrointestinal tract is so small, however, that routine bowel preparations (mechanical and/or antibiotic) are probably not justified. Gastrointestinal, vascular, or urinary tract injuries resulting from laparoscopic trocar insertion should be managed the same as any other penetrating injury to the abdomen.

Another potential complication of trocar placement is arterial or venous injury within the abdominal wall. This may result in bleeding around the cannula and into the peritoneal cavity or the formation of an abdominal wall hematoma. The abdominal wall should be transilluminated with the laparoscope before incising the skin and inserting the trocar. This allows the surgeon to identify and avoid injury to the larger blood vessels within the abdominal wall. If an arterial or venous injury occurs, the cannula should be left in place to tamponade the vessel and allow it to seal. Persistent bleeding around the laparoscopic cannula is generally only a problem in those patients receiving anticoagulation therapy. All trocar insertion sites should be carefully examined prior to and after removal of the cannula. If active bleeding is identified, the skin incision should be enlarged to allow for direct suture ligation of the vessel.

Alternatively, abdominal wall blood vessels injured during the insertion of trocars may bleed into the surrounding tissues and not into the abdominal cavity. This may lead to the development of an abdominal wall hematoma. The insertion of the midclavicular trocar may place the patient at greatest risk for this complication because it is usually placed through the rectus abdominis muscle. A rectus sheath hematoma may be quite painful and should be suspected in any patient complaining of severe abdominal pain following laparoscopic surgery. The tenderness and guarding associated with a rectus sheath hematoma may be confused with localized peritonitis. The diagnosis of abdominal wall hematomas may be confirmed by a CT scan.

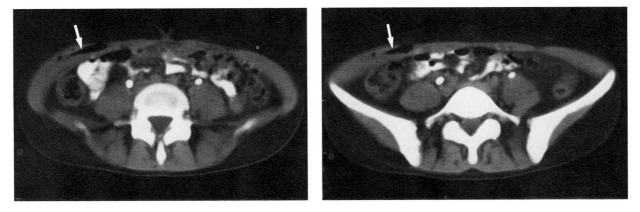

CT scan of abdomen of a 26-year-old woman 5 days after laparoscopic cholecystectomy shows rectus sheath hematoma (arrow) with gas dissecting into muscle.

During the laparoscopic procedure CO_2 may also dissect into the space created by the hematoma. The presence of gas within an abdominal wall hematoma may appear ominous on an x-ray film but will almost always resolve spontaneously. In the absence of fever, leukocytosis, and other clinical signs of severe infection, the surgeon can justify an initial period of conservative management. If there is any evidence that an infected hematoma or a necrotizing fascial process has developed, immediate surgical exploration is recommended.

On completion of the procedure the laparoscopic cannulas are removed from the abdomen. The defects created in the abdominal wall by the trocars are a potential source of hernia formation. The fascial defects from the smaller 5 mm trocars do not need to be closed primarily. These small trocars are usually inserted obliquely through the abdominal wall and are not associated with postoperative hernia formation. Closure of the larger 10 to 12 mm puncture sites, however, is recommended whenever possible. This is especially true for the umbilical fascial defect, which is often enlarged or dilated during the removal of tissues such as the gallbladder. The 10 to 12 mm puncture sites located in the upper abdomen may be left open if the fascial defect cannot be easily visualized and approximated. Overall, the risk of hernia formation is estimated to be less than 0.1%.[33] Herniation, when it does occur, is usually attributable to wound infection rather than improper closure of the fascia.[34]

COMPLICATIONS RELATED TO LAPAROSCOPIC INSTRUMENTATION AND VIDEO IMAGING

The two-dimensional image produced by current laparoscopic video systems results in a loss of depth perception for the surgeon. This handicap can be partially overcome by learning to use specific visual clues to assist in the proper placement and orientation of laparoscopic instruments. The most important factor in overcoming the loss of depth perception is to provide continual visualization of the operating instruments on the video monitor. Coordination of the camera's movements with those of the surgeon and first assistant is essential to the safe completion of any video-directed laparoscopic procedure. This will require the laparoscope and camera to be withdrawn from the operative field and directed toward each cannula where instruments are being introduced. Instruments inserted or manipulated within the peritoneal cavity without direct visual guidance may inadvertently injure the liver or other intra-abdominal structures.

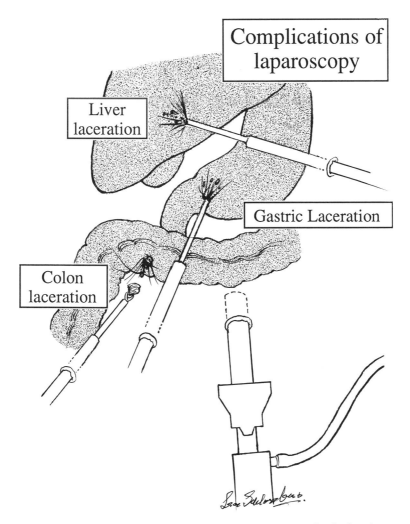

Abdominal viscera can be injured if instrument manipulation is not continuously observed on video monitor.

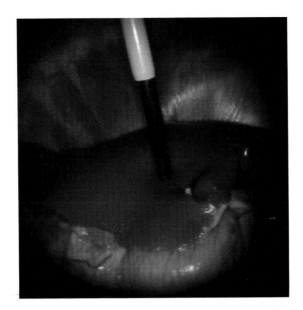

The tip of the grasping forceps has been inadvertently inserted through the surface of the liver.

Laparoscopic instruments are, by necessity, extremely long and thin and therefore can easily penetrate most abdominal organs. As long as the tip of an instrument can be seen by the surgeon, its position can be safely adjusted.

An additional maneuver to help compensate for the loss of depth perception involves touching the tip of the operating instrument (i.e., dissector, scissors, or cautery spatula) to the tissue prior to actual use. Visualization of tissue indentation will permit precise localization of the instrument's position within the operative field. This is especially important when using dissecting or cutting instruments without the benefit of depth perception. Inadvertent placement of such instruments may injure adjacent tissues. The difficulties of working without the benefit of depth perception become apparent even when performing such simple tasks as dividing the cystic duct or artery. Traditional straight scissors are designed so that the tips of the cutting blades come together last. Any tissues within the blades are naturally pushed away as the two jaws of the instrument come together. To compensate, the surgeon naturally advances the scissors to keep the tissues within the blades. Therefore, as attention is often directed to the structure being divided, the surgeon may be unaware of the exact location of the tips of the cutting blades. This may result in injury to nearby tissues such as the liver, right hepatic duct, or hepatic artery. Laparoscopic hook scissors have been designed to lessen this risk. With this instrument the tips of the cutting blades come together first and tissues are not pushed away as the jaws are closed.

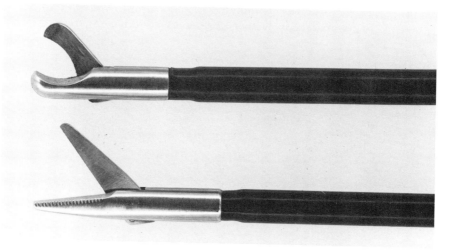

Comparison of laparoscopic hook and straight scissors.

Ligation of blood vessels, nerve bundles, or bile ducts during laparoscopic surgery is usually accomplished with a surgical clip applier. Titanium clips are placed distally and proximally on such structures before transection. Clips must also be placed in a manner that allows precise visualization of both tips of the clip applier prior to its application. It is often extremely difficult to maneuver the clip applier into a position that provides such visualization. This may be facilitated by rotating the clip applier so that the curved head of the instrument allows the clip to be placed perpendicular onto the structure being divided. In this fashion, proper visualization during ligation of critical structures such as the cystic duct and artery is enhanced.

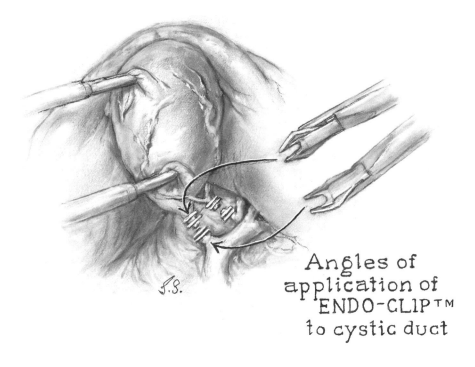

Angles of
application of
ENDO-CLIP™
to cystic duct

An even more serious complication related to the lack of depth perception is injury to the diaphragm resulting in a tension pneumothorax. Such injuries usually result from direct damage to the diaphragm from the electrocautery or laser during cholecystectomy or vagotomy. Cephalad retraction of the gallbladder and right lobe of the liver during cholecystectomy places the operative field in close proximity to the undersurface of the diaphragm. This injury is most likely to occur toward the end of the dissection of the gallbladder from the liver bed. At this point the gallbladder often partially obscures the operative field and may be pushed up against the diaphragm. It is imperative for the surgeon to be aware that the laser or electrocautery energy may come into contact with the undersurface of the diaphragm.

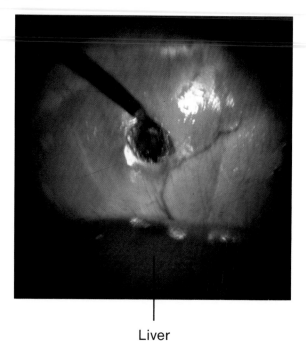

Liver

Electrocautery injury of right diaphragm.

This is of special concern with the use of a free laser beam because the energy effect extends beyond the tip of the instrument. Although less common, the grasping forceps themselves may injure the diaphragm. During upward retraction of the gallbladder these instruments may be pushed directly onto the diaphragm. Perforation may occur from excessive force during retraction or from one of the instruments suddenly slipping off the gallbladder. Once the hole is made in the diaphragm, CO_2 is rapidly forced into the thoracic cavity, resulting in a tension pneumothorax. In this event, insufflation should be halted immediately, all gas removed from the abdomen, a thoracostomy tube placed on the affected side, and the diaphragm repaired.

The development of laparoscopic surgical instruments is still in its infancy. The shortage of laparoscopic instruments has compounded this problem and resulted in the use of various devices for functions for which they were not originally intended. It is important that such instruments be used in ways for which they were designed. Grasping forceps applied directly on tissues such as the stomach, small intestine, or colon may cause severe tissue injury, leading to immediate or delayed perforation. These instruments were not designed to be applied to bowel. Atraumatic laparoscopic bowel clamps (Dorsey intestinal clamp; American Surgical Instruments, Pompano Beach, Fla.) are now available and should be used for this purpose.

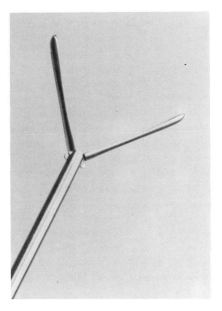

Atraumatic Dorsey intestinal clamp facilitates manipulation of small intestine and stomach during laparoscopic intestinal surgery or vagotomy.

The laparoscope itself may cause significant gastrointestinal tract injury. The high-intensity light source can sometimes make the end of the instrument extremely hot, especially if fluid or blood is allowed to collect on the end. If the tip of the laparoscope is inadvertently allowed to remain against the stomach, small bowel, or colon, a partial or even full-thickness thermal injury may result. This situation is most likely to occur with rapid loss of pneumoperitoneum such as following accidental removal of a laparoscopic cannula from the abdominal cavity. Complete loss of pneumoperitoneum will bring the abdominal viscera into direct contact with the tip of the laparoscope. While attention is being directed toward reestablishing pneumoperitoneum, severe thermal injury may result if the laparoscope is not withdrawn into the cannula.

COMPLICATIONS RELATED TO THE USE OF ELECTROCAUTERY

During the past 20 years several electrocautery bowel injuries have been reported during laparoscopic surgery. In 1981 the Centers for Disease Control (CDC) reported three deaths associated with unipolar electrocautery tubal sterilization procedures.[35] These patients died from overwhelming sepsis following intestinal perforation. The CDC also proposed that unipolar sterilization be abandoned in favor of bipolar or mechanical methods of tubal interruption.

With monopolar electrocautery the energy force is applied through the tip of the instrument and then conducted through the patient via the grounding pad. The dispersion of energy will obviously vary from patient to patient, as will the effect of the electrical energy on various tissues. According to these earlier reports, this variation was more pronounced in the closed abdomen than during open laparotomy. An additional concern was that an electrical charge or capacitance could develop within metallic laparoscopes or cannulas when using electrocautery. This energy could then later discharge onto adjacent tissues and result in severe burns. Because of their concern about uncontrolled electrical energy, many laparoscopic gynecologists condemned the use of monopolar cautery in the closed abdomen and instead urged the use of bipolar cautery, thermocoagulation, or laser energy.

The safety of electrocautery during laparoscopic surgery has been recently studied by a number of contemporary clinical investigators. Soderstrom and Levy[36] reviewed 12 cases of intestinal perforations initially ascribed to monopolar electrocoagulation. A detailed histologic examination of the submitted specimens, however, indicated that in 11 of these patients the injuries were the result of mechanical trauma, not electrical burns. The most likely cause of these injuries was either traumatic perforation during insufflation needle insertion or trocar placement or operative technical errors. Experimental studies in animals also supports the safety of monopolar electrocautery in the closed abdomen.[37] At the University of Maryland Medical Center over 250 patients have safely undergone laparoscopic cholecystectomy without a single injury related to the use of electrocautery. Other institutions that also routinely use electrocautery during dissection of the gallbladder from the liver bed have had a similar experience.[10,38]

Although it appears that earlier reports concerning the complications of electrocautery were largely exaggerated, there are, of course, certain inherent risks in using any sort of energy device (electrical, laser, or thermocoagulation) within the abdomen. The vast majority of the complications associated with these modalities are the result of errors in technique rather than "uncontrolled events."

Electrocautery injuries of the intestine are often not immediately apparent but rather become manifest as long as 4 to 10 days later. Prior experience with laparoscopic injuries suggests that this delayed necrosis of the surrounding tissues may be unique to electrical burns.[36,39] In contrast, patients undergoing traumatic bowel perforation develop symptoms usually within 12 to 48 hours. The most common cause of electrical burns is accidental contact with adjacent bowel during electrocautery dissection or coagulation of bleeding sites. In addition to the lack of depth perception afforded by video imaging, peripheral vision is also limited. Holding the laparoscope 1 to 2 cm from the cautery tip may enhance visualization of the operative field; however, the surgeon may then fail to appreciate the close proximity of adjacent colon or small bowel. Maintenance of abdominal distention is another critical factor in avoiding thermal injury. Inadequate insufflation of the abdominal cavity may severely limit the space surrounding the operative field. Sudden loss of pneumoperitoneum while cauterizing tissue may result in instrument contact against bowel, diaphragm, or major blood vessels. The most common cause of a massive gas leak is accidental withdrawal of one of the laparoscopic cannulas from the abdomen. The use of threaded devices to secure the cannulas to the abdominal wall will help avoid such events (see p. 44). It is also important to ensure that accessory laparoscopic sheaths are well insulated and that the laparoscopic instruments themselves are covered with a nonconductive material to avoid inadvertent transfer of electrical energy to adjacent tissues. The shafts of electrocautery instruments should be inspected on a routine basis to detect defects in the insulation that might lead to arcing and accidental electrical injury.

COMPLICATIONS SPECIFIC TO LAPAROSCOPIC CHOLECYSTECTOMY

The most common laparoscopic procedure performed by general surgeons is undoubtedly cholecystectomy. Therefore the greatest experience with operative misadventures has centered around laparoscopic biliary tract surgery. Although only a limited number of published articles have described such events, they appear to occur with some frequency. Fortunately preliminary reports indicate that the majority of serious complications tend to occur during the initial learning curve inherent as surgeons begin to perform laparoscopic surgery.[10,40] A thorough understanding of the potential operative complications associated with this procedure should help surgeons avoid such mistakes.

Bile Duct Injury

Injury to the extrahepatic biliary tree remains one of the most devastating injuries that can occur during cholecystectomy. It is estimated that such injuries will occur in 1 out of every 200 to 500 open cholecystectomies.[41] Insufficient data currently exist to compare the risk of bile duct injury during traditional and laparoscopic surgery. Operative dissection of the ductal and vascular structures may prove more difficult because of the visual orientation through the laparoscope and the lack of depth perception. The operative view of the gallbladder during open cholecystectomy is from directly above the patient. During laparoscopic cholecystectomy the surgeon views the extrahepatic biliary system from the umbilicus in a horizontal (transverse) plane.

Recognition of the anatomic variations of the extrahepatic biliary and vascular structures is probably the most important factor in preventing intraoperative injury during cholecystectomy.[42] Several of the more common anomalies involving the cystic duct are depicted below.

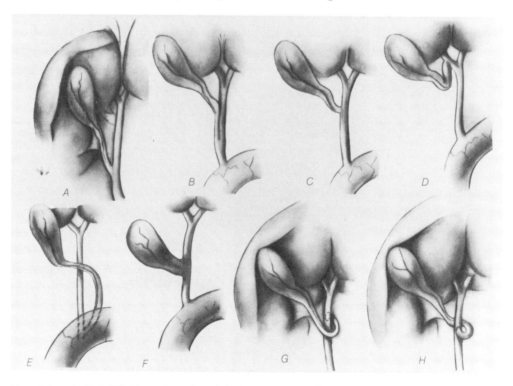

From Schwartz SI. Gallbladder and extrahepatic biliary system. In Schwartz SI, ed. Principles of Surgery. New York: McGraw-Hill, 1984, p 1308. By permission.

A, Low junction between cystic duct and common hepatic duct. **B,** Cystic duct adherent to common hepatic duct. **C,** High junction between cystic duct and common hepatic duct. **D,** Cystic duct draining into right hepatic duct. **E,** Long cystic duct entering common hepatic duct behind duodenum. **F,** Absence of cystic duct. **G,** Cystic duct crossing anterior to common hepatic duct and joining it posteriorly. **H,** Cystic duct coursing posteriorly to common hepatic duct and joining it anteriorly.

The most common variation associated with operative ductal injury is the short cystic duct originating from the right hepatic duct. Incomplete dissection may lead the surgeon to believe that the right hepatic duct is the cystic duct. Thus the right hepatic duct may be clipped, suture ligated, or even completely transected.

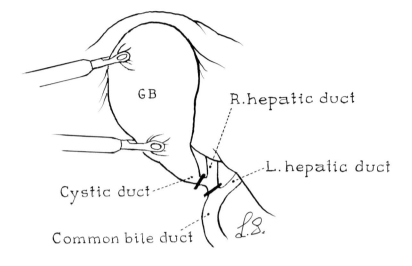

This injury is usually recognized immediately and requires open laparotomy and direct repair. If the duct has been completely transected, a biliary enteric bypass is the procedure of choice. Complete dissection of the cystic and common bile duct junction as well as performing routine intraoperative cholangiography will help avoid this complication. Intraoperative cholangiography may also reveal the presence of accessory bile ducts that were not detected during the operative dissection. Recognition and information concerning the location of such accessory ducts may avoid inadvertent injury and subsequent bile leak.

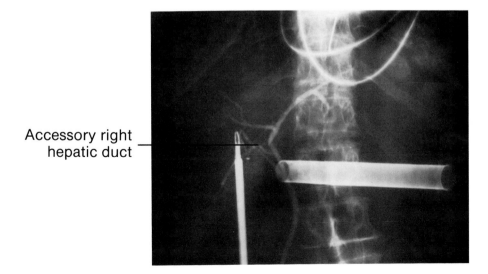

Accessory right hepatic duct

Another important factor associated with ductal injuries is the distortion of the common bile duct that occurs with the cephalad and lateral retraction of the gallbladder and liver during laparoscopic cholecystectomy. This will often result in "tenting up" of the common bile duct, which may lead to some confusion when attempting to identify the cystic and common bile duct junction.

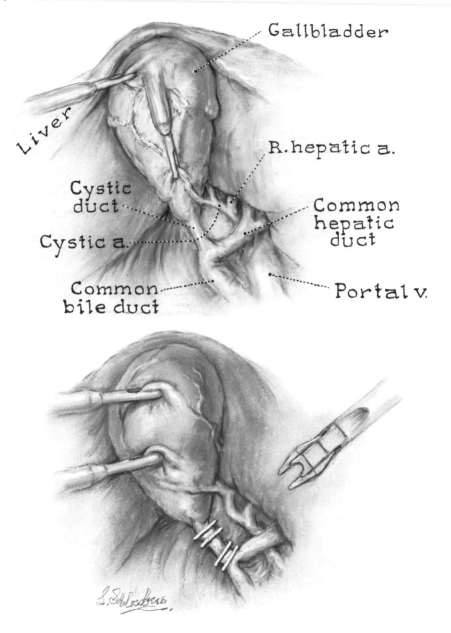

Laparoscopic clips or sutures may then be inadvertently placed right on the cystic and common bile duct junction or across the common bile duct itself. If the duct is only partially occluded, the injury may not be immediately apparent. The patient may be discharged shortly after the procedure only to return within a few days with mild jaundice. If this type of injury is suspected, endoscopic retrograde cholangiopancreatography will visualize the site of partial or complete obstruction. A biliary scintillation scan may also be used to evaluate the extrahepatic bile ducts; however, it may not adequately visualize a partial occlusion of the duct. Once again, complete dissection of the cystic and common bile duct junction as well as an intraoperative cholangiogram will demonstrate the ductal anatomy and help prevent such injuries.

In view of the lack of depth perception, careful attention should be directed to applying clips to the duct. It is extremely important to visualize both tips of the clip applier before activating the instrument. The angle of the clip applier should be used to place the clips perpendicular to the duct (see p. 325). Applying the clips obliquely may also result in a partial occlusion of the common bile duct.

Excessive cephalad traction on the gallbladder combined with vigorous dissection of the cystic bile duct may place considerable tension on the cystic and common bile duct junction. This may lead to a partial or even complete avulsion of the cystic duct from the common bile duct.

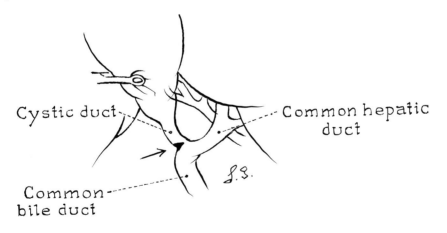

Immediate laparotomy is advised to ensure that the injury is limited to the origin of the cystic duct junction. Primary repair or T-tube drainage through the ductal opening may be performed as indicated.

Electrical burns, similar to those described for the bowel, may also occur to the bile ducts. Lack of depth perception and the limited peripheral vision also appear to play an important role in this type of injury. The most likely cause of such an injury is accidental contact with a ductal structure while cauterizing a bleeding site. As with intestinal electrical injuries, ductal burns may not be immediately apparent. The delayed tissue necrosis may result in the patient being discharged soon after surgery and returning later with abdominal pain and jaundice. Either the cystic or common bile duct may be involved.

Hemorrhage

Significant bleeding during or after laparoscopic cholecystectomy can occur for much the same reasons as during open cholecystectomy. As with the bile ducts, the surgeon must be careful to correctly identify aberrant or accessory right hepatic and cystic arteries so as to avoid injury.

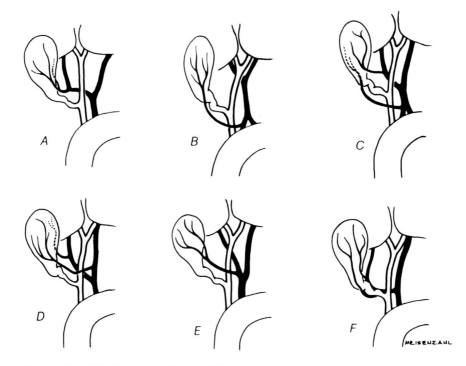

From Schwartz SI. Gallbladder and extrahepatic biliary system. In Schwartz SI, ed. Principles of Surgery. New York: McGraw-Hill, 1984, p 1310. By permission.

A, Cystic artery arises from right hepatic artery in 95% of cases. **B,** Cystic artery arising from gastroduodenal artery. **C,** Two cystic arteries, one arising from right hepatic artery and the other from common hepatic artery. **D,** Two cystic arteries, an abnormal one arising from left hepatic artery and crossing common hepatic duct anteriorly. **E,** Cystic artery arising from right hepatic artery but coursing anterior to common hepatic duct. **F,** Two cystic arteries arising from right hepatic artery, which is adherent to cystic duct and neck of gallbladder. Posterior cystic artery is very short, a common finding.

One specific pitfall that appears to be more common during laparoscopic cholecystectomy is avulsion or injury to a posterior branch of the cystic artery. Branching of the anterior and posterior cystic arteries occurs at variable locations along the medial aspect of the gallbladder.[43] A prominent anterior branch of the cystic artery may be mistakenly identified as the main arterial trunk. The anterior branch alone may be ligated, thereby leaving the posterior branch intact.

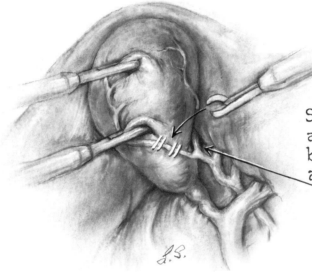

Surgical clips applied to ant. branch of cystic a.-leaving post. branch intact

Later, during the dissection of the gallbladder from the liver, the posterior branch may be divided and bleed into the operative field. Although this can usually be controlled by applying a clip or cauterizing the severed vessel, it is preferable to secure both branches or the main trunk during the initial dissection. Following ligation and transection of the cystic duct and artery, further blunt dissection is recommended until the neck of the gallbladder is free from the underlying liver bed. This will help identify any anomalous ductal or vascular structures.

Bleeding from the gallbladder bed is not uncommon but is usually self-limiting. Electrocauterization of bleeding sites is effective in controlling most hemorrhage. If persistent bleeding from the liver occurs, coagulation current may be increased. If this is not successful, then small amounts of topical thrombin or other coagulation-promoting products can be applied to the site of hemorrhage. The use of such techniques, combined with the patient's inherent coagulation abilities, will control bleeding from the gallbladder bed in almost all circumstances.

Postoperative hemorrhage may occur following laparoscopic cholecystectomy, as it sometimes does following open cholecystectomy. Initial reports tend to support the theory that the incidence of postoperative bleeding should not be greater following laparoscopic surgery.[10,38,40,43] However, it is possible that the presence of a tense pneumoperitoneum (12 to 16 mm Hg) may tamponade venous bleeding within the gallbladder bed. Postoperative hemorrhage may subsequently ensue once the pneumoperitoneum is deflated at the end of the procedure. This question has not yet been definitively answered, but it is unlikely that such bleeding would be clinically significant.

Bile Leakage

Bile leakage may occur as either an intraoperative or postoperative complication. Intraoperatively, spillage of bile may occur from inadvertent gallbladder perforation or bile duct injury. Regardless of the cause, immediate treatment involves irrigation and identification of the source of the bile leak. Gallbladder perforations resulting from the grasping forceps are quite common, especially in the early learning phase. If a perforation occurs, an attempt should be made to gain control of the opening as soon as possible with one of the grasping forceps.

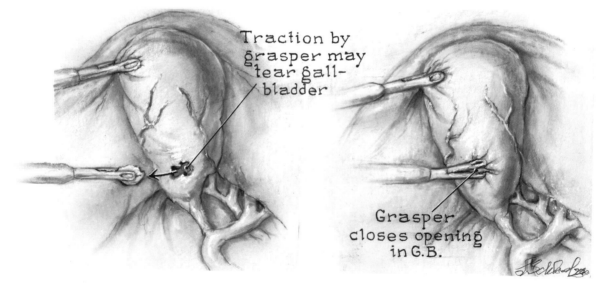

Traction by grasper may tear gallbladder

Grasper closes opening in G.B.

Once temporary control has been established, copious irrigation of the operative field should be performed. The perforation can then be permanently closed with the use of an endoscopic snare or titanium surgical clip.

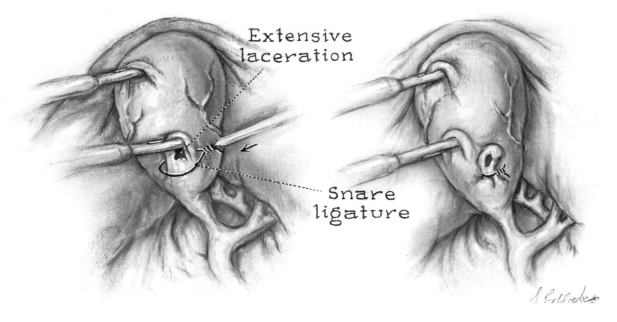

Postoperative bile leakage may result from an unrecognized ductal injury, opening of the cystic duct remnant, or directly from the liver bed. Patients developing delayed bile leaks usually present with abdominal pain and jaundice. Occasionally they may also manifest a mild leukocytosis and low-grade fever. Initial evaluation may include either an endoscopic retrograde cholangiopancreatogram or a biliary scintillation scan (see below).

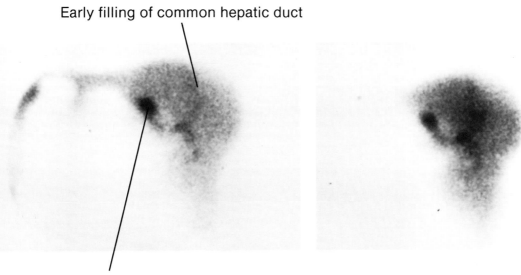

Leakage from the cystic duct remnant may occur if the clips or sutures become dislodged. An unrecognized electrocautery injury may result in delayed tissue necrosis and bile leak from the cystic duct remnant. Initial nonoperative management may include endoscopic sphincterotomy to lower the resistance across the ampulla and possible placement of a biliary stent over the origin of the cystic duct. If these therapeutic modalities fail, the patient should undergo laparotomy and closure of the bile leak. If the ductal structures are intact and the source of the bile leak appears to be from the liver bed, nonoperative management is usually successful. If the bile accumulation is large, it may be drained percutaneously under radiologic or sonographic guidance. Continued bile leakage may require operative intervention, but this is uncommon.

Ductal injuries detected postoperatively should be managed as appropriate for the location and extent of the injury. Right hepatic, common hepatic, or common bile duct injuries usually require laparotomy and a biliary-enteric bypass.

Intra-Abdominal Spillage of Calculi

Loss of stones can also be expected following perforation of the gallbladder. After the opening in the gallbladder is secured, an attempt should be made to remove all or as many of the stones as possible. Smaller calculi may be removed with 5 or 11 mm grasping forceps inserted through one of the accessory cannulas. Large and irregular-shaped stones may prove difficult to grasp with currently available instruments. Endoscopic or ureteral stone baskets have proved effective for retrieving these types of stones.

Despite these efforts, biliary calculi may occasionally be lost within the abdominal cavity. Laparotomy solely for the purpose of stone retrieval is probably not necessary. Lost stones within the abdominal cavity rarely result in complications; however, isolated case reports of postoperative abscess from such retained calculi have been described.

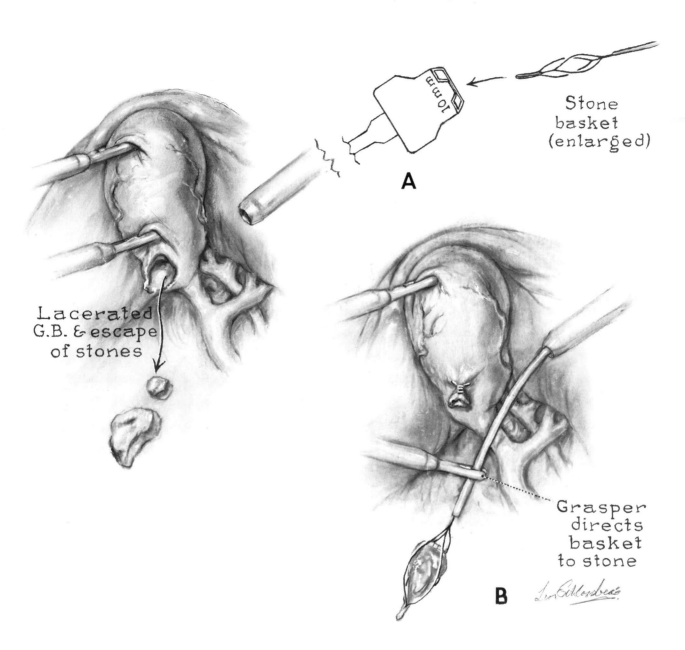

Stone
basket
(enlarged)

A

Lacerated
G.B. & escape
of stones

Grasper
directs
basket
to stone

B

Miscellaneous Complications

Loss of the gallbladder within the abdominal cavity while attempting to pull it through the umbilical fascial opening has also been reported. This can easily occur if a small, atraumatic grasping forceps has been used for extracting the gallbladder. On occasion a lower, midline laparotomy has been necessary to retrieve the gallbladder from the pelvis or from between loops of small bowel. For this reason I recommend the use of a large (11 mm) penetrating "claw" forceps for grasping and pulling the gallbladder through the abdominal wall (see p. 173). Fortunately, in most circumstances, the gallbladder can be identified and retrieved if control is lost. To facilitate removal, it is recommended that the gallbladder be transferred from the 5 mm atraumatic forceps to the larger claw forceps in a region that is readily accessible to laparoscopic visualization. We routinely perform this transfer over the top of the liver near its inferior edge. If the gallbladder is dropped, it will usually remain resting on top of the liver.

Infectious complications following elective cholecystectomy via laparotomy are uncommon.[44] Initial results from clinical series indicate that this is also true for laparoscopic cholecystectomy.[10,38,40,43] No wound or intra-abdominal infections have been seen at the University of Maryland in over 250 procedures performed.

• • •

Although experience with newer laparoscopic procedures such as vagotomy, appendectomy, intestinal resection, hernia repair, and pelvic lymphadenectomy is still limited, complications will undoubtedly occur. As with laparoscopic cholecystectomy, proper training and experience will help prevent serious morbidity.

REFERENCES

1. Levinson CJ, Hulka JF, Richardson DC. Laparoscopy. In Schaefer G, Graber EA, eds. Complications in Obstetric and Gynecologic Surgery. Hagerstown, Md.: Harper & Row, 1981, pp 281-298.
2. Phillips JM. Complications in laparoscopy. Int J Gynaecol Obstet 15:157-162, 1977.
3. Phillips JM, Hulka JF, Keith D, Keith L. Laparoscopic procedures: AASGL membership survey for 1975. J Reprod Med 18:227-238, 1977.
4. Katz M, Beck P, Tancer ML. Major vessel injury during laparoscopy: Anatomy of two cases. Am J Obstet Gynecol 135:544-545, 1979.
5. Newton M. Complications of abdominal operations. In Newton M, Newton ER, eds. Complications of Gynecologic and Obstetric Management. Philadelphia: WB Saunders, 1988, pp 143-174.
6. Kane MG, Kreijs GJ. Complications of diagnostic laparoscopy in Dallas: A 7-year prospective study. Gastrointest Endosc 30:237-240, 1984.

7. Mintz M. Risks and prophylaxis in laparoscopy: A survey of 100,000 cases. J Reprod Med 18:269-272, 1977.

8. Borten M. Laparoscopic Complications. Prevention and Management. Toronto: BC Decker, 1986.

9. Götz F, Pier A, Bacher C. Modified laparoscopic appendectomy in surgery: A report of 388 operations. Surg Endosc 4:6-9, 1990.

10. Zucker KA, Bailey RW, Gadacz TR, Imbembo AL. Laparoscopic guided cholecystectomy. Am J Surg 161:36-44, 1991.

11. Pentecost MP, Curtis EM. Laparoscopy. In Ridley JH, ed. Gynecologic Surgery: Errors, Safeguards, Salvage. Baltimore: Williams & Wilkins, 1981, pp 135-158.

12. Carmichael DE. Laparoscopy: Cardiac considerations. Fertil Steril 22:69-70, 1971.

13. Scott DB, Julian DG. Observations on cardiac arrhythmias during laparoscopy. Br Med J 1:411-413, 1972.

14. Gomar C, Fernandez C, Villalonga A, Nalda MA. Carbon dioxide embolism during laparoscopy and hysteroscopy. Ann Fr Anesth Reanim 4:380-382, 1985.

15. Brantley JC III, Riley PM. Cardiovascular collapse during laparoscopy: A report of two cases. Am J Obstet Gynecol 159:735-737, 1988.

16. Smith I, Benzie RJ, Gordon NLM, Kelman GR, Swapp GH. Cardiovascular effects of peritoneal insufflation of carbon dioxide for laparoscopy. Br Med J 3:410-411, 1971.

17. Lenz RJ, Thomas TA, Wilkins DG. Cardiovascular changes during laparoscopy: Studies of stroke volume and cardiac output using impedance cardiography. Anaesthesia 31:4-12, 1976.

18. McKenzie R, Wadhwa RK, Bedger RC. Noninvasive measurement of cardiac output during laparoscopy. J Reprod Med 24:247-250, 1980.

19. Motew M, Ivankovich AD, Bieniarz J, et al. Cardiovascular effects and acid-base and blood gas changes during laparoscopy. Am J Obstet Gynecol 115:1002-1012, 1973.

20. Endler GC, Moghissi KS. Gastric perforation during pelvic laparoscopy. Obstet Gynecol 47:40-42, 1976.

21. Levinson CJ, Schwartz SF, Saltzstein EC. Complication of laparoscopic tubal cauterization: Small bowel perforation. Obstet Gynecol 41:253-256, 1973.

22. Thompson BH, Wheeless CR. Gastrointestinal complications of laparoscopy sterilization. Obstet Gynecol 41:669-676, 1973.

23. Lynn SC, Katz AR, Ross PJ. Aortic perforation sustained at laparoscopy. J Reprod Med 27:217-219, 1982.

24. Peterson HB, Greenspan JR, Ory HW. Death following puncture of the aorta during laparoscopic sterilization. Obstet Gynecol 59:133-134, 1982.

25. Shin CS. Vascular injury secondary to laparoscopy. NY State J Med 82:935-936, 1982.

26. Baadsgaard SE, Bille S, Egeblad K. Major vascular injury during gynecologic laparoscopy: Report of two cases and review of published cases. Acta Obstet Gynecol Scand 68:283-285, 1989.

27. Deshmukh AS. Laparoscopic bladder injury. Urology 19:306-307, 1982.

28. Georgy RM, Fetterman HH, Chefetz MD. Complications of laparoscopy: Two cases of perforated urinary bladder. Am J Obstet Gynecol 120:1121-1122, 1974.

29. Homburg R, Segal T. Perforation of the urinary bladder by the laparoscope. Am J Obstet Gynecol 130:597-601, 1978.

30. Irvin TT, Goligher JC, Scott JS. Injury to the ureter during laparoscopic tubal sterilization. Arch Surg 110:1501-1503, 1975.

31. Perone N. Conventional vs. open laparoscopy. Am Fam Physician 27:147-149, 1983.

32. Penfield AJ. How to prevent complications of open laparoscopy. J Reprod Med 30:660-663, 1985.

33. Kleppinger RK. Laparoscopy at a community hospital: An analysis of 4300 cases. J Reprod Med 19:353-363, 1977.

34. Fischer JD, Turner FW. Abdominal incisional hernias: A ten-year review. Can J Surg 17:202-204, 1974.

35. Deaths following female sterilization with unipolar electrocoagulating devices. MMWR 30:149, 1981.

36. Soderstrom RM, Levy BS. Bowel injuries during laparoscopy: Causes and medicolegal questions. Continuing Obstet Gynecol 27:41-45, 1986.

37. Soper NJ, Barteau JA, Clayman RV, Becich MJ. Safety and efficacy of laparoscopic cholecystectomy using monopolar electrocautery in the porcine model. Surg Laparosc Endosc (in press).

38. Dubois F, Icard P, Berthelot G, Levard H. Coelioscopic cholecystectomy: Preliminary report of 36 cases. Ann Surg 211:60-62, 1990.

39. Wheeless CR. Gastrointestinal injuries associated with laparoscopy. In Phillips JM, ed. Endoscopy in Gynecology. Downey, Calif: American Association of Gynecological Laparoscopists, 1978, pp 317-329.

40. Peters JH, Ellison EC, Innes JT, Liss JL, Nichols KE, Lomano JM, Roby SR, Front ME, Carey LC. Safety and efficacy of laparoscopic cholecystectomy: A prospective analysis of 100 patients. Ann Surg 213:3-12, 1991.

41. Henry ML, Carey LC. Complications of cholecystectomy. Surg Clin North Am 63:1191-1204, 1983.

42. Lippert H, Pabst R. Arterial Variations in Man: Classification and frequency. Munich: JF Bergmann, 1985.

43. Reddick EJ, Olsen DO. Laparoscopic laser cholecystectomy: A comparison with mini-lap cholecystectomy. Surg Endosc 3:44-48, 1989.

44. Ganey JB, Johnson PA, Jr, Prillaman PE, McSwain GR. Cholecystectomy: Clinical experience with a large series. Am J Surg 151:352-357, 1986.

CHAPTER 17

Training for Laparoscopic Surgery and Credentialing

Anthony L. Imbembo, M.D.
Karl A. Zucker, M.D.

The widespread popularity of diagnostic laparoscopy and laparoscopic-assisted general surgery has prompted a large number of general surgeons to offer these procedures to their patients. Laparoscopic surgery, however, has not been a required component of most general surgery training programs. At the present time most general surgeons are unfamiliar with even the most basic laparoscopic techniques. Widespread adoption of laparoscopic cholecystectomy as well as other laparoscopic-assisted procedures has been hampered by the lack of adequately trained surgeons. The demonstrated efficacy of laparoscopic surgery dictates that this discipline be incorporated into general surgery residency programs. In addition, the training and accreditation of practicing general surgeons have become important medical and legal issues. No federal or local governing bodies currently exist to regulate or advise hospitals, insurance carriers, etc. as to who is qualified to perform such procedures. Individual institutions must establish guidelines defining adequacy of training and experience in order to credential surgeons for these newly developed procedures.

TRAINING OF PRACTICING GENERAL SURGEONS

Practicing general surgeons have had little or no exposure to diagnostic or therapeutic laparoscopy. Therefore formal training programs have been established to provide the necessary clinical and didactic experience. The majority of individuals who have expressed an interest in performing laparoscopic surgery have enrolled in intensive 2- or 3-day courses. Many hospitals have even mandated that surgeons requesting laparoscopic privileges attend such a course. Preliminary instruction in such programs usually consists of formal presentations covering topics such as the history of laparoscopic surgery, principles of general laparoscopy, techniques of laparoscopic cholecystectomy, potential complications, and summation of current clinical results. These presentations may be supplemented by instructional videotapes covering techniques and by reference to an operative atlas. It is essential that all course participants become familiar with the specialized instrumentation, insufflation devices, video cameras and imaging equipment, and irrigation/suction apparatus as well as the safe use of laser or electrocautery energy within the closed abdomen.

Following completion of this introductory program, technical expertise is acquired in phases. These include utilization of simulation devices, experience in the animal laboratory, and hands-on exposure in the operating room in a supervised environment.

Simulation Training

Surgeons must become facile with the handling and control of laparoscopic instruments as well as proficient in the techniques of stapling, suturing, and knot tying that are unique to this type of surgery. The hand-eye coordination required in the performance of video-directed surgery is one of the most difficult tasks to master. This is, to a considerable degree, due to the loss of depth perception afforded by the currently available video imaging equipment. Simulation devices may aid the surgeon in acquiring the necessary coordination. One such apparatus is the Berci-Sackier laparoscopic trainer (Karl Storz Endoscopy, Culver City, Calif.). This apparatus consists of a rectangular container (12 × 18.1 × 8 inches) constructed of solid dark Plexiglas. The top plate contains four fenestrated rubber diaphragms 4 to 12 cm in diameter.

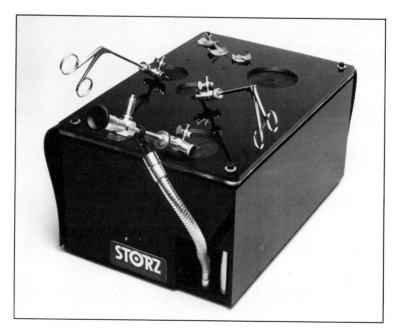

The top plate corresponds to the anterior abdominal wall, and the four rubber diaphragms allow for the introduction of laparoscopic trocars and other instruments into the chamber, simulating actual laparoscopic surgery. Introduction of the laparoscope connected to the video camera permits visualization of the interior of the chamber on the video monitor. Laparoscopic grasping forceps inserted through the separate portals are used to manipulate synthetic materials constructed to simulate viscera such as the gallbladder, uterus, or fallopian tube. Trainees then practice laparoscopic techniques such as placement of suture ligatures and snares as well as knot tying utilizing both intra- and extracorporeal methods.

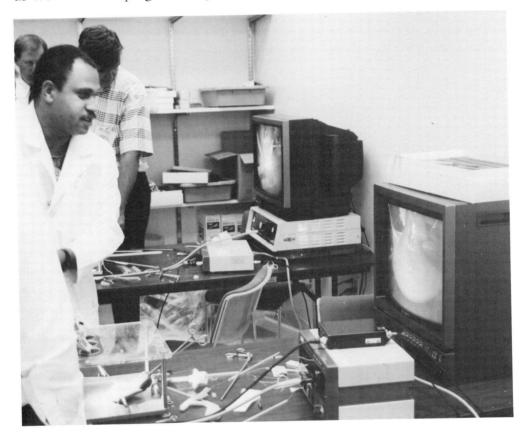

Practice continues until all such tasks can be readily performed. It is also possible to substitute cadaveric animal tissues for the synthetic materials, thereby permitting the novice to practice actual tissue dissection using electrocautery and/or laser.

Animal Experience

Direct operative experience should first be obtained in the animal laboratory under conditions closely resembling the actual clinical setting. All protocols require approval by the institutional body governing animal care. Young swine (25 to 40 kg) are anesthetized and placed on continuous mechanical ventilation. The entire laparoscopic procedure is performed according to the protocols developed for humans. The instructor carefully monitors the progress of each trainee, correcting procedural errors, guiding technique, and commenting on potential complications. Demonstration of anatomic distortions commonly encountered during laparoscopic-assisted surgery is an important aspect of training. Multiple animals are employed until each surgeon is experienced in the roles of surgeon, assistant, and camera operator. The amount of animal practice required to become proficient with laparoscopic procedures will vary among individual surgeons. Opportunities should also be available for surgeons to train on additional animals on an independent basis. This can usually be arranged at the institution that organized the training program.

Unfortunately the many courses that offer such training in surgical laparoscopy vary widely in quality of instruction, the equipment available, and the amount of animal operating experience. Many are organized and conducted by individuals with limited clinical or academic experience. Such programs are often conducted in hotels or other makeshift surroundings and many travel from city to city. Such programs are usually unable to provide additional training such as supplemental animal experience. It is imperative that both the surgeons seeking such training as well as institutions reviewing the credentials of applicants desiring to perform this type of surgery examine carefully the quality of instruction offered.

Clinical Experience

The most important component in the training process is hands-on exposure in an actual operating room environment. Direct clinical experience is best acquired by assisting surgeons who have already been credentialed for laparoscopy and laparoscopic-assisted procedures. The first priority is to become totally familiar with the use and proper handling of the laparoscopic instruments themselves. The trainee should assist on at least 5 to 10 laparoscopic procedures before assuming the role of surgeon. As surgeon, the trainee works under the direct supervision of an accredited laparoscopic surgeon throughout the procedure. Once the trainee has mastered the basic maneuvers performed during laparoscopic-assisted surgery, clinical competency is usually attained rapidly. At our institution a minimum of 5 to 10 procedures must be performed under direct supervision before privileges for independent performance of laparoscopic-assisted chole-cystectomy will be granted.

TRAINING OF RESIDENT SURGEONS

Laparoscopic surgery has been included in the general surgery residency program at the University of Maryland Medical Center since 1989. Although desirable, it has not proved feasible to expose all of our residents to such procedures in the animal laboratory first. Fortunately the longer period of training and the large number of surgical cases they are exposed to allow residents to receive adequate training without this experience. Initial resident participation typically involves manipulation of the miniaturized laparoscopic camera on 10 to 20 separate procedures. In this fashion they become familiar with the intricacies of laparoscopic surgery without impeding the progress of the operation because of their lack of experience. For more senior residents, the next phase of training involves participation as the first assistant. The first assistant's main task is providing adequate exposure of the important anatomic structures. Although this may prove difficult for those individuals with limited laparoscopic experience, the primary surgeon can regulate the level of participation. This can range from static positional assistance to independent manipulation of major structures such as the gallbladder and cystic duct. Again, participation in at least 10 cases is required prior to assuming the role of surgeon.

Resident training as surgeon must proceed carefully and deliberately. Residents who are appropriately prepared are first permitted to establish pneumoperitoneum, introduce the laparoscope, complete the abdominal exploration, and provide initial exposure (e.g., of the gallbladder). At this point the attending surgeon must determine whether or not the anticipated operative dissection appears to be technically appropriate for the level of expertise already attained by the resident in training. Factors such as adhesion formation, inflammation, chronic scarring, or aberrant anatomy must all be considered by the supervisory surgeon. If these potential complicating factors are not apparent, the resident may be permitted to continue with the operative procedure with the attending physician prepared to assume control at any point. This may become necessary if the dissection becomes difficult or, most important, if there is any question as to the proper identification of anatomic structures.

CREDENTIALING ISSUES

It is basic to credentialing that surgeons performing procedures such as laparoscopic-assisted cholecystectomy have the judgment, training, and capability of immediately proceeding to the traditional open procedure. Each institution must develop uniform standards that apply to all hospital staff requesting privileges to perform surgical laparoscopy. The criteria must be clinically sound without being unreasonably restrictive, with the goal of delivering the highest quality patient care and assuring patient safety. Issues such as disturbing local referral patterns and competition must be avoided.

At a minimum the surgeon must have satisfactorily completed an accredited residency training program in general surgery. Completion of a surgical residency or fellowship program that incorporates structured experience in laparoscopic surgery is satisfactory for credentialing. For those surgeons without prior experience in laparoscopic surgery, the Society of American Gastrointestinal Endoscopic Surgeons (SAGES) recommends basic *minimum* requirements for training.

In addition to SAGES' recommendations, the Society for Surgery of the Alimentary Tract has adopted a resolution that also advocates that individuals "provide notification to their patients of the surgeon's experience with, and the status of, the procedure."

At our institution we presently insist on proctoring all applicants requesting privileges in laparoscopic surgery. This is done in recognition of the vagaries of written reports and in recognition of the relative novelty of these procedures for most general surgeons. Once laparoscopic surgery has become a required component of residency training in general surgery, the need for such proctoring should be eliminated. Proctoring should be performed by an experienced, unbiased general surgeon chosen either from the existing medical staff or solicited from academic medical centers or from national surgical endoscopic societies. Proctoring must be done in an unbiased, confidential, and objective manner. A mechanism for appeal must be established for individuals for whom privileges are denied, including the opportunity for repeat proctoring by a newly chosen referee.

TRAINING AND DETERMINATION OF COMPETENCE*

Formal Fellowship or Residency Training in General Surgery

Determination of Competence in Laparoscopic Surgery

1. Completion of a surgical residency/fellowship program which incorporates structured experience in laparoscopic surgery. Competence should be documented by the instructor(s).
2. Proficiency in laparoscopic surgical procedures and clinical judgment equivalent to that obtained in a residency/fellowship program. Documentation and demonstration of competence is necessary.
3. For those without residency training or fellowship which included laparoscopic surgery or without documented prior experience in laparoscopic surgery, the basic *minimum* requirements for training should be:
   a. Completion of approved residency training in general surgery
   b. Credentialing in diagnostic laparoscopy
   c. Training in laparoscopic general surgery by a surgeon experienced in laparoscopic surgery or completion of a university sponsored or academic society recognized didactic course with clinical experience and hands-on laboratory practice
   d. Observation of laparoscopic surgical procedures performed by a surgeon (or surgeons) experienced in the performance of such procedures
4. The applicant's laparoscopic training director should confirm in writing the training, experience (including the number of cases for each procedure for which privileges are requested), and actually observed level of competency. It is recognized that by virtue of completing a residency program in surgery the laparoscopic surgeon will have acquired at least 5 years of cognitive experience in anatomy, physiology, and disease processes combined with the progressive development of visual and psychomotor experience necessary for the performance of procedures in the abdominal cavity. Such experience includes indications, complications, and alternative approaches. The training director's opinion and recommendation should be considered prima facie evidence for the trainee's acceptance as an individual qualified in laparoscopic sur-

gery. Likewise, attendance at short courses which do not provide supervised hands-on training is not an acceptable substitute for the development of equivalent competency.

New Procedures

Self-training in new techniques in laparoscopic surgery must take place on a background of basic surgical and endoscopic skills. The laparoscopic surgeon should recognize when additional training is necessary.

Proctoring

Recognizing the limitations of written reports, proctoring of applicants for privileges in laparoscopic surgery by a qualified, unbiased staff surgeon experienced in general and laparoscopic surgery may be desirable, especially when competency for a given procedure cannot be adequately verified by submitted written material. The procedural details of proctoring should be developed by the credentialing body of the hospital and provided to the applicant. Proctors may be chosen from existing staff or solicited from surgical endoscopic societies. Criteria of competency for each procedure should be established in advance. It is essential that proctoring be provided in an unbiased, confidential, and objective manner. A satisfactory mechanism for appeal must be established for individuals for whom privileges are denied or granted in a temporary or provisional manner.

Monitoring of Endoscopic Performance

To assist the hospital credentialing body in the ongoing renewal of privileges there should be a mechanism of monitoring each surgical endoscopist's procedural performance. This should be done through existing quality assurance mechanisms in the institution. This should include monitoring utilization, diagnostic and therapeutic benefits to patients, complications, and tissue review in accordance with previously developed criteria.

Continuing Education

Continuing medical education related to laparoscopic surgery should be required as part of the periodic renewal of privileges. Attendance at appropriate local or national meetings and courses is encouraged.

---

*From Society of American Gastrointestinal Endoscopic Surgeons. Granting privileges for laparoscopic (peritoneoscopic) general surgery. Los Angeles: The Society, 1990.

SUGGESTED READING

Bailey RW, Imbembo AL, Zucker KA. Establishment of a laparoscopic cholecystectomy training program. Am Surg (in press).

Dubois F, Icard P, Berthelot G, Levard H. Coelioscopic cholecystectomy: Preliminary report of 36 cases. Ann Surg 211:60, 1990.

Society of American Gastrointestinal Endoscopic Surgeons. Granting of privileges for laparoscopic (peritoneoscopic) general surgery. Los Angeles: The Society, 1990.

Society for Surgery of the Alimentary Tract. Resolution concerning privileges to perform laparoscopic cholecystectomy. San Antonio: The Society, 1990.

Zucker KA, Bailey RW. Atlas of Endo Cholecystectomy. Norwalk, Conn.: United States Surgical Corporation, 1990.

Partial Listing of Manufacturers of Surgical Laparoscopy Equipment

American Surgical Instruments
901 E. Sample Rd.
Suite C
Pompano, FL 33064
800-527-5294

Specialty instruments for laparoscopic surgery.

Cabot Medical
110 Cabot Blvd.
Langhorne, PA 19047
800-523-6078

A full line of laparoscopes, video imaging equipment, insufflators, and instruments.

Candela Laser Corporation
530 Buton Post Rd.
Wayland, MA 01778
800-255-1287

A pulsed-dye laser for endoscopic stone fragmentation.

Ethicon, Inc.
P.O. Box 151
Somerville, NJ 06786
800-388-1000

Disposable laparoscopic cannulas and sutures.

Ideas for Medicine
2167 49th St. North
Clearwater, FL 34622
813-576-2747

Special balloon-tipped cholangiogram catheter.

Karl Storz Endoscopy–America, Inc.
10111 W. Jefferson Blvd.
Culver City, CA 90232
800-421-0837

A full line of laparoscopes, video imaging equipment, and instruments.

Laserscope
3052 Orchard Dr.
San Jose, CA 95134-2011
800-356-7600

A KTP/YAG surgical laser.

MPVideo
65 South St.
Hopkinton, MA 01748
508-435-2131

A line of video imaging equipment used for laparoscopic surgery.

Olympus Medical
4 Nevada Dr.
Lake Success, NY 11042
800-950-3636

A full line of laparoscopes, video imaging equipment, and instruments.

Richard Wolf Medical Instrumentation Corporation
7046 Lyndon Ave.
Rosemont, IL 60018
800-323-WOLF

A complete laparoscopic set, including insufflators, video imaging equipment, and instruments.

Solus Endoscopy
6191 Atlantic Blvd.
Atlanta, GA 30071
800-868-8371

A complete laparoscopic set, including laparoscopes, insufflators, video imaging equipment, and instruments.

Surgical Laser Technologies, Inc.
One Great Valley Parkway
Malvern, PA 19355
800-772-5273

An Nd:YAG surgical laser.

United States Surgical Corporation
150 Glover Ave.
Norwalk, CT 06856
800-321-0263

An extensive selection of disposable laparoscopic materials, including trocars, cannulas, converters, multifire clip appliers, GIA staplers, and other instruments.

WISAP USA
14227 Sandy Lane
Tomball, TX 77375
800-233-8448

A complete line of laparoscopic equipment, including insufflators, video imaging equipment, and instruments.

Index